Infectious Pathology of the Respiratory Tract

Vsevolod Zinserling

Infectious Pathology of the Respiratory Tract

With Contributions by
Yulia R. Zyuzya
Vladimir V. Svistunov
Valery V. Varyasin

Springer

Vsevolod Zinserling
Pathomorphology
Institute of Experimental Medicine at V.A. Almazov Research Center
Saint Petersburg
Russia

ISBN 978-3-030-66324-7 ISBN 978-3-030-66325-4 (eBook)
https://doi.org/10.1007/978-3-030-66325-4

This Springer imprint is published by the registered company Springer Nature Switzerland AG
The registered company address is: Gewerbestrasse 11, 6330 Cham, Switzerland

Preface

The importance of respiratory infectious pathology is obvious. Several manuals discuss the fundamental aspects of the pathogenesis of infections [1, 2], and many issues of its diagnostics in routine work of clinical pathologists are excellently presented as well [3–6]. Especially informative are the chapters devoted to tropical infections. Due to quite objective reasons, there are practically no modern publications founded upon autopsy studies. The only exception is a review based upon a limited number of cases including SARS, MERS, pandemic influenza, and Legionella [7]. In 2020, numerous publications appeared presenting autopsy series in COVID-19 (see Chap. 6). Several infections (mycoplasmosis, chlamydiosis, etc.) appeared to lie outside the focus of attention of a majority of pathologists. In Russia, especially in Leningrad/Saint Petersburg, different variants of infectious pathology, including pneumonia, influenza, mycoplasmosis, HIV, and intrauterine infections, have been successfully studied in children, adults, and on experimental models for fast a century in the scientific school of Vsevolod D. and Alexander V. Zinserling [8, 9]. Russian pathology has also outstanding experience in investigating tuberculosis [10, 11]. For certain reasons, having no relation to the professional work, these results were published in English only in a limited number of contributions. In this book, we summarize the experience of our scientific schools presenting the results, which have been achieved in previous decades in comparison with the modern data and literature. It appears necessary to cite Russian publications of the former century, especially when they present reliable results, the topic remains actual, and there are no modern contributions at all. We paid more attention to diseases that are less known and we had the opportunity to study thoroughly. We considered it very important to present a set of numerous original illustrations, mostly demonstrating our own observations. We found it unnecessary to try to perform a complete review of the literature; unfortunately the majority of modern publications do not discuss lifetime and postmortem morphological diagnostics of infectious lung lesions—the main task that we put before us while preparing the manual. Valuable contributions were made by Yulia R. Zyuzya, Dr. Med. Sci. (Russia)—Chapters 7.3, 13, 14.2, 14.6, 15, 18; Vladimir Svistunov, Dr. Med. Sci (Russia)—Chapters 10, 11.6; and Valery Varjasin, Dr. Med. Sci. (Russia)—Chapter 5.3.

Saint Petersburg, Russia Prof. Vsevolod Zinserling

References

1. Mims CA, Dimmock NJ, Nash A, Stephen J. Mim's pathogenesis of infectious disease. 4th ed. Academic Press; 1995. 414 p.
2. Engleberg NG, Rita V, Dermody TS, editors. Shaechter's mechanisms of microbial disease. 4th ed. Lippincott Williams & Wilkins; 2007.
3. Kradin RL, editor. Diagnostic pathology of infectious diseases. Elsevier; 2018. 698 p.
4. Procop GW, Pritt BS, editors. Pathology of infectious diseases. Elsevier; 2015. 706 p.
5. Hofman P, editor. Infectious disease and parasites. Springer Reference; 2016. 343 p.
6. Schmitt BH, editor. Atlas of infectious pathology. Springer; 2017. 255 p.
7. Bradley BT, Bryan A. Emerging respiratory infections: the infectious disease pathology of SARS, MERS, pandemic influenza and Legionella. Semin Diagn Pathol 2019;36:152–9. https://doi.org/10.1053/j.semdp.2019.04.06.
8. Zinserling VD, Zinserling AV. Pathological anatomy of acute pneumonia of different etiology. Gos Izd Med Lit. Leningrad; 1963. 175 p. (In Russian).
9. Zinserling AV, Zinserling VA. Modern infections: pathologic anatomy and issues of pathogenesis: a guide. SPb: Sotis; 2002. 346 p. (In Russian).
10. Strukov AI. Forms of pulmonary tuberculosis in morphological light. M.: Publishing House of the USSR Academy of Medical Sciences; 1948. 160 p. (In Russian).
11. Puzik VI, Uvarova OA, Averbakh MM. Pathomorphology of modern forms of pulmonary tuberculosis. -M.: Medicine; 1973. 215 p. (In Russian).

Contents

1 General Aspects of Infectious Pathology

Infectious pathology is now recognized as one of the most important public health problems worldwide. According to the World Health Organization (WHO), in 2016, the ten most common causes of death are ischemic heart disease, stroke, chronic obstructive pulmonary disease, pneumonia, Alzheimer's disease and other dementias, respiratory cancers, diabetes mellitus, road accidents, intestinal infections, and tuberculosis [1]. Till yet, the more recent data are absent. Among the most important causes of death claiming leadership on a global scale, in addition, we have to mention HIV infection and malaria. In 2020, COVID-19 became one of the most discussed causes of death. If we consider the widely discussed connection of biological pathogens with many noncontagious diseases, including the most common, infections continue to play a crucial role in human pathology. Currently, one of the most discussed issues in the physiology and pathology of a person is the state of his microbiome [2].

Despite the great attention paid by WHO, national health authorities and the media to morbidity and mortality from infections, it should be noted that the statistics, even presented in official sources, has only relative reliability. According to expert estimations, 30–50 million cases of infectious diseases occur in the world, the economic damage from which is not currently calculated. COVID19 pandemic is the most impressive example. Its economic damage currently cannot be calculated exactly, but surely is enormous.

So we are sure that the true significance of infections is much greater than commonly accepted previously. This, of course, is associated with a whole range of factors, among which the failure in many cases to perform qualified autopsy examinations or to underestimate their data is important. It should be noted that, despite a significant number of modern studies devoted to certain aspects, primarily the molecular biology of a number of pathogens, epidemiology, diagnosis, and treatment of the most relevant infectious diseases, some aspects remain as if in the "shadow." This primarily relates to issues of pathology. The literature does not provide a complete morphological characteristic of any of the newly discovered infections.

Paying tribute to the existing approaches to diagnosis, one has to note two issues: (1) in many diseases obviously of an infectious nature, all the tests used can be negative; (2) with the simultaneous use of many diagnostic methods, their results almost never completely coincide. It can be assumed that in some cases we are dealing with pathogens not yet known, in others with poorly known forms of pathogens and their tissue inhibitors. In many cases, imperfection of the methods used, nonoptimal terms and objects of research are of importance. Recently, one has to deal with other situations. The positive results of a lifetime

V. Zinserling, *Infectious Pathology of the Respiratory Tract*,
https://doi.org/10.1007/978-3-030-66325-4_1

study, for example, relied to coronavirus, in the case of a fatal outcome, are automatically considered even without clinical autopsy as a cause of death, which certainly leads to a distortion of statistics, the role of which is not purely medical. It seems that all this indicates that a number of unclear issues of pathogenesis and diagnosis of infectious diseases still exist.

Since ancient times, physicians of various civilizations have described macroscopic changes in diseases whose infectious nature was later established—tuberculosis, chronic viral hepatitis in the cirrhotic stage, pneumonia. During the great microbiological discoveries of the late 19th century, which coincided with the widespread introduction of microscopic studies into practice, the infectious subject became the main one for most pathologists in the world [3]. Later on, due to numerous objective and subjective reasons, interest for the pathology of infectious processes decreased by the middle of XX and only a few researchers continued to study it. In Russia, these are primarily representatives of the Leningrad/St. Petersburg school (V.D. and A.V. Zinserling). Traditionally Russian pathology (primarily in Moscow, Leningrad/Saint-Petersburg, Novosibirsk) has been successfully studying tuberculosis.

It is obvious that a fruitful study and diagnosis of infectious pathology should be comprehensive and must include an analysis of structural changes. Summarizing long-term experience in studying the pathology of infections in our scientific school, it seems appropriate to formulate the following requirements for the morphological study of the infectious process on autopsy and biopsy materials [4]: (1) identification of pathogens and their components in tissues; (2) a broad comparison of morphological data with clinical and laboratory; (3) differentiated assessment of changes caused by individual pathogens; (4) assessment of the characteristics of tissue reactions in different etiology and the form of the infectious process; (5) the widest use of nosological experimental models of infections in order to clarify patho- and morphogenesis and evaluate the effectiveness of therapy; (6) the study of interactions between various pathogens in mixed infections with each other and with the host; (7) the study of peculiarities of infectious processes in different organs and tissues; (8) determination of the immediate causes of death in infections. The listed principles are well known to many experts, but they have been rarely summarized.

Any infectious process can be interpreted as an interaction between macro- and microorganisms. The total number of microorganisms that are simultaneously in different relationships with the host organism can be very significant. It is important to note that all of them should naturally interact with each other. In addition, it should be noted that both macro and microorganisms are influenced by environmental factors (Fig. 1.1).

At present, it is customary to distinguish several forms of the infectious process: acute infection, chronic infection, latent infection, carriage, slow neuroinfection. Their brief clinical and morphological characteristics are presented in Table 1.1.

Commenting on this generally accepted classification, it is appropriate to dwell on several points. The distinction between acute and chronic infections is not always based on the known duration of the disease from the anamnesis. The severity of clinical manifestations usually correlates with the activity of the inflammatory process, but there are often exceptions. In a number of diseases with characteristic chronicity (viral hepatitis B and C, etc.), it is advisable to distinguish subacute forms. The clinical separation of chronic and latent infections is sometimes somewhat conditionally, since it is largely based on such subjective criteria as patient's complaints. In cases of life term morphological studies, very often the "carriage" of one or another pathogen (or its antigen) has to be attributed to a "latent

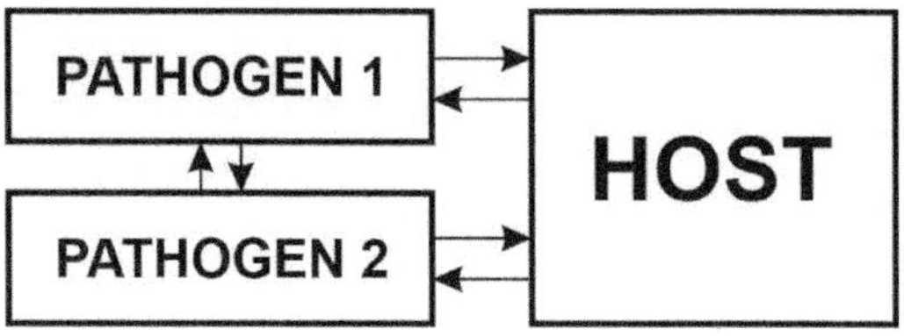

Fig. 1.1 Relationship between pathogens and host

Table 1.1 Clinical and morphological characteristics of the main forms of the infectious process

Form of infection	Clinical manifestations	Nature of structural changes	Outcomes	Note
Acute	Severe	Acute inflammation	Death, recovery, chronicity	More detailed characteristics of outcomes see in Fig. 1.4
Chronic	Severe	Chronic inflammation	Death, recovery, stabilization	Recovery in many diseases is impossible or doubtful
Latent	None	Chronic inflammation	Transition to chronic or convalescence	Manifestations of chronic inflammation usually moderate
Carriage	None	None	Transition to a manifest disease or debridement	Pathogens are detected by laboratory methods
Slow (neuroinfection)	Expressed	Only alterative changes	Death	

infection." Our vision upon the outcome of latent infections and carriage are largely speculative due to a lack of confirmed data. We found it possible to add a new variant of the relationship between macro- and microorganism—a veiled infection, in which the pathogen begins to manifest itself and is determined by clinical methods only when the body is exposed to other factors, such as traumatic brain injury or HIV infection [5]. When formulating the definition of "infectious disease," one should remember the possibility of its occurrence in a subclinical form.

Diagnosis of various forms of infectious diseases is based primarily on the results of a variety of microbiological and molecular biological methods, as well as clinical, laboratory, and epidemiological data. In many typical ("student's") cases, they coincide, but exceptions are not uncommon in clinical practice. The causes of atypical manifestations of infections need a special comprehensive study. A striking and extremely important example of this kind is occult viral hepatitis B, which proceeds without the appearance of HBsAg in the blood.

To date, the laws of the infectious process, especially its initial stages, have been studied quite successfully for many diseases [6, 7], which allows to present its main steps in the acute course: (1) entering the pathogen through the "entrance gate" into the area of the possible onset of the infectious process—in the vast majority cases at mucous membranes of the respiratory system, intestines, genital, and urinary tract; (2) pathogen adhesion on the surface of sensitive cells; (3) reproduction of the pathogen (intra- or extracellularly); (4) local damage and inflammatory reaction; (5) the spread (dissemination) of the pathogen (in some rare cases, may be absent) (Fig. 1.2).

It should be specially noted that the listed general pattern can vary quite significantly depending on the pathogen and the clinical situation. Our information on the sequence of events in chronic, latent, slow infections, and carriage is fragmentary and cannot be summarized. It should only be noted that the condition for the development of a chronic infection is the persistence of the pathogen, which can be associated both with the properties of the biological agent and with defects in the general and/or local resistance of the host. The real time of challenge can often not be established. In some cases, even intrauterine penetration of pathogen cannot be excluded. A pathogen can exist for a long time both extra- and intracellularly. The mechanisms allowing the pathogen's long presence in the body are in most cases unknown. There is evidence that the pathogen can persist in the cells in an inactive form or integrate into the genome.

The study of the pathogenesis of infectious processes is currently most often carried out in vitro on cell cultures. Using the most modern technologies allows us to get valuable information about the interaction of microorganisms and various cell populations. Attention of numerous researchers is attracted to different mechanisms of cell death. According to the recent data, they can be classified as non-permeabilizing (i.e.,

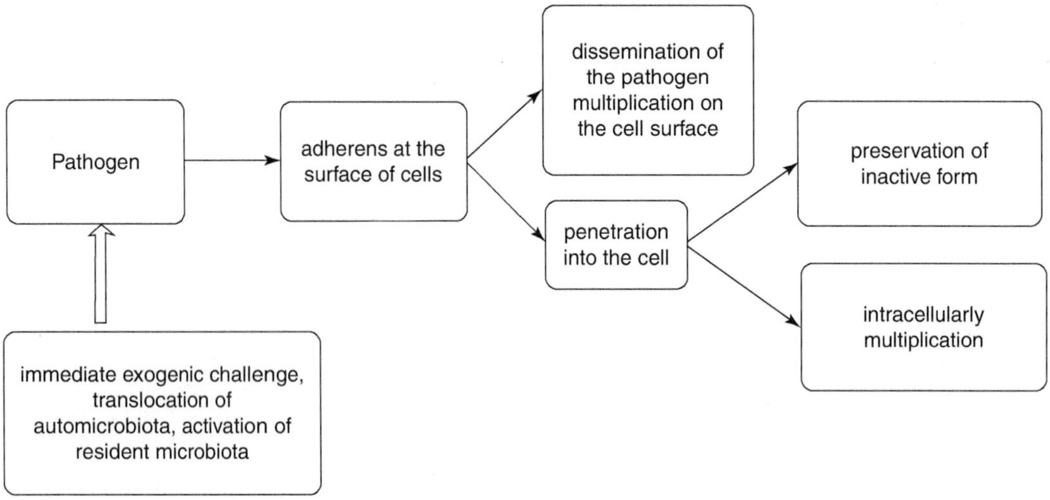

Fig. 1.2 Schema of acute infectious process

without significant rupture of cellular membrane): apoptosis, autophagy, and anoikis; while pyroptosis, necroptosis, ferroptosis are considered to be permeabilizing [8]. Attention of several researchers is drawn also to a relatively new mechanism of cell death—unfolded protein response [9].

However, not all researchers consider that even the primary interaction of the pathogen with the host cells can be different in vivo, and it is impossible to judge about the development of the pathological process in a whole organism during cytological studies. Quite valuable are the currently relative rare experimental studies with modeling infections in laboratory animals, which are now more often used to evaluate the effectiveness of new antimicrobials. When analyzing the results of experimental studies in the field of infectology, one should always evaluate the similarities and differences between the pathological process in animals and humans. Unfortunately, many diseases in animals cannot be reproduced at all, and the clinical and morphological features of a number of experimental infections in men and used animal species can differ seriously.

Question of the entrance gate for the pathogen is not always simply solved. So, the possibility that the pathogen can enter from the nasal mucosa directly into the central nervous system has been supposed but is insufficiently studied [10]. There is little information about lymph–cerebrospinal communication in the cervical spine [10]. Mechanisms of intrauterine infection of the fetus in early pregnancy are still unclear. We have to admit that in many cases the entrance gates and infection paths remain unknown.

One of the most important problems of infectious pathology is autoinfection, which has been the subject of numerous studies [6, 7, 11]. The fact of the obligatory development of the often severe and life-threatening inflammatory process associated with the body's own microbiota is undeniable. The most striking example is the development of diffuse peritonitis with intestinal perforation, for example, in typhoid fever or destructive appendicitis. Obviously, the microbiota of the large intestine even without any special properties, getting into other organs and spaces, especially in large quantities, can cause purulent inflammation. At the same time, the widespread notion that "banal" microflora occupying an unusual niche always leads to serious consequences is not certain. A striking example of this kind is ascending pyelonephritis. Based on the polymorphism of bacteria detected during this disease in urine, with the prevalence of untyped (during routine studies) *Escherchia coli*, it is customary to consider it as the leading causative agent of this autoinfection. Serious corrections of such concepts are to be made by the data that in pyelonephritis, the leading role is played by special strains of *E. coli* with tropism for urothelium (UTEC) [6, 7], and the frequent combination of bacterial microbiota with chlamydia, mycoplasmas, and viruses also is important.

Many people carry yeast-like fungi of the genus Candida (primarily *C. albicans*) on the mucous membranes of the upper respiratory tract. In case of immunodeficiency candidiasis of esophagus and other parts of gastrointestinal tract develops, as well as (currently rare) lung candidiasis.

It is widely and reasonably said that any representatives of the microbiota of the upper respiratory tract when they enter the respiratory parts of the lungs can cause pneumonia. However, at least with respect to pneumococcus, it is known that the development of the most severe form of the disease, croupous pneumonia, is preceded by colonization (carriage) of the pharyngeal mucosa by highly virulent strains of *Streptococcus pneumoniae* [7].

It is also obvious that in many cases the activation of a latent infection and the initiation of the inflammatory process during carriage are taken as autoinfection, as, for example, occurs with actinomycosis. All of the above indicates that the problem of autoinfection is far from being resolved.

From an epidemiological point of view, the source of infection can be a person (patient or carrier), animal, environmental objects. The most important in this case is the stability of the pathogen in the external environment and its ability to spread. A number of infections (vector-borne) require a carrier. It should be noted that in some cases, even with an epidemic increase in the incidence rate, as was the case with dysentery in the early 1990s of the 20th century in Russia, it is impossible to establish the exact path of the circulation of microorganisms. The infectious dose for different pathogens can vary quite significantly. It should also be remembered that in addition to the type of microorganism, its potency to express pathogenicity factors is also extremely important. In addition to the term pathogenicity, it is now customary to use the terms virulence (as a measure of pathogenicity), toxigenicity, and invasiveness. Pathogenicity is primarily determined by the genes that make up the mobile cellular elements (plasmids, transposons) and can vary significantly within the species. Different properties of strains of the same pathogen lead to significant variants of lesions, which can be especially clearly manifested in experimental studies. The most indicative in this regard is the example of *Pseudomonas aeruginosa* [12].

The most important condition for the onset of an infectious process is direct contact of the pathogen with sensitive cells. The body has many different mechanisms to prevent such contact: glycan or proteoglycan mucus, movements of the cilia, acidic environment of the stomach, etc. Pathogen adhesion is currently associated exclusively with ligand–receptor interactions, which suggests congenital sensitivity or resistance (constitutional immunity) to certain pathogens. Currently, interesting studies are being carried out in this regard related to the study of different types of toll-like receptors [6, 7]. With these circumstances, it is possible to explain the encouraging fact that a relatively small part of known microorganisms can act as pathogens (even potential) causing human diseases. Although the receptor apparatus of the host cell used by pathogens is associated with a conservative genotype, incompletely understood are variations in the susceptibility of patients at different ages, in conditions of mixed infection, etc. In such situation, we are able to speak about onset of the first (incubation) stage of the infection (Fig. 1.3).

The next mandatory stage of an acute infectious process (unlike other forms) is the reproduction of the pathogen. It can occur extracellularly (on the surface of cells) or intracellularly. In the latter case, it is preceded by the ingress of a microorganism into the cell. It should also be noted that some microorganisms, in particular mycoplasmas and some others, are capable of both extra- and intracellular reproduction. Some microorganisms with complex developmental cycles (some protozoa, fungi, chlamydia) have both extra- and intracellular forms [6, 7].

The most important task of a pathological study is to identify pathogens directly in the tis-

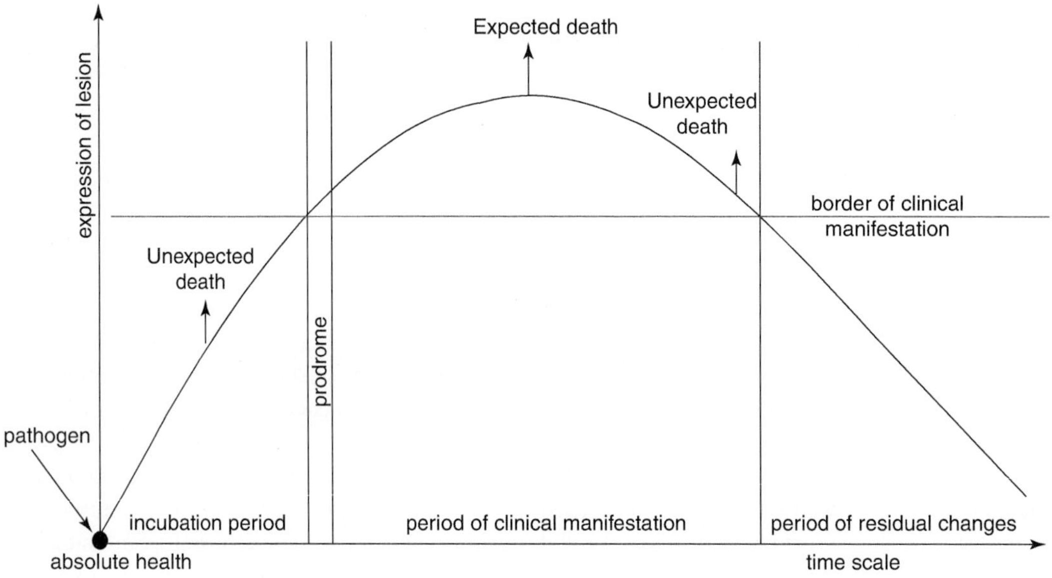

Fig. 1.3 Schema of infectious disease

Fig. 1.4 Outcomes of acute infection

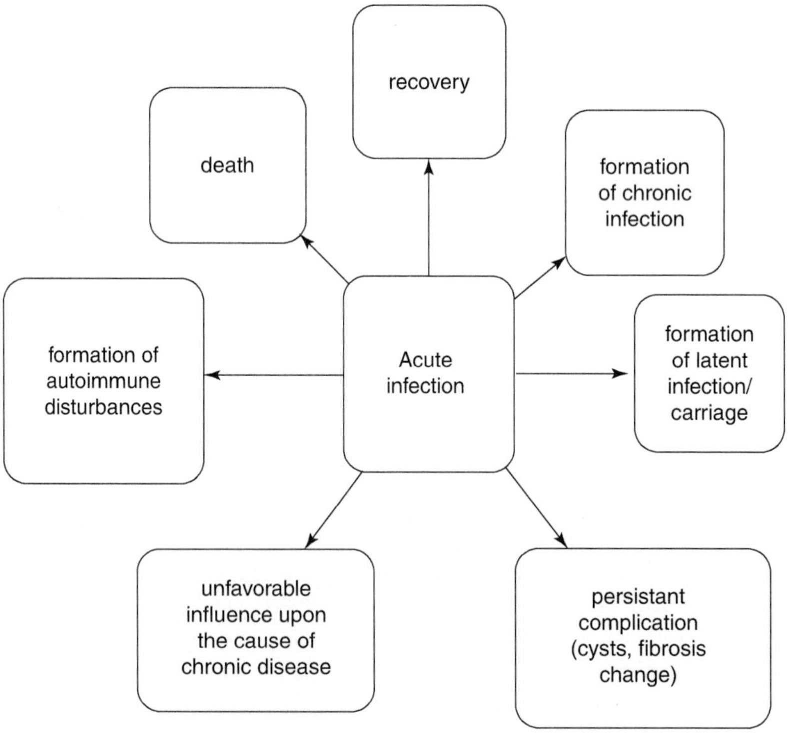

sues and compare the data obtained with the results of various microbiological and molecular biological studies. The greatest experience in this regard is in the diagnosis of bacterial processes when comparing the results of histobacterioscopic examination (when staining paraffin slices stained with azure or Gram in various modifications) with results of bacteriological examination. It should be noted, however, that even with such comparisons, it is not always easy to take into account changes in the shape and size of pathogens as compared to their "reference" species, demonstrated on artificial nutrient media, related both to the microenvironment and the effects of antibiotics and other drugs. New methods for the detection of pathogens (in situ hybridization, mass spectrometry, real-time PCR, and others) are only very limitedly used for the determination of pathogens in tissues and practically inaccessible to the vast majority of pathologists all over the world.

Pathologists of the whole world are very disappointed when they cannot detect acid-resistant rods at all in slices with indisputable tuberculosis when stained according to Ziehl–Neelsen (ZN) or the number of typical pathogens is very small. Our studies of the most recent time have shown that, at least with long-term treated fibrocavernous tuberculosis, and in a combination of tuberculosis with HIV infection mycobacteria revealed by ZN staining, luminescence microscopy when stained with auramine–rhodamine and during IHC studies are located exclusively extracellularly and often have a coccoid or other irregular shape [13, 14]. Obviously, these facts are not only of practical importance for the morphological differential diagnosis of tuberculosis but also justify the need to review some of the fundamental principles of its pathogenesis, based on the postulate that the main localization of mycobacteria is intracellular.

It is not always possible to explain the fact that a microorganism (bacterium or fungus) is determined by laboratory methods and it is impossible to detect it during a microscopic examination. One can only assume that this may be due to a small number of them. Anyway, in most cases, it can be said that the etiological role in the development of pathological processes is played only by microorganisms that are also determined by microscopic examination.

The multiplying pathogen often leads to local damage of individual cells or tissue as a whole, initially reversible (adaptive), and then irreversible (necrotic), the border between which can only be determined conditionally. Various toxins, aggression, and/or pathogenicity factors can act as damaging factors. Currently, it has been shown that the death of many cells in the zone of infection is associated with apoptosis. Other cell death mechanisms (entosis, necroptosis, pyroptosis, netosis, partanotosis, feroptosis, autophagy, etc.) have to be studied, one has to consider that till now they were discovered and described practically only in cell cultures. Various autoimmune factors (cytotoxic lymphocytes, autoantibodies, immune complexes) can be essential for damage even in acute infectious processes, as was recently demonstrated in COVID-19 [15]. The role of these factors increases in chronic infections. The effect of some intracellular pathogens can also provoke changes in the proliferative activity of a viable cell, which is manifested either in their growth or the appearance of giant multinucleated cells, for example, during paramyxovirus and coronavirus infections. The appearance of giant multinucleated cells is typical for several infections including influenza (since 2016) and COVID-19 [16].

Oncogenesis is associated with the incorporation of viral nucleic acid fragments in the host cell genome in many tumors [17]. Most striking examples are papillomaviruses and cervix carcinoma, EBV, and lymphomas. Analysis of the role of biological pathogens in oncogenesis is not among the aims of present issue.

The pathogen is associated with a local inflammatory reaction. The mechanisms of its induction have been studied for a long time. In Russian literature, the concept that inflammation has to be divided into specific and nonspecific (banal) is still preserved. The term "specific inflammation" was apparently for the first time introduced by O. Lubarsch in a textbook edited by L. Aschoff (1909) [18]. It was emphasized that granulomatosis has exceptional diagnostic significance, but nothing was said about banal inflammation. It should be noted that the term "specific inflammation" no longer appears in any modern manual. Currently, in morphological literature and practice, it is often understood as the right of a pathologist to diagnose tuberculosis without any relevance to epidemiological, clinical, and microbiological data. However, this point of view contradicts with all modern approaches to the diagnosis of this disease (requiring mandatory detection of the pathogen) [19], although, of course, in many cases, structural changes in tuberculosis are very characteristic, but not specific.

Currently, it is obvious that the host responds unequally to different pathogens and the local inflammatory reactions are not stereotype. In all textbooks in the world inflammation, as a local reaction, and the immune response, as generalized, are traditionally described separately. At present, the conventionality of their strict distinction has become obvious, since Th17 lymphocytes participate in the formation of the most common purulent inflammation, and therefore, we have to talk about an immune-mediated response. The fact that the most important participant in the inflammation is the macrophage, presenting the antigen at the initial stages of the immune response, provides additional justification for the conditionality of their differentiation. It should be noted that both the protective and pathological components can be found in the inflammatory reaction at the same time, the border between them can be determined only conditionally. Many bacteria and fungi have the ability to induce chemotaxis and the development of purulent inflammation. In most organs and tissues, massive accumulations of neutrophilic leukocytes have both a protective and a damaging role. A significant part of necrotic changes in purulent inflammation is due to the release of proteolytic enzymes from lysosomes of dying polymorphic nuclear granulocytes. Behind the blood–brain barrier, for reasons not yet fully understood, the bactericidal properties of neutrophilic leukocytes, starting from the end of the first day, cease to appear, which leads to the preservation of a large number of viable microorganisms in purulent meningitis with high neutrophilic pleocytosis [10]. Significant peculiarities of protective reactions and inflammation also exist in the placenta [20] and, probably, other organs and tissues.

For the vast majority of acute infectious processes, after the multiplication of the pathogen, its dissemination follows. Fundamentally, there are three main ways—along the length, hematogenous, lymphogenous. In addition, in neuroinfections, the spread of pathogens through the peripheral nerves and cerebrospinal fluid is possible. It should be noted that a number of pathogens do not spread in the human body in a free form, but use either the host's own cells as a Trojan horse—most often macrophages (eg HIV) [6, 7] or other larger eukaryotic microorganisms (e.g., lamblia). The establishment of a mechanism for the passage of a microorganism through the vessel wall is also very important. Fundamentally, three options are possible: transcytosis, passage through intercellular spaces, destruction of the endothelial lining [6, 7]. Despite the intensive studies that are currently provided for many infections, many issues still stay unclear.

During the period of active reproduction and spread of pathogens, the reactions of the host are maximally expressed, as well as the clinical manifestations of the disease. The main importance for their development plays numerous cytokines, primarily tumor necrosis factor, interleukin 1, 6, and acute-phase proteins. In addition, it is customary to attribute a significant role to general neurohumoral reactions (stress). Nowadays appeared even the term "cell stress" [8]. These reactions are largely nonspecific, which determines the similarity of the initial clinical manifestations of many acute infections. Currently, pronounced manifestations of a systemic inflammatory reaction are usually associated with sepsis or septic shock [21]. The highlighting of these conditions is extremely important in the practice of resuscitators, but needs a more thorough study of the etiology, pathogenesis, and structural features.

Later on, in the case of the effectiveness of general and local protective reactions and successful treatment, the number of viable pathogens decreases, the severity of the inflammatory reaction reduces, the clinical signs of the disease disappear, and after, as a rule, unspecified duration of the postclinical stage of the disease, a somewhat abstract complete recovery occurs (see Fig. 1.3). With an unfavorable course of the disease, the onset of a "predictable" or sudden fatal outcome is possible. A frequent outcome of an acute infectious process is the formation of a chronic infection, which can have both a relatively favorable low-symptom and a progressive course leading to death. Obviously, the outcomes of an infectious disease depend on many factors: species and strain properties of the pathogen, its quantity, general and local resistance of the host, its hereditary predisposition, and certainly the treatment, first of all. In many cases, it is impossible to determine reliably the causes of a particular outcome.

Long-term infection of the host with a microorganism can lead to a change in their properties. On the part of the host are described, both different variants of acquired immunodeficiency, as well as stimulation of immune reactions, including due to sensitization immunopathological (allergic) ones. Microorganisms can both enhance and weaken their virulence, often changing their structure, including determined by histobacterioscopic study [4]. It should be noted that this question remains little studied.

As already mentioned above, a thorough analysis of the etiology of infectious processes often reveals several biological pathogens in the body of a sick person, which in many cases leads to a mixed infection. This fact was first seriously studied in the works of A.V. Zinserling [4], still remains relevant today, especially in the terminal stage of HIV infection, in which the number of identified infectious processes can reach 10. Variants of the interaction of various pathogens as part of a mixed infection: (1) activation of infectious processes caused by both (all) pathogens; (2) preferential activation of one of the infectious processes; (3) the manifestation of antagonism between pathogens—the activation of the infectious process does not occur.

The spatial relationships between microorganisms may also be different: (1) pathogens can be localized in different organs; (2) microbes can be in one organ, but have different targets; (3) pathogens can simultaneously affect the same cell without directly coming into contact with each other; (4) pathogens can come into contact with their external surfaces, for example, viruses adhere to the surface of bacteria and mycoplasmas; (5) one microorganism is in another, for example, viruses in fungal cells; (6) pathogens can form a common biofilm. It should be noted that many aspects of mixed infections need special study. In Chap. 16, mixed infections in respiratory organs are discussed specially.

An important issue of infectious pathology is pathomorphism [4] (term predominantly used in Russian literature), by which we mean changes in the course of both individual diseases and their panorama as a whole. While the obvious sharp decrease in the incidence of mortality from "controlled infections"—such as smallpox, measles, poliomyelitis does not need special comments, then significant fluctuations in the frequency of other infections, such as dysentery, meningococcal infection, and escherichiosis remain unclear [4]. We can also state unexplained changes in the clinical and morphological manifestations of individual infectious diseases. The most striking example is meningococcal infection, which initially (XIX and the first half of the XX century) caused mainly cerebrospinal meningitis, while the role of meningococcemia, which was primarily described as casuistic observation, significantly increased in the 70th of the XX century [19]. On the other hand, the analysis of a large number of autopsy observations of diphtheria in adults in the first half of the 90th of the XX century showed that clinical course of the disease and its structural changes remained practically the same as in classical descriptions of the first half of the century [4]. It should be noted that in many cases we do not know exactly the causes and mechanisms of pathomorphosis.

In modern literature, some new promising directions in the study of infectious processes are widely discussed, first of all: analysis of biofilms from various bacterial, mycoplasma, fungal, protozoal microorganisms on the surface of mucous membranes under physiological and pathological conditions [22]; study of the morphology and molecular biological characteristics of tissue forms of microorganisms, taking into account the age of the patient, his immune status, treatment, localization of the lesion in different organs; clarification of the possible etiological and/or pathologic role of biological pathogens in the occurrence and course of a number of common not communicable diseases.

Further research is related to solve a number of issues. Firstly, these are the most obvious problems associated with the need to clarify many aspects of the pathogenesis and diagnosis of certain diseases. We have no reason to consider the pathogenesis of any infectious disease to be completely known. Secondly, this is the streamlining of terminology. Obviously, many historical terms require more precise definitions. One of the most obvious examples is related to lesions by biological pathogens of the respiratory tract. A certain confusion is noted when using the terms "pneumonia," "alveolitis," "pneumonitis," "diffuse alveolar damage," "generalized infection with lung involvement."

Recently, one can note rising interest to the problem of pneumonias. In the manual on practical pulmonary pathology in 2011 appeared very informative chapters on acute lung injuries (including those caused by infections) and lung infections [23]. In 2018 appeared a fundamental review "Integrative physiology of pneumonia," based upon 574 publications in English, where numerous questions of its pathogenesis are discussed in detail [24]. The only substantial gap is absence of any mention of morphological changes and their peculiarities related to etiology of pneumonia. It is not strange, because in the literature of the last 50 years, there are no serious contributions on histopathology of pneumonias, as if there is no topic for study.

The junction between microbiology, molecular biology, and pathology has to be promoted. Obviously, despite the outstanding achievements of modern research carried out at the cellular level, they are not able to answer all the urgent questions that medical practice poses. Among the necessary approaches, morphological studies are of great importance. A harmonious combination of traditional, well-established methods and the latest technologies, such as immunohistochemistry, in situ hybridization, in situ PCR, molecular genetic analysis after laser microdissection with the use of confocal microscopy, are required. It is gratifying that the methodological capabilities of tissue studies are rapidly improving. In addition to the appropriate technologies, the correct choice of research objects with the formulation of adequate tasks is very important.

References

1. The top 10 causes of death. https://www.who.int/news-room/fact-sheets/detail/the-top-10-causes-of-death
2. Patricia Marques. Human microbiota and microbiome. p. 275, 2018
3. van den Tweel JG, Gu J, Taylor CR, editors. From magic to molecules. An illustrated history of disease. Beijing: Peking University Medical Press; 2016.
4. Zinserling VA. School of infectious pathology of A.V. Zinserling: achievements and perspectives. Arkhiv Patologii. 2014;76(1):3–9. (In Russian)
5. Vaynshenker YI, Ivchenko IM, Zinserling VA, et al. Low manifested infections with CNS lesions in patient with longterm unconciency state of non inflammatory etiology. Zh Microbiol Epidemiol Immunobiol. 2011;88(6):85–9. (In Russian)
6. Mims CA, Dimmock NJ, Nash A, Stephen J. Mim's pathogenesis of infectious disease 4th Ed. Cambridge, MA: Academic Press 1995 414 p.
7. N.G. Engleberg, V.Rita, T.S. Dermody Shaechter's mechanisms of microbial disease. 4th Ed. Philadelphia, PA: Lippincott Williams & Wilkins, 2007.
8. FitzGerald ES, Luz NF, Jamieson AM. Competitive cell death interactions in pulmonary infection: host modulation versus pathogen manipulation. Front Immunol. 2020;11:814. https://doi.org/10.3389/fimmu.20.00814.
9. Mehrbod P, Ande SR, Alizadeh J, et al. The roles of apoptosis, autophagy and unfolded protein response in arbovirus, influenza virus, and HIV infections. Virulence. 2019;10(1):376–413.
10. Zinserling VA, Chukhlovina ML. Infectious Lesions of nervous system. Issues of etiology, pathogenesis and diagnostics. Saint-Petersburg: ElbiSPb; 2011. p. 583. (In Russian)
11. Anichkov NN, Zakharyevskaya MA. Experimental studies on autogenic infectious processes in lungs. Vest Khir. 1954;113(5):19–25. (In Russian)
12. Zinserling VF, Moroz AF. Comparative estimation of pathological process on the model of experimental pneumonia in rats caused by strains of Pseudomonas aeruginosa of different origin. Zh Microbiol Epidemiol Immunobiol. 1984;61(12):68–75. (In Russian)
13. Zinserling VA, Agapov MM, Orlov AN. The informative value of various methods for identifying acid-fast bacilli in relation to the degree of tuberculosis process activity. Arkhiv Patologii. 2018;80(3):40–5. (In Russian)
14. Agapov MM, Zinserling VA, Semenova NY, et al. Pathological anatomy of tuberculosis in the presence of human immunodeficiency virus infection. Arkhiv Patologii. 2020;82(2):12–9. (In Russian)
15. Ehrenfeld M, Tincani A, Andreoli L, et al. COVID-19 and autoimmunity. Autoimmun Rev. 2020, 2020; https://doi.org/10.1016/j.autrev.2020.102597.
16. Skok K, Stelzl E, Trauner M, et al. Post-mortem viral dynamics and tropism in COVID-19 patients in cor-

relation with organ damage. Virchows Arch. 2020; https://doi.org/10.1007/s00428-020-02903-8.
17. Krump NA, You J. Molecular mechanisms of viral oncogenesis in humans. Nat Rev Microbiol. 2018;16(11):684–98. https://doi.org/10.1038/s41579-018-0064-6.
18. Aschoff L. Hrg Pathologische Anatomie/ Ein Lehrbuch für Studierende und Ärzte Jena 1909 Verlag von Gustav Fischer
19. Achkar JM, Lawn SD, Moosa M-YS, et al. Adjunctive tests for diagnosis of tuberculosis: serology, ELISPOT for site-specific lymphocytes, urinary lipoarabinomannan, string test, and fine needle aspiration. J Inf Dis. 2011;204(4):1130–41. https://doi.org/10.1093/infdis/jir450.
20. Zinserling VA, Melnikova VF. Perinatal infections: issues of pathogenesis, morphological diagnostic and clinic-pathological correlations. Manual for doctors: Elbi-SPb; 2002. p. 351. (In Russian)
21. Wiersinga WJ, Seymour CW, editors. Handbook of sepsis. New York: Springer; 2019. p. 267.
22. Tolker-Nielsen T. Biofilm development. Microbiol Spectr. 2015;3(2) https://doi.org/10.1128/microbiolspec.MB-0001-2014.
23. Leslie K.O., Wick M.R. Eds Practical pulmonary pathology. A diagnostic approach. 2nd Ed. 2011, 828 p.
24. Quinton LJ, Walkey AJ, Mizgerd JP. Integrative physiology of pneumonia. Physiol Rev. 2018;98(3):1417–64. https://doi.org/10.1152/physrev.00032.2017.

2 Microbiology, Molecular Biology, Immunology, and Microscopy in Diagnostics

The leading role in the accurate etiological diagnosis of bacterial infections belongs to the bacteriological study of autopsy, biopsy, surgical materials, and afterbirths. It should be noted that a prerequisite for the correct interpretation of the results is not only the correct sterile sampling of the material for the study but also using an adequate set of nutrient media. Otherwise, many microbes, especially anaerobic ones, and some aerobic such as pneumococci and hemophilic bacilli, practically stop sowing. In practice, for various reasons, the effectiveness of postmortem bacteriological studies is often insufficient [1].

It should be noted that during postmortem bacteriological research, valuable information can be obtained even in relation to those microbes, for example, meningococcus, which, according to popular belief, are not sown from corpses. The main factor leading to a sharp decrease in the seeding rate of this pathogen is even short term and clinically ineffective antibiotic therapy. The elapsed time between death and autopsy, as well as ambient temperature, does not play a significant role.

It was also shown that the quantity and quality of the detected microbes do not differ significantly depending on the timing of the autopsy after death. Naturally, the corpse of the deceased should be kept in the refrigerator. Otherwise, there will be a sharp increase in the seeding of bacteria, mainly conditionally pathogenic—"false positives," i.e., without clinical importance. It is not possible to reliably explain them in all cases, but as a working hypothesis we can suggest—a violation of the permeability of histohematogenous barriers in the agonal period. It is important that according to our observations, a clinically significant pathogen is always determined not only bacteriologically but also histobacterioscopic and there must be a tissue reaction to it. Quite often one can meet with the "false negative" results of the postmortem bacteriological study. This fact, of course, can be associated with operating defects in the pathological department or the bacteriological laboratory, but in most cases, it is associated with objective reasons. Treatment, even short term, with antibiotics can lead to the formation of "non-sowing forms" [2–4]. It should be noted that this process in modern bacteriology has been studied extremely insufficiently. In addition, in mixed bacterial infection, antagonism between individual pathogens can affect.

Microscopic examination of smears taken from the surface of lesion with probable inflammatory changes due to bacteria and fungi was introduced in practice of pathologists at the beginning of the XXth century, in spite of the approximating results, such study appeared to be extremely effective even in the field conditions (Fig. 2.1) and can be useful nowadays as well (Fig. 2.2).

Isolated bacterial cultures are preferably typed as accurately as possible. If it is necessary to

V. Zinserling, *Infectious Pathology of the Respiratory Tract*,
https://doi.org/10.1007/978-3-030-66325-4_2

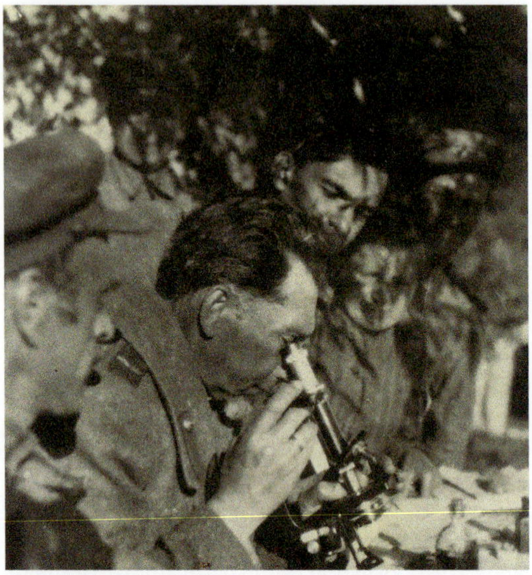

Fig. 2.1 Chief pathologist of Leningrad front lieutenant-colonel V.D. Zinserling provides (1944) cytological examination of smears after the autopsy directly at the battle field

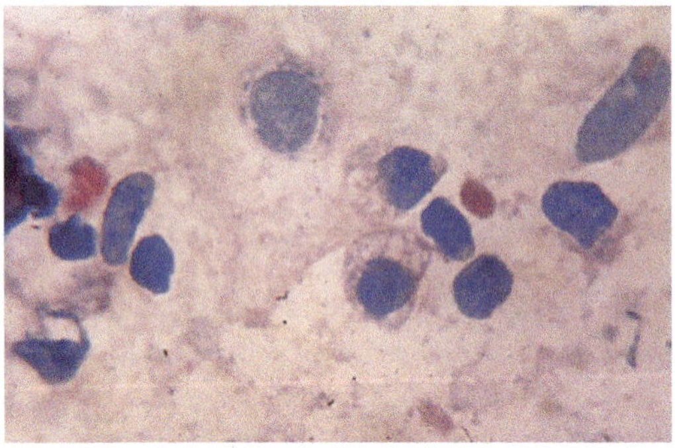

Fig. 2.2 Different cell types in a smear from the surface of lung cut at the autopsy. Stained after Seller. ×800

prove the fact of nosocomial (hospital) infection, it is necessary to use several methods of intraspecies typing with the determination of immuno-, piocin-phagotypes, etc. [5]. Can we expect differences in the clinical and morphological manifestations of the disease depending on the immunotype (serovar) of the pathogen? Although such judgments have repeatedly been presented in the literature related to several pathogens, a definite answer to this question cannot be given. Of course, correlations between surface antigens that determine the immunotype and the expression of pathogenicity factors that determine the virulence of the pathogen are possible. However, the pathogen's immunotype does not affect directly its pathogenic properties.

It is extremely important to emphasize that such a widely used division of bacteria into "conditionally" and "unconditionally" pathogenic is very relative. The virulence of the microorganism varies greatly in individual strains of the same species and depends on the set and degree of expression of pathogenicity factors. As a very illustrative example, the results of our comprehensive study of *Pseudomonas aeruginosa* strains of different origin can be presented. Strains isolated from organs of children who died from severe necrotic pneumonia due to *P. aeruginosa* expressed a greater number of enzymes of pathogenicity and caused incomparably more severe changes during intratracheal challenge of laboratory rats compared with strains obtained from asymptomatic patients [5].

In many cases, for a detailed characterization of the pathogen properties, along with the determination of pathogenicity enzymes, it is desirable to determine the plasmid profile, conduct genotyping, and determine the production of various types of toxins [2–4]. It is regrettable to note that many of the existing methods are often either not used at all or only in research.

It is fundamentally possible to identify bacteria by using luminescent sera according to the Coons method. We are aware of such studies regarding pneumococcus and meningococcus. However, the difficulty in obtaining diagnostic sera that do not give a cross reaction with related microorganisms, as well as the ability of such a widespread pathogen as staphylococcus to adsorb nonspecifically all sera, impede the widespread introduction of this method into practice. For the same reasons, the system for IHC did not find wide application for the detection of many bacterial pathogens. Only the diagnosis of chlamydial infection can be very effective. It is most successfully used in clinical practice in the study of smears, and the results obtained with its help are often more informative than PCR. We have some positive experience with its use also in paraffin sections, provided that nonspecific lighting is suppressed (Fig. 2.3). When examining paraffin sections without a special treatment in a luminescent microscope, a nonspecific luminescence, especially strong in the walls and lumens of blood vessels, is naturally revealed. To detect acid-resistant bacteria (primarily mycobacteria), fluorescence microscopy with staining by auramine–rhodamine can be successfully used studying not only smears, as in bacteriological laboratories but also in tissue slices (Fig. 2.4). The use of this method in the practice of pathologists is extremely limited.

Currently, PCR is widely used to diagnose a number of bacterial infections, especially poorly

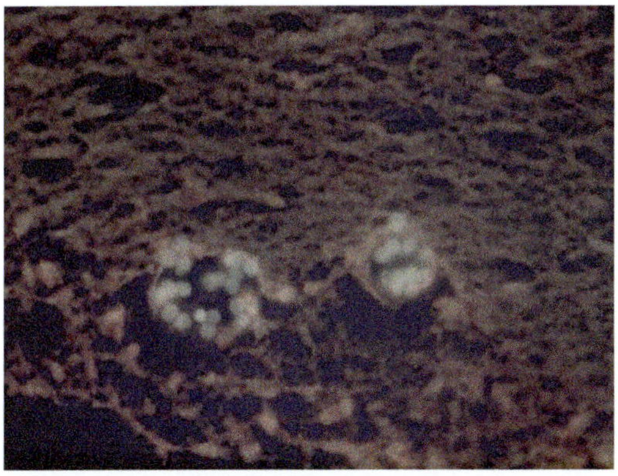

Fig. 2.3 Antigen of *Chlamydia trachomatis* in paraffin slice of the lung of newborn child. Luminescent microscopy. ×1000

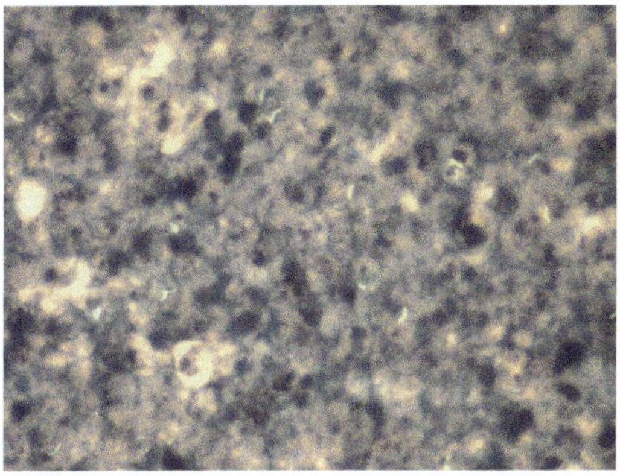

Fig. 2.4 Acid-fast Mycobacteria in paraffin slice of lungs deceased from tuberculosis. Stained by auramine–rhodamin. Luminescent microscopy. ×650

growing on nutrient media, primarily tuberculosis and atypical mycobacteriosis [6]. Moreover, the DNA necessary for its performance can also be obtained from small volumes of tissue fixed in formalin and embedded in paraffin. Despite the exceptional value of this method, especially if it is set up according to the "real-time" method, which allows quantitative determination of the DNA of the desired pathogen, both literature data and our own experience do not allow us to exclude both false-positive and false-negative results. Currently, a very promising method is being considered for the detection of all bacteria during sequencing of ribosomal RNA with determination of 16S rRNA and fungi by 18S rRNA [7]. Unfortunately, due to the lack of our own experience, it is not possible to assess the real sensitivity of this method.

In certain bacterial infections, for example, salmonellosis and staphylococcus, serological examination of postmortem taken blood in RBC and RBH may be informative. In other diseases, which are characterized by a rapid development of the disease, for example, meningococcal infection, serological studies are usually negative. It should also be noted that in the serological diagnosis of infections belonging to the Enterobacteriaceae family and having numerous common antigens, a cross-reaction between different pathogens is possible. Determination of antibodies against a number of pathogens, for example, pneumococcus, is uninformative for diagnosis. Serodiagnostics of many bacterial infections has not been developed.

For the posthumous diagnosis of a number of infections, a number of auxiliary methods developed for clinical practice can be used: latex agglutination, coagglutination, etc. However, their use has never been officially legalized and was carried out only in the framework of research.

The significance of virus isolation in the postmortem diagnosis of infections is incomparably less than the seeding of bacteria. This is due to the complexity, high cost, as well as lower productivity of this method. In addition, for a number of viruses, primarily human immunodeficiency virus, hepatitis B, C, D viruses, JCV, and a num-

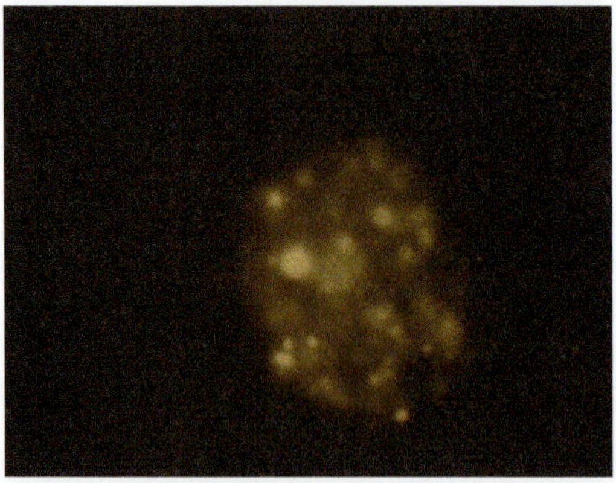

Fig. 2.5 Antigen of influenza A in smear from the surface of lung cut. Luminescent microscopy. ×900

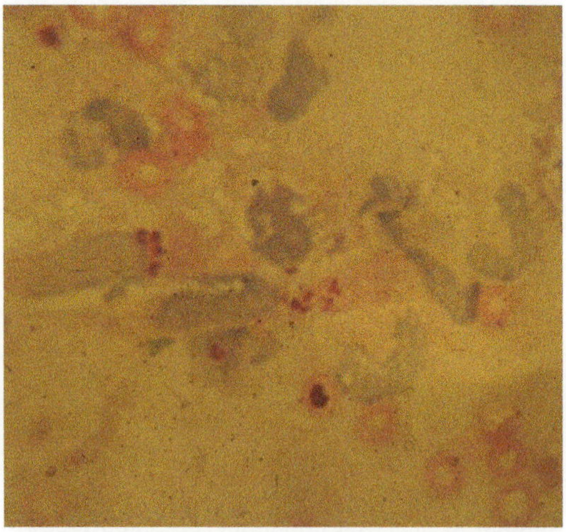

Fig. 2.6 Fuchsinophilc inclusions in cytoplasm of ciliary epithelial cell in a smear from the surface of lung cut at the autopsy. Stained after Seller. ×800

ber of others, such methods are generally absent. It should also be held in mind that in some cases it is possible to isolate a virus, for example, herpes simplex or enterovirus, in the absence of any distinct structural changes in the investigated organ. When assessing the possibilities of virology research, it is necessary to take into account the thermal lability of viruses. Obtaining viral cultures is of practical importance only with in-depth virology research, preparation of vaccines, although many problems in modern virology are solved using molecular biological methods in the study of nucleic acids.

In the world practice usually are used simpler, cheaper, and more informative methods. Historically, the most widely used method was IF microscopy (Fig. 2.5). As objects of research, smears or scrapings from the respiratory tract, lungs, meninges, brain, kidneys, liver, and other organs, as well as cryostat and even paraffin sections (especially with special processing), can be used. In the past, high-quality diagnostic sera for all respiratory and herpes simplex viruses were widely available. It should be noted that the effectiveness of this method to a large extent depends not only on the quality of the applied sera, relevance of the strains used, but also on the experience of the specialist conducting the research.

We have also quite positive experience in using for immediate diagnostics smears (scrapings) stained with methylene blue–fuchsine according to Seller (or in other modifications) [1]. In such cytological smears, one can find intracytoplasmic fuchsinophilic inclusions (typical for influenza and other RNA–viral respiratory infections) (Fig. 2.6), intranuclear basophilic inclusions in DNA viral infections, typical for Mycoplasma and Chlamydia vacuolization, bacterial and fungal microbiota. It is obvious that this method can be considered only as preliminary and its results highly depend upon the qualification of technician and pathologist.

Detection of virus antigens in sections using an IHC study, its DNA during in situ hybridization (Fig. 2.7), detection of viral particles with various modifications of electron microscopy is usually carried out by pathologists. One has to note that the reliable results can be obtained only in case of the use of appropriate diagnostic tools, strictly following the technology with all necessary controls.

Among the most rapidly developing technologies at present is the PCR method. Currently, it is widely used to detect almost all viruses. For research, especially DNA-containing viruses, archival paraffin-embedded material is also suitable for a storage period of no more than 5–7 years. The possibility of sequencing (determining the sequence of nucleotides) of the selected segment of the nucleic acid of the virus

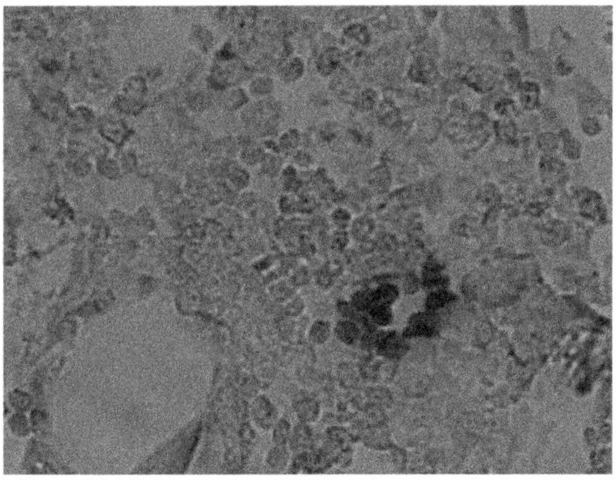

Fig. 2.7 DNA of Herpes simplex in bone marrow slice in newborn rabbit with generalized infection after intraperitoneal challenge. In situ hybridization. ×600

is also very valuable, which allows us to judge the individual properties of the pathogen. One of the first works in this regard, devoted to the diagnosis of CMV infection was a study performed in our laboratory [8].

Of the other laboratory methods, serological is very informative with the determination of the level of antibodies to different viruses in ELISA, as well as today considered as obsolete reaction of complement binding (RCB) and reaction of indirect hemagglutination (RIH). For these reactions can be used not only blood but also CSF and amniotic fluid. If the pathologist has at his disposal the results of even a single postmortem examination, it has diagnostic value, including for determining the duration of the disease, especially when detection of the immunoglobulin fractions is provided and when comparing its results with methods that detect the pathogen itself or its antigen and histological study.

In the last decade, in practical virological diagnostics, including the study of autopsy materials, commercial systems for enzyme immunoassay have been used, aimed both at determining antigens and antibodies in blood serum. This method is very technological and economical. We have a positive experience in its use for the diagnosis of infections caused by herpes simplex viruses, cytomegaly, Epstein–Barr, HIV, hepatitis B and C, tick-borne encephalitis, ECHO viruses, rotaviruses.

Diagnosis of mycoplasmosis can be based on their isolation on special feeding media (*Ureaplasma urealyticum*, *Mycoplasma hominis*), but in some cases (with *Mycoplasma pneumoniae*), its effectiveness is extremely low. Different specialists have an ambiguous attitude to the IF microscopy method used in many cases due to the possibility of cross reactions. We have a positive experience in using RBC. Today, PCR is considered as the most informative method, although even with these infections, we have no reason to absolutize the results obtained with its help. There are no commercial systems for IF and IHC diagnostics; fundamentally for tissue diagnostics, it is possible to use an indirect method.

Approaches to laboratory diagnosis of chlamydia are similar. There are no doubts about the reliability of the IFM (see Fig. 2.3). Both monoclonal serum for certain types of pathogen and polyclonal are commercially available. There are also commercial systems for IHC diagnostics. It is possible to use PCR, however, due to incompletely clarified reasons (most likely related to the presence of inhibitor proteins), the results of this study may be falsely negative [9].

For the accurate diagnosis of mycoses, pathogen isolation is important. Mushrooms of the genus Candida and Cryptococcus can grow on ordinary nutrient media. Isolation of other fungi requires special media that are used to a limited extent. Methods of isolation of Pneumocystis on artificial nutrient media are generally absent. Serological reactions in the pathological diagnosis of practical application are not found. Commercial serum for IHC studies does not exist. To a limited extent, PCR diagnostics is used. Recently, the use of ribosomal RNA sequencing to detect 18sRNA has begun. Of particular importance is microscopic examination in many cases requiring the use of additional staining methods: PAS, impregnation according to Grokkott, and Gram.

In the diagnosis of diseases caused by protozoa, the detection of pathogens by sowing is practically not carried out. Available serological reactions in most cases are absent with exception of toxoplasmosis. An enzyme-linked immunosorbent assay for class G antibodies only confirms the very frequent infection with this pathogen. Only the presence of serum IgM has diagnostic value, indicating an acute form of the infectious process. For diagnostics of toxoplasmosis, IHC is successfully used. Of great importance is the identification of structures typical for various protozoa (toxoplasma, plasmodium, amoeba, balantidia, etc.) in the tissues. In most cases, additional stains cannot help; the only exception is toxoplasmosis, in which the pathogen stains well during the PAS reaction.

Immunological methods are used in the study of autopsy material only in a very limited volume. In blood of the deceased, in principle, practically all modern immunological studies can be carried out, naturally making some corrections for postmortem changes. Individual lymphocytes capable of blast transformation can be detected even 3 days after death [1]. Our own experience with immunologists confirms the fundamental possibility of determining in blood taken 2–4 h after the death of B and T lymphocytes.

It is quite realistic to determine the content of the main classes of immunoglobulins (G, M, A) in blood taken during autopsy. For these studies, blood taken on an autopsy performed at the usual time is quite suitable. In this case, serums stored in the freezer of a virology or bacteriological laboratory can be used. It is also possible to determine immunoglobulins in other biological fluids.

The posthumous determination of interferon, which can be determined both in biological fluids and tissues of various organs, provides valuable information about the body's resistance. It should be noted that both its total content and individual properties can be studied.

It is also possible to determine in the posthumous blood circulating immune complexes (CIC) that play a significant role in the pathogenesis of many infectious and infectious-allergic diseases. For this purpose, the most widely used method of deposition of CIC in polyethylene glycol can be used with their subsequent quantitative determination on a spectrophotometer.

The concept of infectious diseases as the interaction of macro- and microorganisms developed in the 19th century. It was obvious for all researchers involved in this problem that there is the need to study the response of the host to the defeat and the microbial aggression (see Fig. 1.1).

In recent decades, especially great progress has been made by specialists involved in immunology, allergology, and inflammation mechanisms. Presentation of these issues at the current molecular biological level represents the content of many very significant manuals [10, 11]. Almost all studies of this kind were performed either in experimental animals, or on cell cultures, or in blood obtained from sick and healthy people.

A study of the reactions of a host based upon investigation of tissues (in autopsies, surgical, biopsy materials, and afterbirths) is rarely carried out. There are practically no works in which comparisons were made between clinical–immunological and immunomorphological data. Assessment of the state of the immune system after death is usually based on a study of the thymus gland (in children and adolescents), the spleen, tonsils, and peripheral lymph nodes by morphological methods. In this case, as a rule, detailed comparisons with the results of clinical and immunological studies are not carried out. This circumstance significantly complicates the clinical and morphological comparisons in primary and secondary immunodeficiency, "thymus–lymphatic status," etc.

In many cases, it is highly desirable to assess the nature of the cellular response in the lesion. Certain information can also be obtained during routine staining with hematoxylin–eosin. One should only beware of taking zones with pronounced karyorrhexis for neutrophilic infiltration, which sometimes happens when a slice is studied at a low magnification. For more reliable detection of eosinophilic leukocytes and mast cells in tissues, the importance of which is often underestimated, stains with azure–eosin (in any of many modifications) and/or toluidine blue are very informative. The most valuable results can be obtained by IHC analysis of cell infiltrate. The identification of various populations of macrophages (CD68, CD14), T (CD3, CD4, CD8), B (CD20), NK (CD56) lymphocytes, and dendritic cells is of greatest importance. The list of sera can certainly be significantly expanded; however, we do not always have the opportunity to reliably interpret the detected morphological picture. The determination of proliferative activity of the cells (Ki-67), expression of apoptosis factors (p53, FasR, FasL, tunnel test, caspasa3 and several others) is also important for understanding the essence of the infectious process. Other mechanisms of cell death (NETosis) may be of importance as well [7].

IHC studies with a detailed determination of the phenotype of cells in world practice are carried out almost exclusively on biopsy material. Most fully, such fairly expensive studies are carried in diagnostics of tumors.

It is important to emphasize that the analysis of cell populations using IHC sometimes gives significantly different results compared to those obtained using routine histological techniques. So, for many decades, it was believed that in the stroma of the chorionic villi of the mature placenta, macrophages (Hoffbauer–Kashchenko cells) are absent. With IHC, they are detected, although having atypical for macrophages morphology. Certain information can also be obtained by morphometric studies of the thymus gland, spleen, lymph nodes, and tonsils with the measurement of their zones.

In previous decades, histochemical reactions were often used for immunomorphological characterization, which allows differentiation of T, B lymphocytes, monocytes, and macrophages by the activity of acid phosphatase, nonspecific esterase, and alkaline phosphatase. Currently, this method is practically not used.

Valuable information can also be obtained by staining a section with a foci of purulent inflammation by fast green in a lysosomal cationic test (Fig. 2.8). When staining smears or paraffin sections by semiquantitative calculations of green granules of cationic proteins of neutrophilic granulocytes, their potential bactericidal activity can be determined, and the number of green-colored microbes can be used to detect dead ones under the influence of cationic proteins [12].

Useful information can also be obtained using the method of luminescent microscopy, due to which immunoglobulins of various classes and fixed immune complexes can be detected in tissue slices.

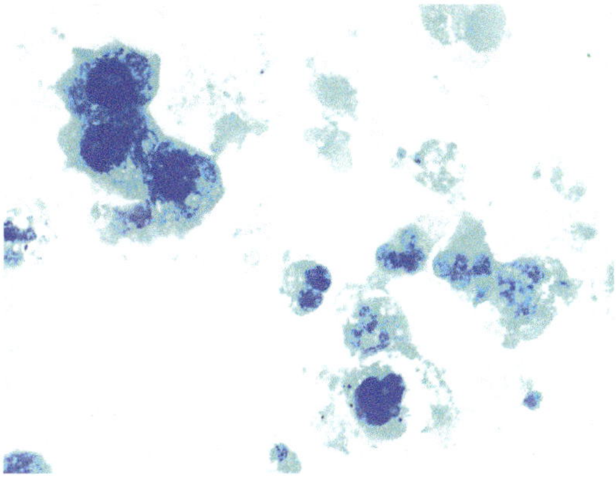

Fig. 2.8 Smear from the cut surface of the lung of the patient with secondary pneumonia. Note mixed exudate and single free and phagocyted cocci. Lysosomal cationic test. Stained by fast green. ×1000. Courtesy of Yu.A. Mazing

Of particular interest are the data that can be obtained by lectin histochemical study. In particular, much attention is paid to the detection of the Thomas–Fredenreich antigen, which is credited with a significant role in the pathogenesis of hemolytic–uremic syndrome and autoimmune lesions of a number of internal organs. Normally, this antigen is not determined, but appears after exposure to derivatives of sialic acid in the surface structures of cells of neuraminidases of bacterial and viral origin. The detection of this antigen is associated with its specific affinity for peanut agglutinin, which can be detected using a fluorescent or enzyme label in both frozen and paraffin sections.

An electron microscopic autoradiographic method is very valuable for studying the function of phagocytosis and the bactericidal activity of neutrophilic leukocytes. It allows to identify in detail the microbial population labeled with H3 thymidine, to trace in detail all the stages of the relationship of microbes, in particular autostrains, with neutrophilic leukocytes [13].

Analysis of the ultrastructure of lymphocytes allows us to identify large granular lymphocytes (LGL), which by their functional properties and IHC characteristics can be divided into cytotoxic

(CD8+) and natural killers (CD57+). The role of these cells in the cytolysis of target cells infected with viruses or bacteria has been proven. All phases of their cytotoxic effect are traced. In this case, the activation of LGL is accompanied by a change in their shape from spherical to elongated with a concentration of granules in the cytoplasmic region adjacent to the target cell. Activated LGLs are characterized by a sharply eccentric arrangement of the nucleus with elongation of the cytoplasm and the formation of one or several outgrowths completely covered with villi.

In immunodeficiency, ultrastructural rearrangements of immunocompetent cells with the appearance in their cytoplasm or nucleus of unusual tubulo-reticular inclusions, crystalloid structures, cylindrical, or amorphous globules have also been described. Opinions were expressed that such changes are directly related to the defeat of HIV cells, but there is a view that their appearance is due to a disruption in the production of interferon and cytokines.

In the nuclei of the cells be detected PML–nuclear bodies (inclusions containing regulatory protein—ProMyelocytic Leukemia protein) (Fig. 2.9). Formation of PML–nuclear bodies is nowadays considered as a hallmark of activation of unspecific antiviral response related with expression of interferon genes [14].

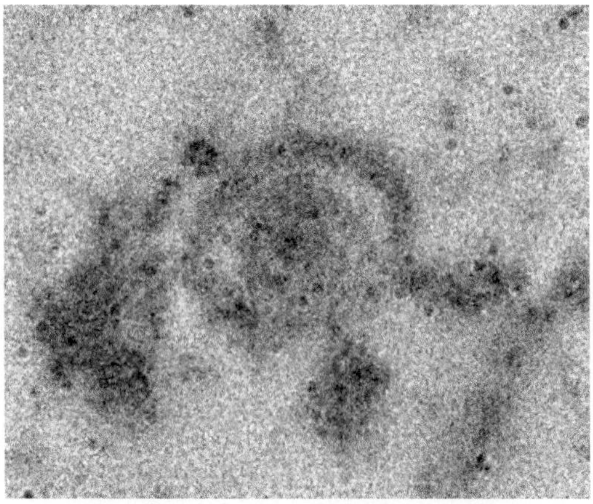

Fig. 2.9 ProMyelocytic Leukemia antigen in brain vessel wall. Specimen from early autopsy. Electron microscopy ×20,000

References

1. Zinserling AV, Zinserling VA. Modern infections: pathologic anatomy and issues of pathogenesis: a guide. SPb: Sotis; 2002. 346 p. (In Russian).
2. Morris JA, Harrison LM, Partridge SM. Postmortem bacteriology: a re-evaluation. J Clin Pathol. 2006;59(1):1–9. https://doi.org/10.1136/jcp.2005.028183.
3. Barer MR, Irving W, Swann A, Perera N. Medical microbiology. 19th ed. Elsevier Science; 2018. p. 800.
4. Goering R, Dockrell HM, Zuckerman M, Chiodini P. Mims' medical microbiology and immunology, International Edition. 6th ed. Elsevier Science; 2018. p. 568.
5. Zinserling VF, Moroz AF. Comparative estimation of pathological process on the model of experimental pneumonia in rats caused by strains of Pseudomonas aeruginosa of different origin. Zh Microbiol Epidemiol Immunobiol. 1984;61(12):68–75. (In Russian).
6. Zimina VN, Alvares Figueroa MV, Degtyareva SY, et al. Diagnostics of mycobacteriosis in HIV-positive patients. Infectious diseases. 2016;14(4):63–70. (In Russian).
7. Kradin RL. Diagnostic pathology of infectious diseases. Elsevier; 2018. 698 p.
8. Popov SD, Tsinzerling VA, Vinogradskaia GR, et al. Cytomegalovirus infection in autopsy material using molecular biologic methods. Arkh Patol. 1993;55(4):69–72. (In Russian).
9. Chen H, Wen Y, Li Z. Clear victory for Chlamydia: the subversion of host innate immunity. Front Vicrobiol. 2019;10:1412. https://doi.org/10.3389/fmicb.2019.01412.
10. Abbas AK, Lichtman AH, Pillai S. Basic immunology. 6th ed. Elsevier Science; 2019. p. 336.
11. Rich Robert R, et al. Clinical immunology: principles and practice. 5th ed. Elsevier Science; 2018. p. 1328.
12. Bryazhnikova TS, Aleshina GM, Isakov VA, Mazing YA. Functional activity of neutrophilic granulocytes in patients with relapsing herpes. Bull Exp Biol Med. 1995;120(3):968–9. (In Russian).
13. Sarkisov DS, Pal'sin AA, Kolker II, et al. RNA synthesis during neutrophil activation. Arkh Patol. 1986;48(12):6–13. (In Russian).
14. Lallemand-Breitenbach V, de Thé H. PML nuclear bodies. Cold Spring Harb Perspect Biol. 2010;2(5):a000661.

3 Local Immunity of Respiratory Tract in Different Age Groups

Air contains a variety of different suspended particles, including microorganisms. Inside buildings, there are 400–900 microorganisms per cubic meter, mostly nonpathogenic bacteria, viruses, or fungi. Thus, the average man inhales at least eight microorganisms per minute or about 10,000 per day [1]. Efficient cleaning mechanisms do exist and infection of respiratory tract has to be related with their disturbances. A mucociliary blanket covers most of the surface of the lower and upper respiratory tract. It consists of ciliated cells, single goblet cells, and subepithelial mucus-secreting glands. Foreign particles deposited on this surface are entrapped in mucus and moved upwards by ciliary action, called mucociliary escalator. The average person produces 20–200 mL mucus both from nasal cavity and respiratory tract. Alveoli are lined by alveolocytes (partly playing a defensive role as well) and macrophages. IgG and secretory IgA antibodies are produced in the lower and upper respiratory tract (Fig. 3.1) [2, 3]. There are also data related to the production of different types of interferon. We have to assume that in infants the defensive mechanisms are immature.

The development of inflammatory changes in the lungs is also facilitated by the intensive blood supply to the organ. For the spread of pathogens throughout the lung tissue, the presence of a message between the individual alveoli, the so-called Kohn pores.

Inflammatory changes in the respiratory system can be caused by many pathogens, the most important among which in Europe and North America are viruses, bacteria, mycoplasma and, to a lesser extent, fungi, as well as protozoa. Viruses, protozoa, and most other pathogens enter the human body during exogenous infection. Nevertheless, there is limited evidence of the ability of some viruses to persist with the activation of a process that may clinically manifest itself as an acute infection [4]. Less definitively we can judge about entrance gates for bacteria and fungi. Many researchers consider pneumonia, especially in debilitated patients, for example, in the postoperative period, as an auto-infectious disease. Pulmonary candidiasis is often considered as autoinfection associated with irrational antibiotic treatment. However, a number of clinical and morphological studies indicate the possible role of exogenous infection in pneumonia with pneumococcal, klebsiella, candida and, especially, pseudomonas etiology.

Pathogens from the external environment most often enter the proximal parts of the respiratory system, in particular the nasopharynx. Fine particles containing the pathogen, resulting from severe coughing and sneezing, are able to enter directly into the respiratory departments. In the nasopharynx, at first, it is possible to establish a temporary equilibrium between macro- and microorganisms, which is commonly called carriage. It should be noted that its mechanisms

V. Zinserling, *Infectious Pathology of the Respiratory Tract*,
https://doi.org/10.1007/978-3-030-66325-4_3

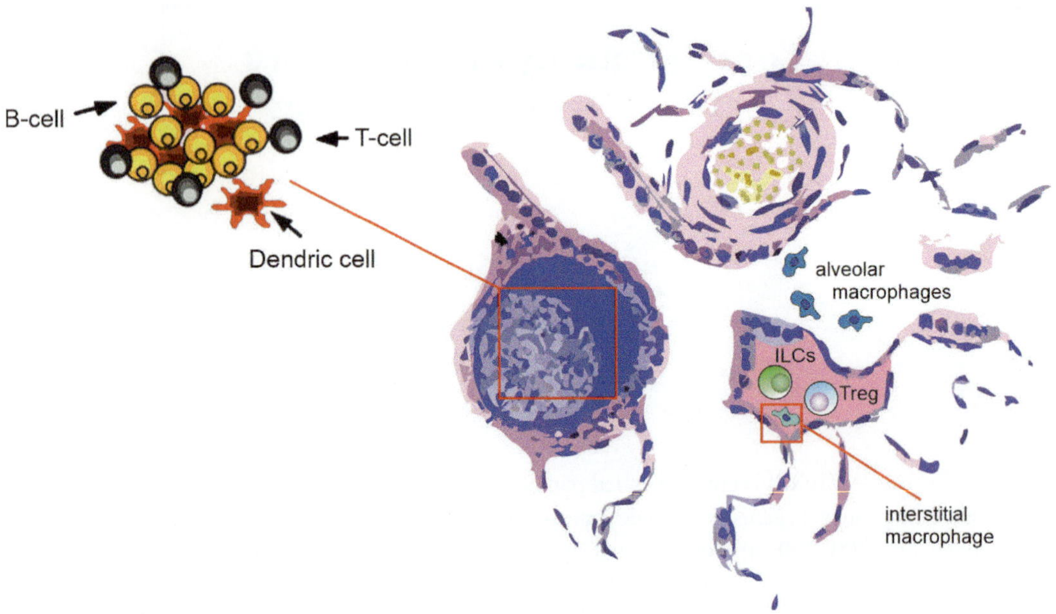

Fig. 3.1 Schema of local lung defense

remain largely unclear. If this balance is disturbed as a result of cooling, trauma, including surgical operation associated with inhalation anesthesia, alcohol intoxication, concomitant diseases, especially viral ones, microorganisms accumulate in the nasopharynx and then spread them to the respiratory departments and develop an inflammatory process there.

In individual clinical situations (in newborns with asphyxia and in people of any age with congenital or acquired, usually traumatic, disorders of the swallowing center of the medulla oblongata), aspiration becomes the leading pathogenetic mechanism. In addition, with generalized intrauterine infections and sepsis, hematogenous infection is observed. Very rarely lymphogenous infection is possible as well.

Further spread of pathogens through the respiratory system can occur in various ways. First of all, there is an intracanalicular dissemination as a result of the receipt of contents from infected bronchi to other, previously intact ones. The bacterial process, especially with pneumococcal and Klebsiella lesions, can spread over the length—by spreading through the lungs through the interalveolar pores. This is possible only in adults or older children, in which there is no more expressed segmental structure with wide intersegmental connective tissue layers. Lymphogenous spread is also possible, especially typical for streptococcal lesions and lymphohematogenous, mainly with pseudomonas.

Naturally, only a small number of all the microorganisms present in the upper respiratory tract enter the respiratory parts of the lungs. Particularly important for the occurrence of pneumonia is a violation of the cleansing mechanisms.

Among the protective mechanisms of the respiratory tree, the leading role is usually assigned to the ciliated ciliary epithelium. Local damage in clinical practice can most often be associated with viral infections, harmful fumes, including inhalation anesthesia, alcoholic intoxication, and tobacco smoke. A violation of the mobility of the cilia can also be congenital, for example, with Kartagener syndrome, the true frequency of which is unknown due to the objective difficulties of its diagnosis [2]. Important role is also played by tight cell junctions formed between epithelial cells and underlying stroma.

Similar conclusions can be made when analyzing numerous experimental works carried out mainly in the middle of the last century. Thus, the introduction to a healthy animal of foreign masses or microbial cultures suspended in a solution of sodium chloride usually does not cause pneumonia. Meanwhile, it naturally arises if the microorganism is introduced into a viscous liquid. The classical studies of N.N. Anichkov and M.A. Zakharyevskaya (1951–1961) [5], which studied the effect of various effects on the respiratory tract: narrowing or closing of the bronchi, the introduction of foreign bodies into their lumens, and various injuries of the mucous membrane. Under all these circumstances, there is a violation of the evacuation function, and bronchopneumonia develops without additional infection. It should be noted that there are numerous data on the frequent pneumonia of animals kept in vivarium under inappropriate conditions.

Assessing the importance of aspiration, it is impossible, of course, to think that the particles themselves that enter the lungs (food, squamous epithelium, etc.) themselves are capable of causing pneumonia, which occurs only when microorganisms are simultaneously present. Without pathogen the only reaction observed is foreign body granuloma.

Very important is the immune defense of the lungs. It is carried out primarily at the body level due to synthesis of antibodies and other immunoglobulins, complement, interferon, various inhibitors, properdin, and other substances that are intensively flowing through the lungs within the blood.

Along with these, much attention is currently being paid to the system of local resistance, which includes both humoral and cellular components. The functioning of the humoral mechanism can be judged by the detection of albumin, transferrin, antitrypsin, IgA and its free secretory component, IgG, lysozyme, and interferon in the washings of the bronchi.

It is customary to consider as immunocompetent tissue in the lung: (1) bifurcation lymph nodes; (2) broncho-associated lymphoid tissue (BALT–bronchi-associated lymphoid tissue); (3) macrophages and lymphocytes of the pulmonary parenchyma (Fig. 3.1). BALT is represented by single lymphoid follicles and their groups located in the wall of the bronchi, as well as lymphocytes diffusely scattered in their tissues. Lymphoid follicles consist mainly of B-lymphocytes—the precursors of plasmocytes capable of the synthesis of IgA, IgG, IgM. These immunoglobulins act as the first immune barrier, causing agglutination of microorganisms, neutralizing toxins, and decreasing the adhesion of ligands of microorganisms to mucosal receptors.

Particular attention is paid to IgA. Its molecule is synthesized in monomeric form. When passing through the epithelium of the bronchi and glands, monomeric IgA polymerizes and binds to the secretory S-component. As a result, dimeric secretory IgA appears in the contents of the respiratory tract.

The main role in cellular defense is played by alveolar macrophages that perform a variety of functions [6]. Currently, it is generally accepted that they are of bone marrow origin. They recognize and are activated by pathogen-associated molecular patterns (PAMPs) and damage-associated molecular patterns (DAMPs). More than 50 factors (lysozyme, hydrolases, proteases, interferon, interleukins, etc.) with protective value have been found in the cytoplasm of macrophages. Of great importance is their ability to phagocytosis, including the immune, in favor of which evidence is found for IgG receptors and various complement components found on their surface. In addition, alveolar macrophages modulate immune and inflammatory responses. In certain situations, we assume that being infected alveolar macrophages start to overproduce cytokines, thus causing "cytokine storm" with the clinics of systemic inflammatory syndrome, which may be considered as sepsis. Other innate immune cells that are important in the lung immune response are interstitial macrophages and dendritic cells. In addition to myeloid cells, their small numbers of lymphocytes are also present in different lung compartments. Among the new important for lung defence cytokines are described IL22 and IL15. Pulmonary immune response is reviewed in detail in several papers [2].

Interferon synthesized by T-lymphocytes and macrophages also plays a significant local protective role in the lungs. The protective role of this factor was clearly shown in the experimental studies of A.V. Zinserling with collaborators [7].

Respiratory epithelial cells and lung resident immune cells perform immune surveillance with diverse repertoire of pattern recognition receptors (PRRs), such as toll-like receptors, C-type lectin receptors, cytoplasmic retinoid acid-inducible gene-I-like receptors (RLR), and NOD-like receptors. These PRRs are responsible for the detection of microbes in the respiratory system by binding PAMPs and DAMBs. Appropriate signaling leads to activation of reactive oxygen species production (ROS), phagocytosis, secretion of mucus, and bactericidal proteins in epithelial cells. PAMP-sensing cells can also induce different mechanisms of regulated cell death such as apoptosis or proinflammatory pyroptic cell death, driving immune activity. Phagocytes engulf pathogens, dead and dying host cells by efferocytosis.

Recently new subpopulation of lymphocytes was detected, such as innate lymphoid cells (ILCs), which were divided into three groups, first of which includes NK cells [8]. Research in ILCs and lung infection is in early stages and there are no data related to human tissues. Among NK cells nowadays are distinguished invariant natural killer T (iNKT) cells and mucosa-associated invariant T (MAIT) [8]. Both of them are not completely characterized till yet.

It will be of interest to determine whether megakaryocytes in the lung and the differentiation of stem-like precursors into megakaryocytes are induced by and in turn influence pneumonia [8, 9].

A recently identified anti-inflammatory role of pulmonary neuroendocrine cells also suggests neural regulation of lung immunity [8].

Afterward, respiratory and immune cells in the lung participate in resolution of inflammatory response and start to contribute in the repair and remodeling of the lung tissue.

There are data that defense mechanism of the respiratory system can be modulated by environmental factors, the role of cooling is well known from medical and everyday practice, probably due to inhibition of leucocytes migration.

Certain role has to play starvation. In conditions of the siege (blockade) of Leningrad (1941–1944) during the Second World War, the frequency of tuberculosis and lobar pneumonias on autopsy material increased as expected, but influenza and other respiratory infections, on the contrary, inexplicably decreased [9].

Infants, young children, and elderly persons suffer and die from pneumonia more frequently than in other age groups. With children, it can be at least partly explained by lack of heterotypic immunologic memory, altered phagocyte function, and cytokine production by their AMs, preponderance of T reg cells in their lungs. With elder patients is supposed the negative influence of smoldered inflammation [3].

Serious impact upon development and course of infectious lung lesions possess many factors such as smoking, alcohol consumption, and numerous concomitant diseases [3].

References

1. Mims CA, Dimmock NJ, Nash A, Stephen J. Mim's pathogenesis of infectious disease. 4th ed. Academic; 1995. 414 p.
2. Leslie KO, Wick MR, editor. Practical pulmonary pathology. A diagnostic approach. 2nd ed. 2011. 828 p.
3. Quinton LJ, Walkey AJ, Mizgerd JP. Intergrative physiology of pneumonia. Physiol Rev. 2018;98(3):1417–64. https://doi.org/10.1152/physrev.00032.2017.
4. FitzGerald ES, Luz NF, Jamieson AM. Competitive cell death interactions in pulmonary infection: host modulation versus pathogen manipulation. Front Immunol. 2020;11:814. https://doi.org/10.3389/fimmu.20.00.
5. Anichkov NN, Zakharyevskaya MA. Experimental studies on autogenic infectious processes in lungs. Vest Khir. 1954;113(5):1–25. (In Russian).
6. Allard B, Panariti A, Martin JG. Alveolar macrophages in the resolution of inflammation, tissue repair, and tolerance to infection. Front Immunol. 2018;9:1777. https://doi.org/10.3389/fimmu.2018.01777. Published 2018 Jul 31.

7. Zinserling AV, Zinserling VA. Modern infections: pathologic anatomy and issues of pathogenesis: a guide. SPb: Sotis; 2002. 346 p. (In Russian).
8. Branchfield K, Nantie L, Verheyden JM, et al. Pulmonary neuroendocrine cells function as airway sensors to control lung immune response. Science. 2016;351:707–10. https://doi.org/10.1126/science.aad7969.
9. Bazan OI. Pathology service in sieged Leningrad. Scientific analysis and reminiscence of specialist. 2nd ed. Moskwa, "Prakticheskaya meditsina"; 2020. 159 p. (In Russian).

4 Influenza

Influenza is usually an acute respiratory viral infection caused by different influenza viruses affecting both upper and lower airways, as well as alveoli, which may generalize and lead to extrapulmonary lesions.

Influenza has been a serious public health problem for many centuries; the most famous was the pandemic of 1918. In the last 50 years, despite the progress in the field of its treatment and prevention, a number of pandemics have occurred. Among these one can mention the pandemic of 1957–1958 (so-called Asian flu), pandemic of 1968–1969 (so-called Hong-Kong flu) and, most recently, the pandemic of so-called swine flu in 2009–2011. Several lethal cases due to influenza we had the opportunity to investigate in the following years as well. Thus, the problem still remains relevant.

4.1 Etiology, Pathogenesis

Influenza virus is a single-stranded RNA virus of the *Orthomyxoviridae* family. There are four types of influenza viruses: A, B, C, and D. Most cases of influenza are attributable to influenza A viruses, which are divided into subtypes based on the structure of their surface proteins hemagglutinin (HA) and neuraminidase (NA). Designation of different influenza viruses usually includes their type (A, B, C, or D), place (geographical) of their isolation, strain number, year of isolation, and virus subtype. Thus, novel virus of so called "swine flue" (or swine origine influenza (SOI-)) nis designated A/California/04/2009 (H1N1). In the 70th, we observed in children several lethal cases due to B virus as well. There are no data related to lethal outcomes in influenza C and D.

Genome of influenza virus comprises eight gene segments, which encode 11 proteins. Virus is enveloped in lipid membrane, containing HA, NA, and transmembrane protein M2 (ion channel). Under this outer membrane is the layer of matrix protein M1, surrounding the core that contains viral RNA [1].

Influenza virus diversity is due to the segmentation of its genome, which allows frequent recombination with constant change of viral surface markers, HA, and NA, resulting in new virus subtypes. Although minor changes in virus genome can also be of relevance.

Among the mechanisms of virus pathogenicity is mentioned their ability to increase apoptosis, autophagy, and unfolded protein response in target cells [2].

Since the 30th of XX-century existence of neurotropic strains is well known, some of them (such as WSN) were retained as experimental. The existence of strains with a special affinity to intestine and placenta tissues is highly probable as well.

Influenza is mainly airborne and the lungs usually are primary site of infection. Incubation period is several days. Viral replication initially

V. Zinserling, *Infectious Pathology of the Respiratory Tract*,
https://doi.org/10.1007/978-3-030-66325-4_4

takes place in the epithelium of lower airways and alveoli and then may spread throughout respiratory system, affecting also alveolar macrophages and endothelium. In severe cases, generalized viral infection can develop, which leads to viral lesions in central nervous system (CNS), heart, intestine, kidneys, spleen, liver, and lymph nodes [3–5]. Certain data allow us to suppose, at least in some cases, the possibility of transplacental challenge of the fetus (see Sect. 17.2).

4.2 Pathology

Macroscopic features of influenza on autopsy are nonspecific. Laryngeal; tracheal; and bronchial mucosa is thickened and swollen, local cyanosis and hemorrhages can be seen (Fig. 4.1). Affected areas of the lung are indurated, often with dystelectases and edema. We consider that widely discussed in the literature as specific for influenza necrotic tracheitis cannot be regarded as its hallmark, but were only frequently observed in certain epidemics, being not obligatory complication related to overinfection by staphylococci. Macroscopic changes in other organs are minimal [5–7].

Microscopic features include changes of mucosa in larynx, trachea and bronchi is swollen with mixed infiltration and desquamation of epithelial cells. Sometimes necrotic changes can be seen.

In lungs, serous pneumonia is common (Fig. 4.2). Alveolar walls are usually thickened due to edema and inflammatory infiltration and thromboses in its blood vessels. In alveoli, desquamated cells (epitheliocytes and alveolar macrophages) can often be seen, most of them with cytopathic changes caused by influenza virus (Fig. 4.3) [5–7].

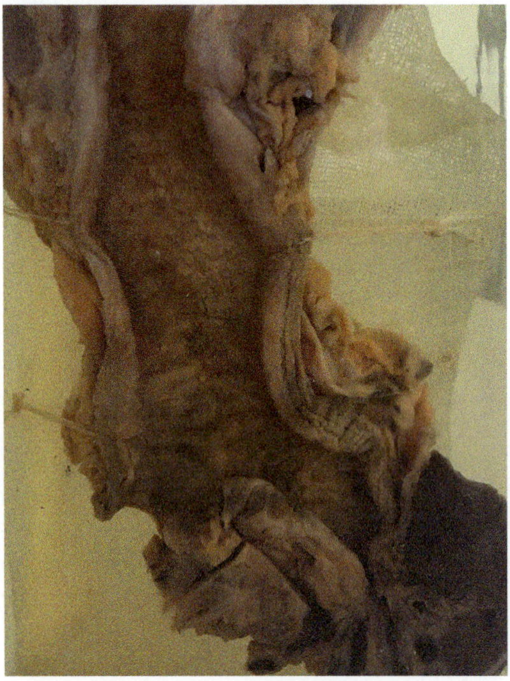

Fig. 4.1 Hemorrhagic tracheobronchitis in an adult deceased from influenza in 70th of XX century. Macropreparation from museum of pathology department of SP Botkin Infectious Hospital, Saint-Petersburg, Russia

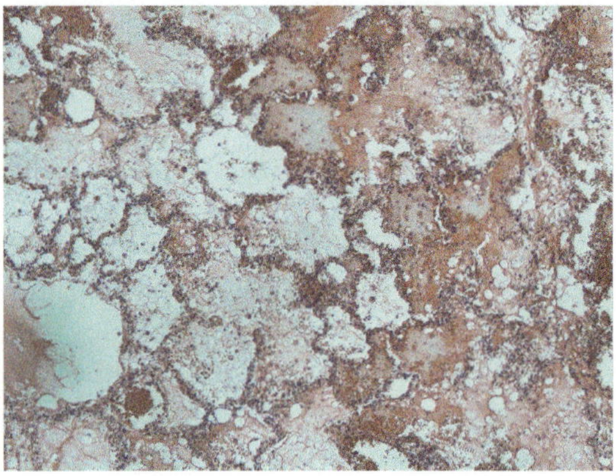

Fig. 4.2 General view on lung lesions in a child deceased from influenza in 70th of XX century. H.-E. ×40

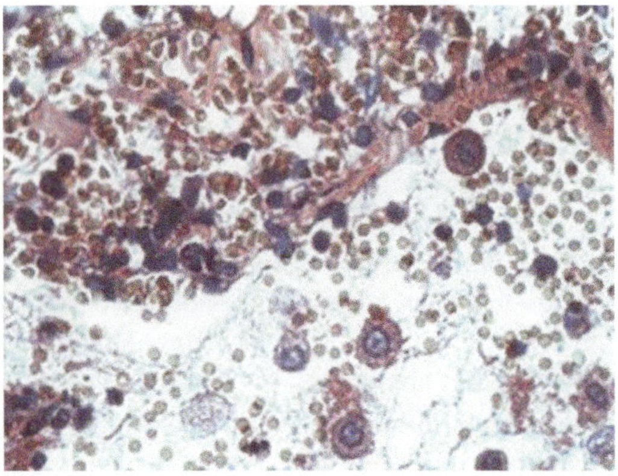

Fig. 4.3 Typical cell changes in influenza in a child deceased from influenza in 70th of XX century. H.-E. ×800

Table 4.1 Age and sex distribution of the patients

	N	%	Male		Female	
Age groups			*N*	% of the group	*N*	% of the group
<25	7	21.2	2	28.6	5	71.4
26–35	10	30.3	7	70	3	30
36–45	8	24.2	4	50	4	50
46–55	7	21.2	5	71.4	2	28.6
>56	1	3	0	0	1	100

In severe cases, destructive changes involve large areas of lung tissue and are often referred as diffuse alveolar damage (DAD). Clinical equivalent of that is acute respiratory distress syndrome (ARDS). Secondary bacterial infection often occurs as can be seen by neutrophilic infiltration. Bacterial pneumonia can be community as well as hospital acquired.

Influenza can also be associated with extrapulmonary lesions [4, 8]. In central nervous system, serous meningitis can develop with cytopathic changes in capillary endotheliocytes. Similar changes can be seen in brain blood vessels, ependymocytes, and choroid plexuses. Interstitial myocarditis with primarily mononuclear cell infiltration can sometimes be seen. Similar cytopathic changes can be found in lymph nodes, liver, kidneys, and intestine. Detection of the virus in fecal specimen indicates involvement of the gastrointestinal tract.

It should be noted that morphological features and severity of influenza are variable and depend on patient general state and susceptibility, as well as virus type. Thus, so-called H5N1 avian influenza virus is considered to be the most dangerous as it causes generalized infection with more than 50% lethality. There are no detailed descriptions of its pathology. Seasonal H3N2 and H1N1 influenza viruses that have been circulating in recent years tend to cause primarily localized respiratory infection, although extrapulmonary lesions may occur in severe cases [5–7].

Morphological changes in the lungs at the early stages of influenza, particularly A/H1N1/California, have been described by many authors [8–13]. Most papers describe only the signs of diffuse alveolar damage and secondary bacterial superinfection. More rarely virus antigen has been revealed in different cell types of the lungs.

Table 4.2 Concomitant diseases of the patients

Concomitant disease or state	% of the patients
Obesity	48
Arterial hypertension	33
Combination of obesity and arterial hypertension	24
Chronic alcoholism	18
Chronic bronchitis	15
Pregnancy	12
Coronary heart disease	9
Chronic viral hepatitis	6
Aplastic anemia	3
HIV infection	3
None	15

4.3 Own Data

We had the opportunity to provide own investigation [14, 15]. The study included 33 lethal influenza cases. In 30 cases, diagnosis of influenza was confirmed by PCR. Medical and autopsy records and sections stained by hematoxylin and eosin, as well as using PAS-reaction, were studied. Patients' age, sex, concomitant diseases, therapy, and death causes were analyzed. Histological changes in lungs, brain, and heart were evaluated with particular attention to the cells regarded as virus affected. In six cases, immunohistochemistry with monoclonal antibodies against hemagglutinin (HA) and nucleoprotein (NP) with Novolink visualization system (Novocastra) was performed. Age and sex distribution of the patients are shown in Table 4.1. The data show that most of cases studied are represented by young (26- to 35-year-old) individuals.

Concomitant diseases are summarized in Table 4.2. Most common concomitant diseases are obesity and arterial hypertension (often in combination).

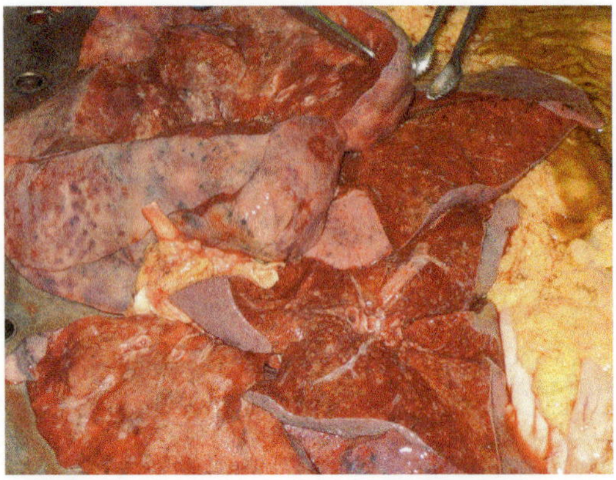

Fig. 4.4 Lungs of patient deceased from "swine" influenza in 2009

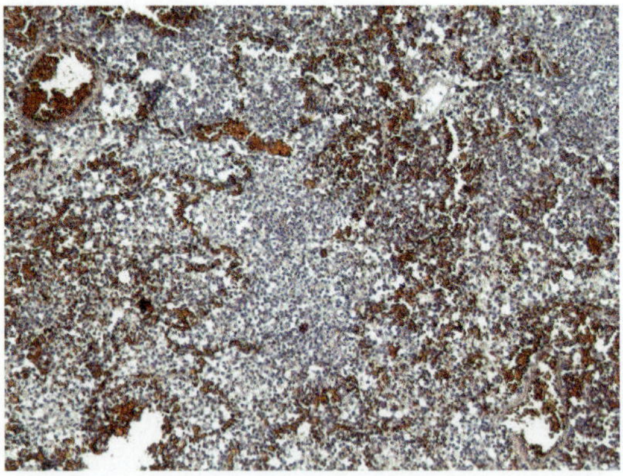

Fig. 4.5 General view of lung of an adult deceased from "swine" influenza in 2009. DAAD H.-E. ×40

Less than half of patients (42.4%) received specific antiviral therapy ("Tamiflu") and almost all patients (97%) received antibiotics. All patients were treated in intensive care units with artificial lung ventilation.

Macroscopically the lungs appeared to be "red, big, heavy" as described in DAD (Fig. 4.4).

Morphological changes in trachea and bronchi included desquamation with proliferative changes; sometimes with metaplasia, necrosis was seen only in three cases (9%).

Considering histological changes in the lungs, they can be divided into five types: (1) massive serous hemorrhagic edema (9% of cases); (2) serous and desquamative viral pneumonia (6%); (3) viral pneumonia with acute phase of diffuse alveolar damage (DAD) clinically corresponding to acute respiratory distress syndrome (ARDS) (18%); (4) viral pneumonia with the prevalence of regenerative and hyperplastic changes (27%); (5) mixed viral and bacterial pneumonia (36%) (Fig. 4.5). Also, two types of virus-affected cells were seen. In the first type, both nuclei and cytoplasm are enlarged, cytoplasm being slightly basophilic (Fig. 4.6). In the second type, cells become polynuclear forming simplasts-like structures with big hypochromic nuclei (Fig. 4.7).

In brain samples, necrobiotic changes of neurons (10 cases (30.3%)), lymphoid infiltration of pia mater (6 cases (18.2%)), and perivascular lymphoid infiltration and satellitosis (4 cases (12.2%)) could be seen. In pia mater cells, similar to the first type, virus-affected cells seen in the lungs were present.

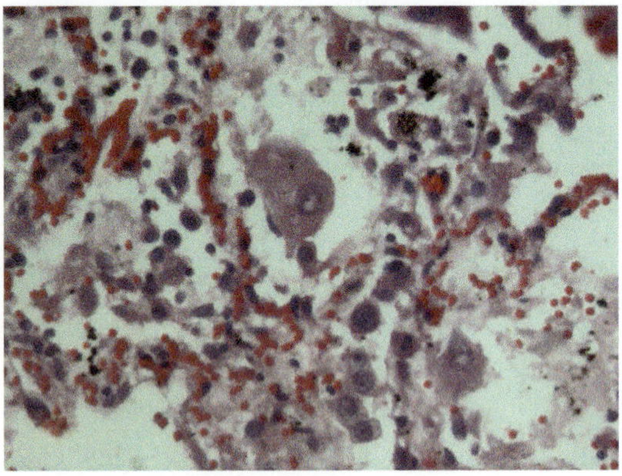

Fig. 4.6 Typical cell changes in influenza in an adult deceased from "swine" influenza in 2009 H.-E. ×800

In the heart, in all samples, interstitial edema, hyperemia, and diapedesis were present. In seven cases (21.2%), interstitial infiltration was seen. Again, some cells of that infiltrates were similar to virus-affected cells in the lungs.

In 16 cases (48.5%), thrombosis of small and medium blood vessels of the lungs and other organs was present, clinically it corresponds to disseminated intravascular coagulation syndrome.

In all six cases, where immunohistochemistry was used viral proteins were detected in the lungs (in respiratory epithelium, alveolocytes, alveolar macrophages, and endothelium). In some cases,

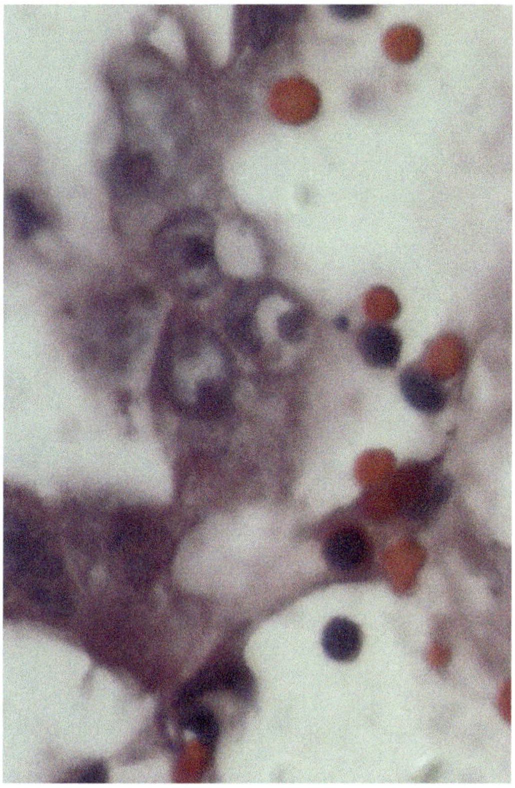

Fig. 4.7 Binucleated alveolocyte in an adult deceased from "swine" influenza in 2009 H.-E. ×1000

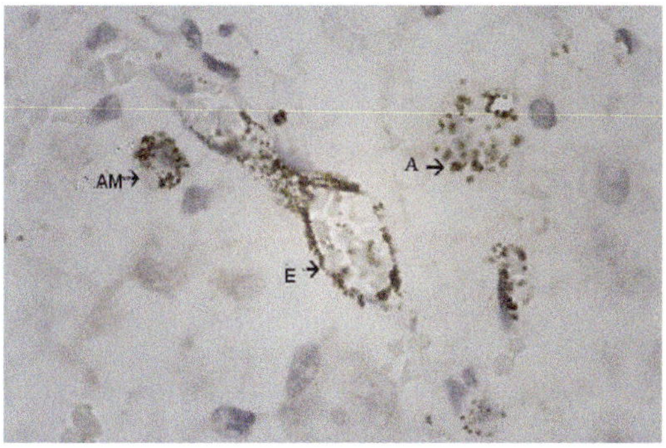

Fig. 4.8 Nucleoprotein of influenza A virus in lung tissue. AM-alveolar macrophage. A—alveolocyte. E—endothelial cell. IHC. ×800

HA and NP were detected in the heart and brain (Fig. 4.8). All these data strongly indicate the possibility of generalized influenza infection.

We confirm that virus-induced lesions in lungs during the last epidemic are similar to those described previously, but we noted that they were

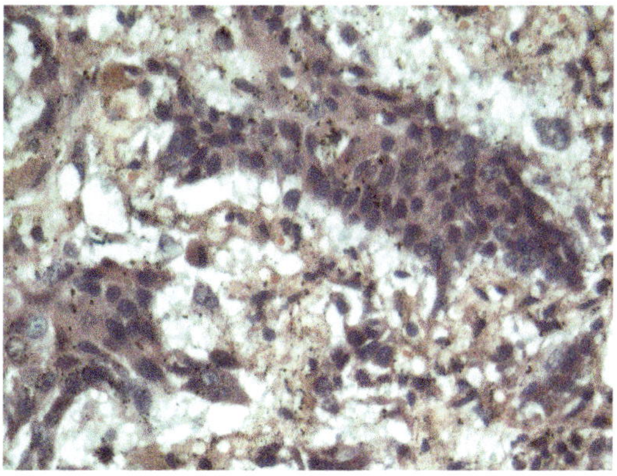

Fig. 4.9 Simplast in an adult deceased from "swine" influenza in 2011 H.-E. ×800

present for a much longer time (till the 21st day of illness) and were characterized by more expressed nuclear changes as well as proliferative changes and formation of symplasts-like structures. It is possible that such changes depend on the properties of the circulating virus.

Later on (2016), we had the opportunity to investigate several lethal cases due to the same influenza virus [16]. Nearby to the changes similar to those described before, we observed also giant multinuclear cells and even metaplasia (Fig. 4.9).

4.4 Conclusion

Influenza has different epidemiological, clinical, and pathological forms depending on different properties of the circulating virus, not only its antigenic formula.

In the majority of publications, no special attention is paid to the cytopathic changes, which can be directly induced by the influenza virus. Only in the works of A.V. Zinserling is the important diagnostically role of typical transformation of epithelial and other virus-affected cells emphasized with proposal to call them "influenza" cells (see Fig. 4.3). The fact that influenza facilitates the development of secondary infections, especially bacterial pneumonias, is widely known. The role of secondary bacterial superinfection during different epidemics varies strongly. In the majority of analyzed lethal outcomes, they were expressed relatively weakly, either due to the effectiveness of the treatment by antibiotics or antagonism with the virus.

The problem of extrapulmonary lesions in influenza has been discussed in the literature with quite confronting views for more than 100 years. Our recent data allow to support our previously published opinion about the reality and clinical importance of such lesions with direct affecting on endothelial cells in different organs, especially brain and heart. It is also obvious that certain questions relating to this problem are still to be solved.

Immediate death causes in influenza differ related to the virus strain and age of the patients and include DAAD, generalized virus infection with brain involvement, secondary necrotic pneumonia as a local complication, and exacerbation of preexisting diseases [17].

There are several animal models of influenza, in which different strains are used for the challenge of different species [7, 18, 19]. One has to note that nearby certain common features with human pathology, there are no ideal nosological models [20].

There are also clinical and experimental data supporting the opinion about the existence of chronic influenza [21–23].

Many issues of influenza require further complex study.

References

1. Boctor SW, Hafner JW. Influenza. In: StatPearls Treasure Island (FL): StatsPearls Publishing; 2020.
2. Mehrbod P, Ande SR, Alizadeh J, et al. The roles of apoptosis, autophagy and unfolded protein response in arbovirus, influenza virus, and HIV infections. Virulence. 2019;10(1):376–413.
3. Zinserling AV, Aksenov OA, Melnikova VF, Zinserling VA. Extrapulmonary lesions in influenza. Tohoku J Exp Med. 1983;140(3):259–72.
4. Bhatnagar J, Jones T, Blau DM, et al. Localization of pandemic 2009 H1N1 Influenza A virus RNA in lung and lymph nodes of fatal influenza cases by situ hybridization: new insights on virus replication and pathogenesis. J Clin Virol. 2013;56(3):232–7.
5. Zinserling AV. Etiology and pathologic anatomy of acute respiratory infections. L.: Meditsina; 1977. 170 p. (In Russian).
6. Zinserling AV. Peculiarities of lesions in viral and mycoplasma infection of respiratory tract. Virchows Archiv A. 1972;356:259–73.
7. Zinserling VA. Chapter: Pathology of influenza. In: Influenza—therapeutics and challenges. p. 17–30. ISBN 978-1-78923-715-3. https://doi.org/10.5772/intechopen.76309.
8. Nakajima N, Hata S, Sato Y, et al. The first autopsy case of pandemic influenza (A/H1N1pdm) virus infection in Japan: detection of a high copy number of the virus in type II alveolar epithelial cells by pathological and virological examination. Jpn J Infect Dis. 2010;63:67–71.
9. Capelozzi VL, Parra ER, Ximenes M, et al. Pathological and ultrastructural analysis of surgical lung biopsies in patients with swine-origin influenza type A/H1N1 and acute respiratory failure. Clinics (Sao Paulo). 2010;65(12):1229–37.
10. Gill JR, Sheng Z-M, Ely SF, Guinee DG Jr, et al. Pulmonary pathologic findings of fatal 2009 pandemic influenza A/H1N1 viral infections. Arch Pathol Lab Med. 2010;134:235–43.
11. Mauad T, Hajjar LA, Callegari GD, et al. Lung pathology in fatal novel human influenza A (H1N1) infection. Am J Respir Crit Care Med. 2010;181(1):72–9.
12. Rosen DG, Lopez AE, Anzalone ML, et al. Postmortem findings in eight cases of influenza A/H1N1. Mod Pathol. 2010;23:1449–57.
13. Lucas S. Predictive clinicopathological features derived from systematic autopsy examination of patients who died with A/H1N1 influenza infection in the UK 2009-10 pandemic. Health Technol Assess. 2010;14(55):83–114.
14. Zinserling VA, Vorob'ev SL, Zarubaev VV, et al. Pathogenic aspects of influenza during the epidemics caused by H1N1v virus in 2009-2010 according autopsy data. Arkh Patol. 2011;73(6):21–5. (In Russian).
15. Gladkov SA, Zinserling VA, Shtro AA, et al. Postmortem diagnosis of influenza during its epidemic and interepidemic periods. Arkh Patol. 2015;77(2):22–7. (In Russian).
16. Zinserling VA, Yakovlev AA, Vasilyeva MV, et al. Morphological changes of the cells due to different strains of influenza A virus clinical and experimental morphology. 2018;(1):4–11. (In Russian).
17. Yakovlev AA, Zinserling VA, Esaulenko EV. Lethal outcomes in influenza: clinic-pathological approach to immediate death outcomes. J Infectol. 2017;9(4):53–8. (In Russian).
18. Zinserling AV, Soldatova VM, Platonov VG. Essence of metainfluenza stage of influenza. Arkh Patol. 1980;42(3):46–50. (In Russian).
19. Prokopyeva EA, Zinserling VA, Bae Y-C, et al. Pathology of A(H5N8) (Clade 2.3.4.4) Virus

in experimentally infected chickens and mice Hindawi interdisciplinary perspectives on infectious diseases. 2019;2019:4124865. https://doi.org/10.1155/2019/4124865.
20. Thangavel RR, Bouvier NM. Animal models for influenza virus pathogenesis, transmission, and immunology. J Immunol Methods. 2014;410:60–79. https://doi.org/10.1016/j.jim.2014.03.023.
21. Melnikova VF, Zinserling VA, Aksenov OA, Zinserling AV. Chronic course of influenza with extrapulmonary involvement. Arkh Patol. 1994;56(1):33–8. (In Russian).
22. Zuev VA, Mirchink EP, Khavitova AM. Experimental slow influenza infection in mice. Vopr Virusol. 1983;28(1):24–9. (In Russian).
23. Mirchink EP, Zuev VA. Influenza and congenital pathology. Vopr Virusol. 1992;37(5–6):226–9. (In Russian).

5 Paramyxovirus and other RNA virus infections

Paramyxovirus family includes many pathogens causing diseases in several species and is divided into six genus: orthopneumovirus, respirovirus, rubulavirus, morbillivirus, henipavirus, and pneumovirus. The nomenclature basing upon the results of molecular virology studies is periodically revised. Nowadays, among the human pathogens are mentioned: human parainfluenza virus, respiratory syncytial virus, metapneumovirus, measles virus, mumps virus, hendra virus, nipah virus. In the present chapter, we are going to discuss lesions caused only by those that cause respiratory infections with known pathology and we have certain own experience. The latter (hendra and nipah) are transmissible from infected animals such as bats, pigs, and horses.

5.1 Parainfluenza

According to traditional nomenclature, the pathogen has been named Parainfluenza virus being divided into four serotypes. Nowadays, virologists distinguish: human respirovirus 1, human respirovirus 3, human rubulavirus 2, and human rubulavirus 4. There are no data concerning the clinical relevance of the new taxonomy.

Parainfluenza viruses as other relative viruses have a nonsegmented ssRNA genome that measures approximately 15 kbp in length and forms complexes with viral structural proteins to produce helical nucleocapsids. Nascent particles bud from cytoplasmic membrane, during which they are enveloped. The resulting particles may be either spherical or filamentous [1].

Parainfluenza virus, as other human viruses causing respiratory infections, is transmitted via aerosolized respiratory secretions and fomites. Clinically they usually cause mild-to-severe upper and lower respiratory tract infections, including false croup. The latter has to be explained by certain immunopathological reactions. Lethal outcomes are rare. In infants was described generalized parainfluenza. The morphological descriptions given below are based upon unique investigations of A. Zinserling in the 60th–80th of the XX century when numerous children and infants died in Leningrad (SU) due to different viral respiratory infections [2, 3].

Macroscopically, the most characteristic is catarrhal laryngotracheobronchitis with the greatest changes in the larynx. In the lungs, mainly in their posterior lower divisions, small reddish cyanotic, moderately dense foci are detected, often subsiding in the section.

The walls of the respiratory tract, mainly their layers adjacent to the epithelium, are somewhat swollen, full-blooded, focal lymphocytic infiltrates are visible in them. As the most typical was considered the overgrowths of epithelial cells, forming "pillowlike" structures (Fig. 5.1). The lumens of the bronchi contain desquamated cells of the ciliated epithelium, lying alone or in layers. There is also serous fluid, individual

V. Zinserling, *Infectious Pathology of the Respiratory Tract*,
https://doi.org/10.1007/978-3-030-66325-4_5

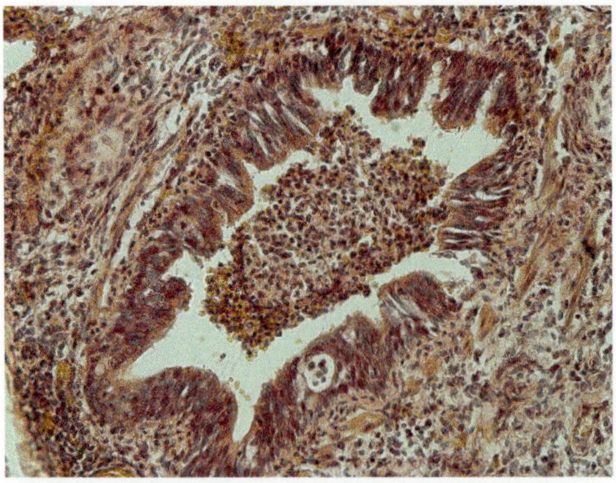

Fig. 5.1 "Pillow-like" overgrowths of bronchiolar epithelium typical for parainfluenza. H.-E. ×200

leukocytes, macrophages, and red blood cells. Peribronchial edema and lymphoid infiltration are often noted.

In children, mainly during the first weeks of life, changes in the alveolar epithelium are observed, similar to changes in the ciliated epithelium. In such cells, inclusions are also found. Subsequently, the cells are rounded and desquamated. In addition, individual two to three nuclear cells, usually alveolar macrophages and single neutrophilic leukocytes, as well as serous fluid, are identified in the lumens of the alveoli, some of the children have hyaline membranes. In adults, we did not observe pronounced lesions of the respiratory departments.

Usually, quite significant changes in the small blood vessels of the lungs are observed. Their walls are thickened, with swollen epithelium; sometimes, perivascular edema and slight lymphoid infiltration are observed.

The diagnosis has to be based upon virological, serological, and molecular–biological data first of all in comparison with described histopathological changes. We have quite positive experience in using IF microscopy of smears from lung surface.

Similar changes in the respiratory system were found in the experiment on cotton rats, goats, and Guinea pigs [4, 5]. With parainfluenza, as well as with other acute respiratory viral infections, in most of the organs, it is possible to identify manifestations of generalization. As a result of this, changes resembling those that occur in the respiratory system may develop. They are, first of all, in the growths of the epithelium. Mild circulatory disorders, dystrophic, and minor inflammatory changes are also observed. On our material, most fully studied were lesions of the central nervous system. We have several observations allowing to suppose the parainfluenza virus persisted in plexus choroideus [6].

We did not observe the expressed manifestations of generalized parainfluenza in adults; with them, we noted parainfluenza only as a concomitant infection.

5.2 Respiratory Syncytial Infection

General characteristics of the virus and clinical manifestations of the infection caused by it were given previously. One has to note only that antigenic diversity of RS virus is not described. Clinical and epidemiological data demonstrate that the frequency and severity of this infection vary dramatically. Severe cases, including lethal ones, appeared after a long pause [7]. Morphological description is based upon the works of A. Zinserling as well [2, 3].

Macroscopically, the mucous membrane of the larynx, trachea, and large bronchi can be either unchanged or somewhat hyperemic. The lumen of these organs contains a few foamy, mucus-rich light semiliquid masses. The lungs are full blooded, mainly in their posterior lower regions small foci of moderate compaction of a dark red color with a smooth cut surface are revealed, with which a little unclear bloody fluid is separated when pressed. In the anterior sections, the lungs are emphysematous. The pleura is smooth, shiny, sometimes with punctate hemorrhages.

Changes in the respiratory system: During histological examination, the presence of peculiar growths of the epithelium of small bronchi, bronchioles, and alveolar passages is especially characteristic in the dead (most often children). These growths have the appearance of papillae or protrusions, consisting of three to eight rather

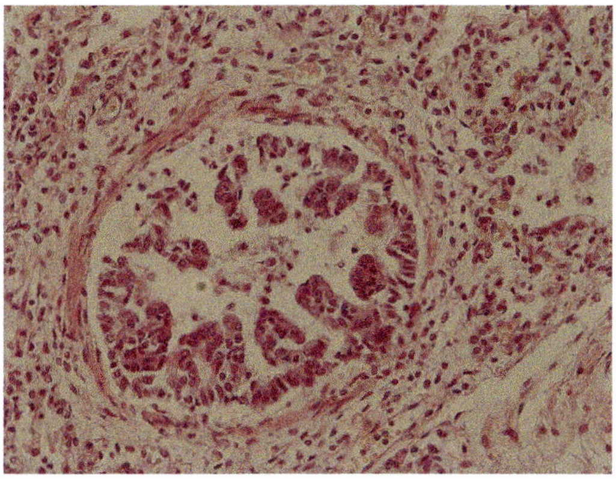

Fig. 5.2 "Papilla-like" overgrowths of bronchiolar epithelium typical for respiratory-syncytial infection. H.-E. ×200

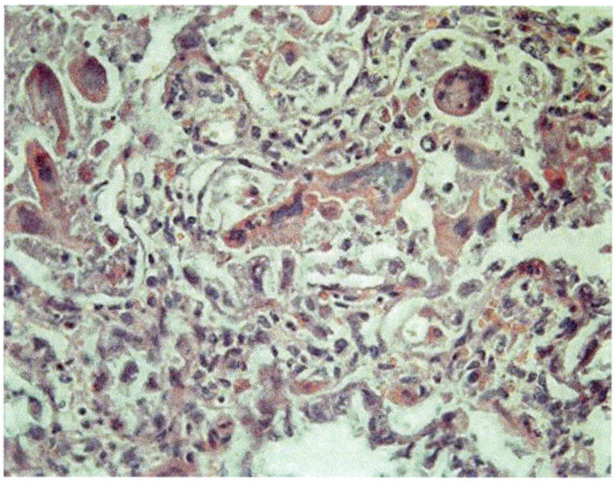

Fig. 5.3 Numerous giant multinuclear cells in the lung of a child deceased from RS infection. Courtesy of V.E. Karev H.-E. ×400

large cells with light nuclei of oval or round shape (Fig. 5.2). During the study, the virus antigen is detected in the cytoplasm of such cells, and with light microscopy, individual small rich RNA inclusions and fuchsinophilic inclusions are found. Isolated inclusions are also present in the cytoplasm of some unmodified epithelial cells. Around the larger caliber bronchi, small lymphocytic infiltrates are often determined. Similar changes can occur and the trachea, in particular, in its glands. Of the other changes in the trachea, homogenization of its own membrane and small lymphoid infiltrates in the deep sections of its wall can be noted.

The alveoli sometimes contain a rather thick exudate, consisting mainly of cells such as macrophages with fairly bright nuclei. These cells are partly small with an oxyphilic cytoplasm, partly larger with a foamy light cytoplasm. Occasionally, large multinucleated cells are found. Nowadays, the presence of virus in them can be documented by IHC (Fig. 5.3). A few neutrophilic white blood cells and fine-grained protein masses are usually mixed with these cells. Individual exudate cells undergo karyorrhexis. The lumen of the bronchi and bronchioles also contains cells of desquamated bronchial epithelium, including in the form of layers. In addition, plethora, small hemorrhages, small focal atelectasis, and emphysema are observed.

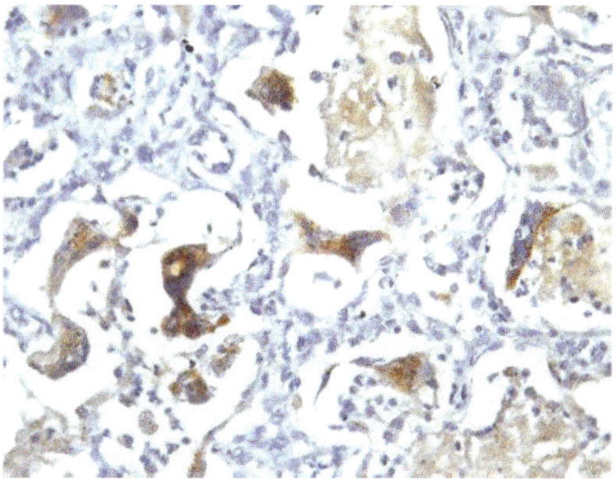

Fig. 5.4 Antigen of RS virus in the same case. IHC. ×400

Due to the clinical importance of RS infection and the necessity to test vaccines recently, several experimental models were approbated [8]. Infection most resembling human was induced in the chimpanzee.

Extrapulmonary lesions. The possibility of generalization of RS infection, mainly in children of the first months of life, with the development of characteristic structural changes, has been proved by the works of A. Zinserling and his collaborators. The greatest diagnostic value is the overgrowth of the epithelium.

In adults, we have seen RS infection only as a concomitant disease without hallmarks of generalization (Fig. 5.4).

5.3 Metapneumovirus Infection

The last two decades have been characterized by the discovery of numerous new viruses, including those causing acute respiratory infections. Among them, metapneumovirus, discovered in 2001, is given particular importance in world literature. At present, the structure of this pathogen, which belongs to the paramyxovirus family, the genus of pneumoviruses, has been studied in some detail, its certain properties determining virulence have been detected. It is shown that it is a very common causative agent of viral respiratory infections, especially in children [9]. Clinically, there is a similarity of the manifestations of this infection with the caused by RS virus. There are several descriptions of cases with the involvement of the central nervous system. In adults, metapneumovirus infection is very rarely diagnosed, deaths are not described. Information about the structural changes caused by this pathogen is minimal. The literature cites only a few experimental studies with infection of mice [10]. In the brief descriptions of microscopic changes, only the development of bronchitis and peribronchial lymphocytic infiltration is indicated. However, in some micrographs related to the monkey experiment [11], small overgrowth of bronchial epithelium are present but the authors did not include them in their description.

Our own observation [12], which, apparently, is the only described case of a fatal outcome from metapneumovirus infection in an adult with a characteristic of structural changes in it.

Patient I.K., 51 years old, was admitted to the hospital in critical condition a week after the onset of signs of acute respiratory viral infection, characterized by increasing shortness of breath. In the outpatient card, there are no indications of severe background pathology; ELISA for the presence of HIV infection is negative. Upon admittance, the temperature is normal, breathing in the lungs is weakened, rales of various sizes were heard. Heart rate: 112/min, respiratory rate: 29/min, blood pressure: 100/60 mm. In analysis of blood: leucocytosis—14,000, thrombocytopenia—89,000, in the analysis of urine—protein 1 g/l. The patient was intubated, therapy included infusions, antibacterial, mucolytic drugs, measures to prevent of thromboembolic complications were started 8 h after admission, against the background of continuing intensive care, cardiac arrest occurred, resuscitation was unsuccessful. The final clinical diagnosis: Community-acquired bilateral severe pneumonia, complicated by pulmonary edema, respiratory and heart failure, and cerebral edema.

With postmortem autopsy (1.5 days after death), increased fatness of the deceased (thickness of subcutaneous fat in the navel 4 cm), clean pale skin was noted. In the pleural cavities, free fluid was not detected. The mucous membrane of the trachea and large bronchi is full blooded, shiny, grayish mucus in the lumen of the main bronchi. Lungs in almost all sections are compacted (except for the part of the apex of the right lung), slightly airy, dark red in color, without distinct focal changes, weighing 1300. A strangulation groove in the tonsils of the cerebellum, flaccid brain tissue (weighing 1300), slit-like form of the brain ventricles, numerous point hemorrhages in a white matter. In addition, there was an increase in the liver (weight 2900), which has a tan color. On the part of other organs, no significant changes were detected.

A postmortem virological study using real-time PCR (at Institute of Virology named after D.I. Ivanovsky) revealed metapneumovirus in lung tissue, bronchi, and trachea. Influenza A and B viruses, parainfluenza types 1,2,3,4, corona-, adeno-, rino-, and bokaviruses were not found. Cytological examination of a smear imprint from the surface of the lungs revealed a few non-neutrophilic leukocytes (2–4 p/v), gram-positive rods, and cocci.

Microscopic examination of the lung revealed sharp plethora, in the lumens of the alveoli, serous fluid, dense protein masses, and in some places hyaline membranes (Fig. 5.5). Were noted numerous overgrowths of the bronchial epithelium of various calibers (Fig. 5.6), individual binuclear pneumocytes, and alveolar macrophages; some of the cells had irregularly shaped nuclei (Fig. 5.7). Peribronchial small lymphocytic accumulations. In isolated limited areas, loose neutrophilic infiltration.

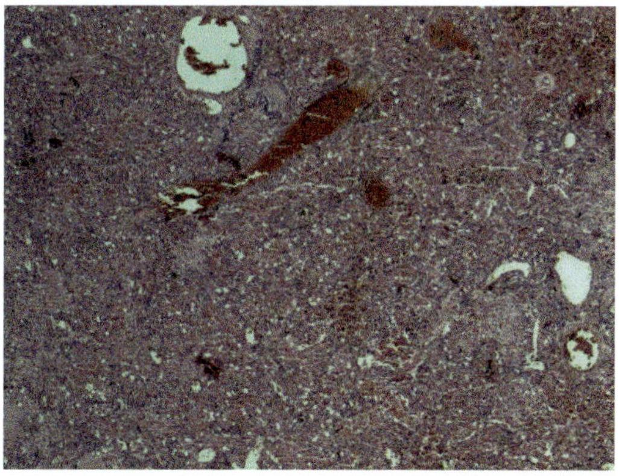

Fig. 5.5 General view on lung lesions in an adult deceased from metapneumovirus infection. H.-E. ×40

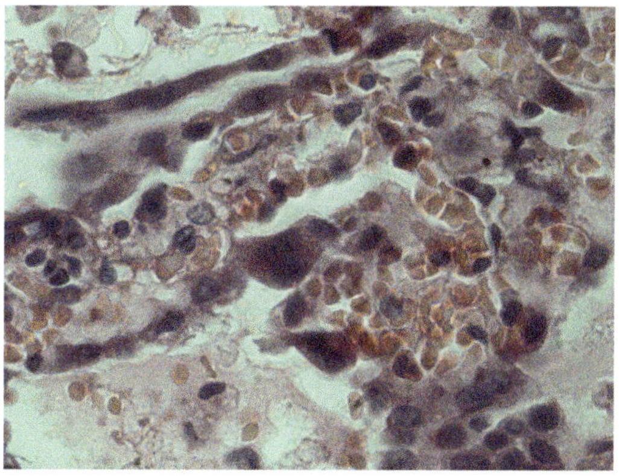

Fig. 5.7 Binucleated cells of irregular form in the same case. H.-E. ×400

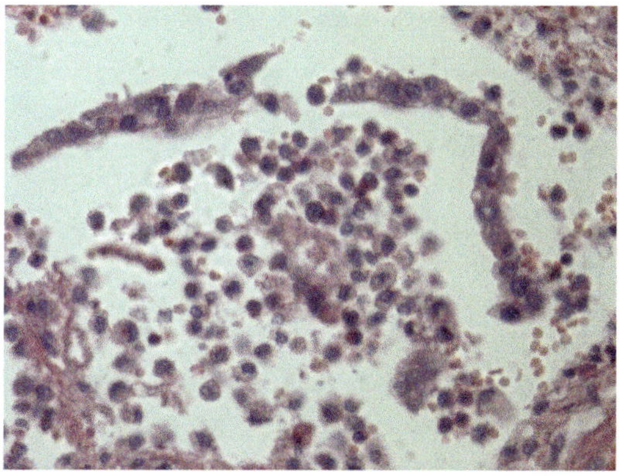

Fig. 5.6 Overgrowths of ciliary epithelium in the same case. H.-E. ×200

In the soft meninges, focal growths of meningocytes, signs of edema, and moderate fibrosis were observed. In the substance of the brain, endothelial swelling of small blood vessels, perivascular edema, and focal hemorrhages was observed. Neurons with signs of ischemic and severe changes were seen. In the kidneys, plethora, numerous fibrin thrombi in the capillaries of the renal glomeruli, focal interstitial lymphocytic infiltration, dystrophic changes in the epithelium of the convoluted tubules, partly with the formation of small growths. In the pancreas, fibrosis and stromal lipomatosis, proliferation (excretory epithelium) was present. In the intestine, venous congestion, autolytic changes, and proliferation of epithelial cells in the glands of the small intestine were observed. In the liver, large-droplet fatty degeneration of individual hepatocytes, chologenous pigmentation of hepatocytes, moderate lymphocytic infiltration in the region of the portal tracts. In the remaining organs, moderately pronounced dystrophic changes were seen. Reactive changes in the spleen and lymph nodes. Bone marrow without pathology was seen.

The final pathological diagnosis was formulated as metapneumovirus pneumonia.

The given observation is the first case of a lethal outcome from metapneumovirus infection in an adult without signs of immunodeficiency described in the literature. The leading significance for the onset of death was severe lung lesions of the type of diffuse alveolar damage and DIC syndrome with severe thrombosis of the renal glomerular capillaries. Bacterial layering was minimally expressed. Considering the presence of protein F in metapneumovirus, which leads to cell fusion, as well as the affinity of the pathogen with parainfluenza and respiratory syncytial viruses, we can consider the epithelial growths revealed by us in the respiratory organs as a characteristic cytoproliferative effect of this pathogen. It is impossible not to note their similarity to the growths described by A. Zinserling for parainfluenza and RS infection. Identification of similar changes in the pia mater, kidney, pancreas, and intestine suggests, by analogy with other paramyxovirus viral infections, the possibility of generalization. Very remarkable is the development in this deceased of severe diffuse alveolar damage, similar to that described in fatal cases from "swine" flu, which in this observation was excluded according to the results of a virological study. Judging by the analysis of the course of metapneumovirus infection in children in the clinical observations described in the literature, this severe and life-threatening complication was not observed in them.

5.4 Measles

Acute viral highly contagious infection is predominant in children. Measles virus belongs to the paramyxovirus family; it probably arose at a later stage from the closely related rinderpest virus that infects cattle [13].

Measles virus contains an RNA genome that encodes eight proteins and forms its envelope from the infected cell. The genome is complexed in a helical nucleocapsid with the nucleocapsid protein and phosphoprotein. Alternate open reading frames within the phosphoprotein gene encode two additional proteins designated V and C, which may have roles in virus replication and pathogenesis. Matrix (M) protein localizes at the inner face of the viral envelope and is necessary for virion assembly. Measles has two important membrane glycoproteins embedded in the viral envelope and displayed on the outer surface of virions. Hemagglutinin (H) serves as the attachment protein that binds to host cell receptors, and the F protein mediates fusion of the viral envelope with the host cell membrane to facilitate genome entry into the cell. The F protein also mediates cell-to-cell fusion of infected cell to adjacent uninfected cell, forming giant cells or syncytia, a hallmark of measles virus cytopathic effect in tissue culture and in vivo. Although mutations do occur in measles virus that circulates in humans, only one serotype of the virus exists. Therefore, a single vaccine strain has proved to be effective in practice.

Measles has a tremendous historical impact because of its highly contagious nature and the significant morbidity and mortality associated with this infection.

Measles is one of the classical diseases of antiquity. It is thought that measles virus became endemic within human populations when concentrated masses of people began living in urban areas. It was first described by the 10th-century Persian physician al-Rhazes, who called the illness by its Arabic name, *hasba* (meaning "eruption"). It was so common that he thought measles was a natural occurrence of childhood, like losing baby teeth, instead of an infectious illness. The most important outbreaks of measles in history are as follows: in central Mexico, the native population dropped from about 30 million to 3 million in just 50 years; 800 children died of measles in the Charlestown area of Boston in 1772, in Fiji, in the 19th century, a quarter of the population died—some 30,000 people; when a single person with measles landed in Greenland in 1951, all but 5 of the 4300 never before exposed natives came down with the disease.

In fact, its present name appeared in the 14th century and was derived from the Arabic word miser, typical for the unhappiness of lepers.

Humans are the only host for the measles virus. Infection leads to lifelong immunity. The persistence of measles virus in the population requires a certain number of susceptible humans (being not infected or vaccinated in the past). That number has been estimated to be 250,000 at a minimum.

Growth of measles virus in tissue culture was obtained in 1954 by J. Enders and T. Peebles, which allowed the development of a live, attenuated vaccine.

The host immune response is important for clearance of measles virus infection. The onset of rash coincides with the appearance of measles-specific antibodies in the normal host, initially of the IgM serotype. Over the next few weeks to months, IgG isotype antibodies appear and persist at low levels for life. Antibodies specific to measles virus are important for protection against disease and may play a role in clearance of acute infection. However, cellular immunity appears to be more important than humoral immunity for clearance of acute infection. Immunocompromised patients can develop giant cell encephalitis, which is distinct from the encephalitis that can occur in normal hosts.

The most important feature of the interaction of measles virus with the immune system is immunosuppression following the infection. There is a very high rate of secondary infections following measles, particularly bacterial pneumonias, but also other bacterial and protozoan intestinal infections. The exact mechanisms of immunosuppression following measles are not known. Two receptors for measles virus have been identified: CD46 (membrane cofactor protein, expressed primarily on the apical surface of polarized epithelial cells) and SLAM (signaling lymphocyte activation molecule, expressed on B cells, T cells, and dendritic cells). Both molecule transducer powerful signals on binding their normal ligands and interactions with measles virus might lead to the attenuation of the immune response. In addition, measles virus nucleocapsid protein binds to an inhibitory immunoglobulin receptor on B cells (Fcλ receptor II) to inhibit antibody production. The initial T-cell response includes CD8+ and Th1 CD4+ cells important for control of the infectious virus. It is possible that other mechanisms also contribute to the immunosuppression following measles.

Immunologically normal, sane people usually do not get complications or long-term consequences from measles even in cases with severe course. In most individuals, the immune response is successful in eventually clearing measles virus infection and in establishing lifelong immunity.

Remarkable progress has been made in reducing measles incidence and mortality as a consequence of implementing the measles mortality-reduction strategy of the World Health Organization (WHO) and United Nations Children's Fund (UNICEF). The revised global measles mortality reduction goal set forth in the WHO-UNICEF Global Immunization Vision and Strategy for 2006–2015 is to reduce measles deaths by 90% by 2010 compared to the estimated 757,000 deaths in 2000. The possibility of measles eradication has been discussed for almost 40 years, and measles meets many of the criteria for eradication. Global measles eradication will face a number of challenges to achieving and sustaining high levels of vaccine coverage and population immunity, including population growth and demographic changes, conflict and political instability, and public perceptions of vaccine safety. To achieve the measles mortality reduction goal, continued progress needs to be made in delivering measles vaccines to the world's children.

Persons infected with measles virus are most contagious 2–3 days before developing a rash, but they remain infectious until approximately 4 days after the rash appears. The virus is easily spread by aerosolized droplets, which can transmit infection during a brief contact. The contagiosity is extremely high.

Measles has always been a typical children's infection with the highest morbidity from the sixth month till 5 years [14]. After the worldwide introduction of vaccination in majority of countries, there are only sporadic cases among nonimmunized persons of different ages registered. An increase in morbidity has been reported among medical students coming for the first time in the children's infectious clinic.

The route of infection is usually by inhalation or conjunctival inoculation, and virus initially replicates in respiratory epithelial tissues. Primary viremia spreads the virus to lymph nodes, tonsils, lungs, gastrointestinal tract, and spleen. A few days later, a second wave of viremia coincides with the onset of major systemic symptoms and rash. Incubation period for measles lies between 10 and 14 days.

Clinical picture is rather typical. A 2- to 3-day prodrome of fever, cough, coryza, and conjunctivitis followed by a rash, and enantema (Koplik spots—small bright red spots with bluish centers on the buccal mucosa) are pathognomic for measles (Fig. 5.8). The rash that follows the prodrome has cephalocaudal progression and transforms from discrete maculopapules to confluence. Manifestations may be altered in previously immunized persons or immunocompromised.

Measles virus infection is often accompanied by leucopenia. Organ-specific complications such as pneumonia, diarrhea, and encephalitis

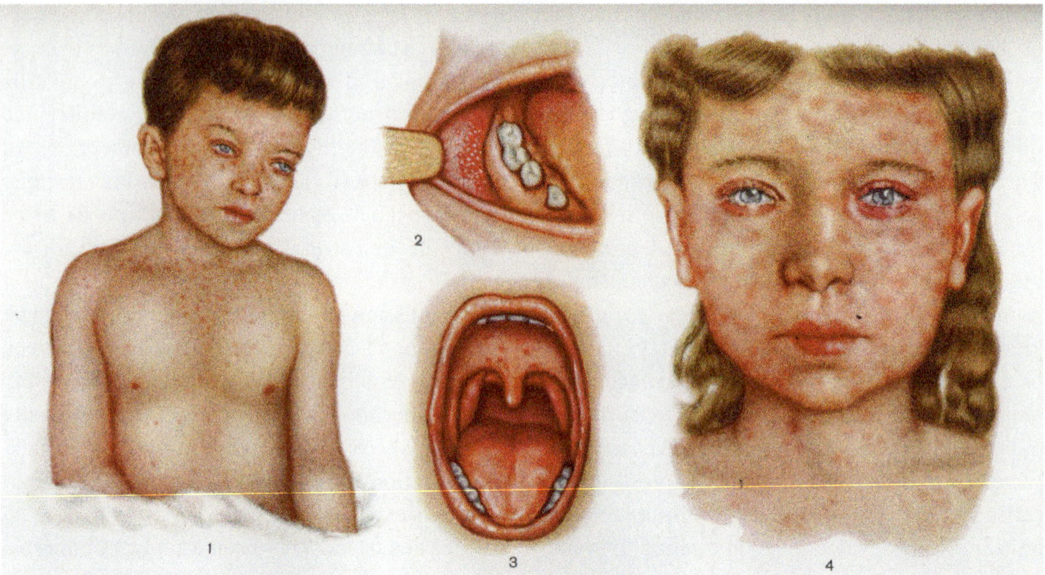

Fig. 5.8 Typical rash and enanthema in children with measles. Picture from M.G. Danilevich's textbook "Childrens infections." Leningrad, 1949

can occur. It is extremely important to notify that such lesions can be caused either directly by measles virus or by other pathogens.

The most frequent complications are respiratory superinfections, such as pneumonia (especially necrotic), laryngotracheobronchitis, and otitis. In developing countries, diarrhea is also common, even as a cause of mortality, it can be due to lesions caused directly by measles virus or different superinfections. Very rare approximately 1 in 1000 cases acute disseminated encephalitis (encephalomyelitis) can develop. The disease has usually an abrupt onset of the fever and altered mental status within 2 weeks following rash. Many authors regard it as autoimmune demyelinating disease, but there are also data proving the possibility of direct lesion of brain tissue by measles virus. In the literature, the possibility of the role of measles in the development of subacute sclerosing panencephalitis has been discussed. Probably this disease is associated with measles virus particles with defects in the envelope-associated proteins.

Among the lesions of other organs, catarrhal colitis must be mentioned. In several cases, acute appendicitis in the incubational period of measles with appearance in the mucous membrane of multinuclear giant cells was described [15].

After the introduction of vaccination in the wide clinical practice, the number of death-threaten cases has dramatically reduced. There are no commonly accepted antiviral drugs; bacterial complications are treated with antibiotics. In a susceptible host exposed to measles, administration of measles virus-specific immune globulin ameliorates the course of the disease.

Nowadays, the prognosis in the majority of countries is quite favorable, but according to the estimation of WHO, the number of deaths related to measles in 2008 was 160,000. According to our experience, the most severe cases with rare lethal outcomes were observed in 70–80th of the last century in young people (medical students and pregnant). Sometimes outbreaks of measles still occur, but without lethal outcomes. In the literature, the possibility of virus persistence after the recovery and its role in the development of subacute sclerosing panencephalitis are discussed.

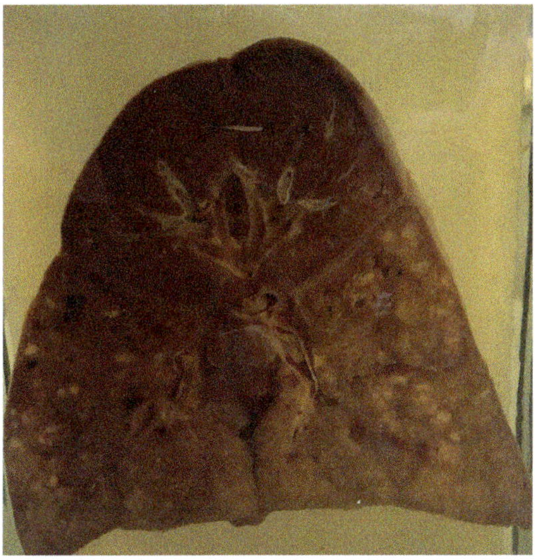

Fig. 5.9 Necrotic bronchitis and pneumonia in measles. Macro-preparation from museum of pathology department of SP Botkin Infectious Hospital, Saint-Petersburg, Russia

Macroscopical diagnostics is based first of all upon evaluation of typical rash and enantema (see Fig. 5.8). In the uncomplicated measles in the internal organ, only catarrhal tonsillitis, laryngitis, and tracheobronchitis can be noted. Changes in the brain are unremarkable.

The development of secondary infectious complications of bacterial or viral origin is extremely typical for measles [16]. In such cases, the macroscopy becomes similar to the observed concomitant disease. The most severe lesions have been observed in the cases when measles has been complicated by staphylococci infection (Fig. 5.9). In the lethal outcomes at this stage of the disease, the typical giant cells may be absent. One must consider also probability of more severe course of preexisting diseases (tuberculosis as example).

Infection of epithelial cells leads to the formation of giant cells, similar to that seen in tissue culture. They can be observed in different organs including tonsils (Fig. 5.10), lungs, appendix, and intestine. Epithelial giant cells are present in nasal secretions and conjunctivae also. The pathognomic mucosal eruption (enanthem)—Koplik spots, consists of epithelial giant cells with surrounding mononuclear cell infiltrates in

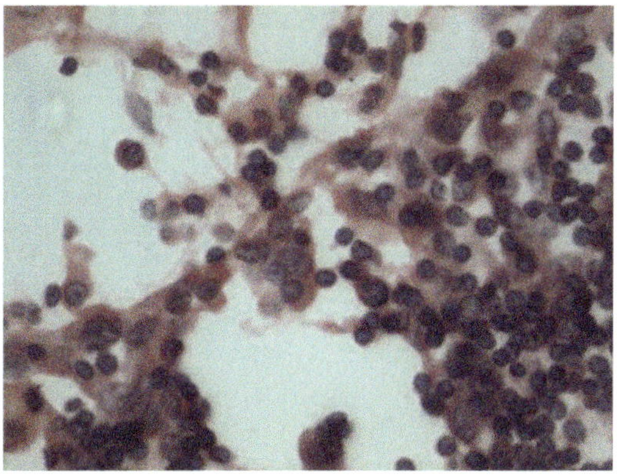

Fig. 5.10 Giant multinuclear cells typical for measles in tonsils. H.-E. ×400

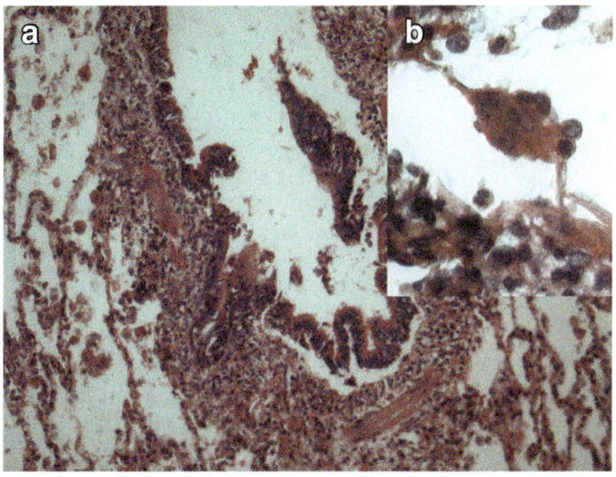

Fig. 5.11 Viral bronchitis in measles. H.-E. (**a**) General view. ×100. (**b**) Detail of the previous picture. Multinucleated cell. ×400

the submucous glands. Viral bronchopneumonia, usually with bacterial superinfection, is regarded as extremely typical for measles (Fig. 5.11). Although at later stages of the disease, giant cells may be absent. Many of the clinical manifestations of measles can be attributed to direct damage of the host. Epithelial and endothelial cells, in spite of the absence of available commercial systems allowing detecting virus or its specific antigens in paraffin-embedded slices, certainly represent the site of viral replication.

Infection of endothelial cells causes vascular dilatation and increased vascular permeability. In the infected sites, intense inflammation and mononuclear cell infiltration are present. As a

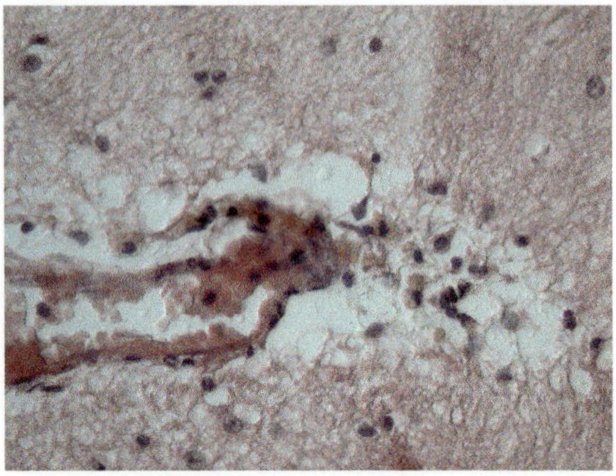

Fig. 5.12 Brain vasculitis in a lethal case of measles in a young woman. H.-E x200

rare occasion, an intrauterine measles with typical rash in the newborn is also described.

From our experience in the lethal cases in generalized measles in brain, one can observe vasculitis with the proliferation of endothelial cells and modest mononuclear infiltration (Fig. 5.12); perivascular demyelination is remarkable.

Initially, the only existing model was the challenge of monkeys, due to ethical and economic reasons, such studies were not provided since the middle of 20th century. The lack of a suitable animal model has greatly hindered the research into the pathogenesis of measles. Identification of two human receptors for the measles virus, CD46, and CD150 has opened new perspectives in this field. During the last decade, numerous transgenic animal models have been developed in order to humanize mice and use them to study measles infection and virus–host interactions. Despite their limitations, these models have provided remarkable insights into different aspects of measles infection, providing a better understanding of virus-induced neuropathology, immunosuppression, mechanisms of virus virulence, and contribution of innate and adaptive immune response in viral clearance.

Definite diagnosis is made by virus isolation in culture from respiratory or conjunctival secretions, blood, or urine. In practice, for diagnostics, serology is usually used, looking for fourfold rise in measles-specific serum IgG level, IgM antibodies in enzyme immunoassay. Polymerase chain reaction (RT-PCR) is sensitive and specific, but not widely used. In certain cases, there are difficulties in differential diagnosis with German measles (rubella) in the clinic.

5.5 Lung Lesions Due to Other RNA-Viruses

It is widely accepted that lungs can be affected by different RNA-containing viruses including those belonging to Enterovirus genus. Although in our certain observations, such changes due to Enteroviruses and Coxsackie viruses were suspected; hence, we had no opportunity to prove them.

Rhinovirus is considered as one of the most common pathogens causing mild respiratory infections. No lethal cases were documented and, therefore, there are no descriptions of histopathology of rhinovirus infections. In collaboration with V.V. Svistunov, we recently got the opportunity to study the changes in three lethal cases where rhinovirus infection was a concomitant disease diagnosed by PCR from lung tissue. We considered to associate with this pathogen the overgrowth of bronchial epithelium (Figs. 5.13 and 5.14).

HIV infection leads to the development of numerous secondary infections, including those with lung involvement (see Chaps. 7, 13–16), but it is less known that RNA-containing HIV virus itself having proved tropism to alveolar macrophages can cause their peculiar changes (Fig. 5.15).

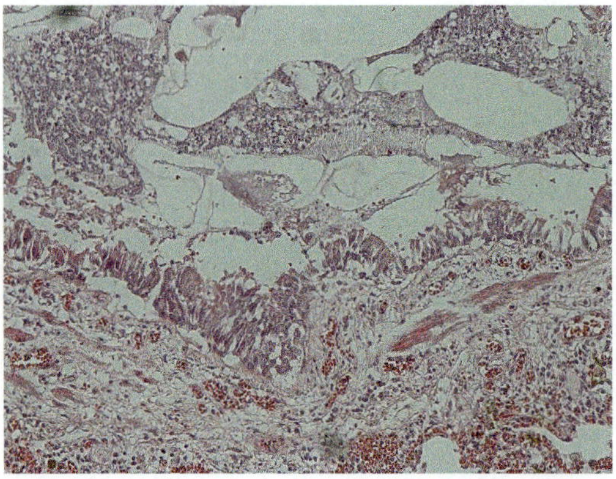

Fig. 5.13 Overgrowth of bronchial epithelium in rhinovirus infection. Courtesy of V.V. Swistunov. H.-E. ×100

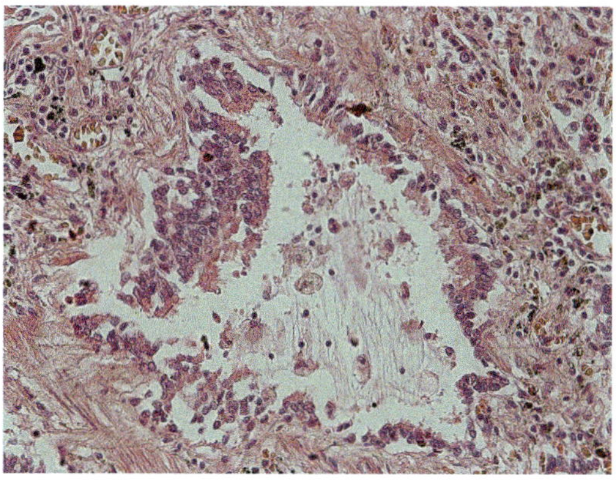

Fig. 5.14 Similar changes. H.-E. ×200

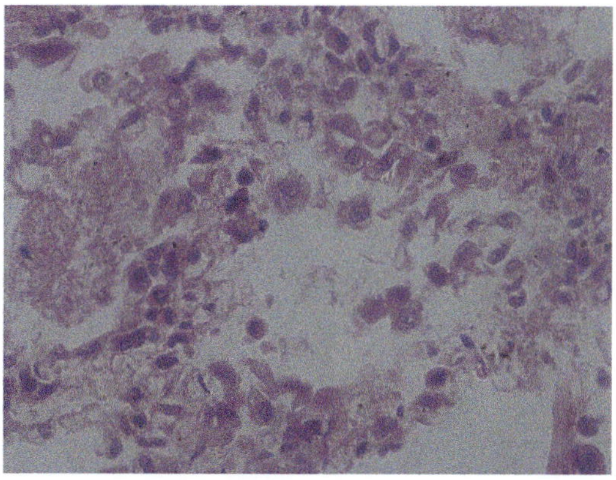

Fig. 5.15 Typical changes of alveolar macrophages in HIV infection. H.-E. ×400

References

1. Branche AR, Falsey AR. Parainfluenza virus infection. Semin Respir Crit Care Med. 2016;37(4):538–54. https://doi.org/10.1055/s-0036-1584798.
2. Zinserling AV. Etiology and pathologic anatomy of acute respiratory infections. L.: Meditsina; 1977. 170 p. (In Russian).
3. Zinserling AV. Peculiarities of lesions in viral and mycoplasma infection of respiratory tract. Virchows Arch A Pathol Pathol Anat. 1973;356:259–73.
4. Murhy TF, Dubovi EJ, Clyde WA. The cotton rat as an experimental model of human parainfluenza virus type 3 disease. Exp Lung Res. 1981;2(2):97–109.
5. Hao F, Wang Z, Mao L, et al. The novel caprine parainfluenza virus type3 showed pathogenicity in Guinea pigs. Microb Pathog. 2019;134:103569.
6. Zinserling VA, Chukhlovina ML. Infectious Lesions of nervous system. Issues of etiology, pathogenesis and diagnostics. Saint-Petersburg, ElbiSPb; 2011. 583 p. (In Russian).
7. Johnson JT, Gonzales RA, Olson SJ, Wright PF, Graham BS. The histopathology of fatal untreated human respiratory syncytial virus infection. Mod Pathol. 2007;20(1):108–19. https://doi.org/10.1038/modpathol.3800725.
8. Taylor G. Animal models of respiratory syncytial virus infection. Vaccine. 2017;35(3):469–80.
9. Panda S, Mohakud NK, Pena L, Kumar S. Human metapneumovirus: review of an important respiratory pathogen. Int J Infect Dis. 2014;25:45–52.
10. Hartmann S, Sid H, Rautenschlein S. Avian metapneumovirus infection of chicken and turkey tracheal organ cultures: comparison of virus–host interactions. Avian Pathol. 2015;44(6):480–9.
11. Kuiken T, van den Hoogen BG, van Riel DA, et al. Experimental human metapneumovirus infection of cynomolgus macaques (Macaca fascicularis) results in virus replication in ciliated epithelial cells and pneumocytes with associated lesions throughout the respiratory tract. Am J Pathol. 2004;164(6):1893–900. https://doi.org/10.1016/S0002-9440(10)63750-9.
12. Varyasin VV, Zinserling VA. Metapneumovirus in adult. Arkh Patol. 2016;78(3):53–6. https://doi.org/10.17116/patol201678353-56.
13. Moss WJ. Measles. Lancet. 2017;390(10111):2490–502. https://doi.org/10.1016/S0140-6736(17)31463-0.
14. Caroline F. Pediatric infections: diagnosis and management. Foster Academics; 2019. p. 248.
15. Kradin RL, editor. Diagnostic pathology of infectious diseases. Elsevier; 2018. 698 p.
16. Hofman P, editor. Infectious disease and parasites. Springer Reference; 2016. 343 p.

6 Infections Due to Coronaviruses

Coronaviruses are a large family of RNA single-stranded enveloped viruses 80 nm in size with helical nucleocapsid viruses able to cause lesions of different animals and men. Several strains known since 1965 can cause light forms of respiratory infections [1–4].

In 2002, a new form of zoonotic coronavirus infection causing acute respiratory syndrome (SARS) with high mortality appeared. In 2002–2003, outbreak originating in Asia resulted in more than 8000 cases and 744 deaths in 29 countries worldwide. No cases reported since 2004. Virus infects tracheobronchial and alveolar epithelial and immune cells; other targets were not reported. Virus binds angiotensin-converting enzyme 2 (ACE2).

Early symptoms consist of fever, headache, and myalgia, at days 2–7, nonproductive cough and dyspnea are typical, later on develop radiographically confirmed pneumonia. Overall, lethality was reported as 10%, predominantly in persons over 60.

There are few pathological descriptions in the literature [4], according to which, at early stage (<11 days), the disease was characterized by diffuse alveolar damage with edema, hyaline membranes, alveolar collapse, desquamation of alveolar epithelial cells, the appearance of scattered multinucleated giant cells of uncertain diagnostic significance. Virus antigen was detected in alveolar epithelial cells and macrophages during IHC and viral particles as nucleocapsid inclusions and typical double-membrane vesicles during EM [2]. After 10–14 days, interstitial/airspace fibrosis and pneumocyte's hyperplasia were described. No extrapulmonary lesions were reported. No pathognomic autopsy features have been identified. We had no opportunity to see such cases our self.

In 2012, a new coronavirus infection—Middle East respiratory syndrome (MERS) has been described in Saudi Arabia, other neighbor countries, and Korea [3]. In spite of high mortality, histopathology was reported only in single cases [4]. The primary finding at autopsy was viral-mediated lung damage with features of Dad. Infected were pneumocytes, multinucleated epithelial cells, and bronchial submucosal glands. These infected cells expressed DPP-4 surface antigen which serves as the cell receptor of MERS-CoV. Viral inclusions were demonstrated by EM in respiratory epithelium and renal proximal tubules. We have no our own experience in study of this infection as well.

6.1 COVID-19

At the end of 2019, a new form of coronavirus SARS-covi2 appeared in China, which caused an epidemic later regarded as a pandemic. Disease became the name COVID-19 [5, 6]. Main clinical symptoms include lesions of respiratory tract beginning with mild respiratory infection till

V. Zinserling, *Infectious Pathology of the Respiratory Tract*,
https://doi.org/10.1007/978-3-030-66325-4_6

total damage of the lungs with high lethality. Most common severe forms are typical for elder patients having diabetes and/or overweight. Extrapulmonary lesions have been noted clinically and morphologically as well [7–9].

Specific macroscopic features of COVID-19 are absent. In observations, the signs of severe respiratory failure strongly prevail, a pattern of respiratory distress syndrome ("shock lung," DAD) is observed—sharp plethora and diffuse lung compaction, almost indistinguishable from that observed with "swine" influenza A/H1N1pdm (2009 and subsequent years). The mass of the lungs is increased, the lungs are of a doughy or dense consistency, low-air or airless; lacquer appearance from the surface, dark red (cherry) color, when pressed from the surface of the cuts, a dark red liquid flows, which is hardly squeezed out. In certain cases, such lesions may be focal. Sometimes, there may be large hemorrhagic infarctions, obstructing blood clots, mainly in the branches of the pulmonary veins. Significant lesions of the trachea are not observed in this case; occasionally serous-purulent exudate detected in intubated patients is most likely associated with nosocomial infection. In cases where COVID-19 joined another severe pathology, a combination of changes characteristic of various diseases is naturally observed. A component that can be associated with the effect of the 2019 virus is observed in the form of focal lower lobe pneumonia with severe plethora.

The dynamics of changes in ARDS associated with COVID-19 can only be judged by analogy with SARS and influenza A/H1N1pdm. In the late (productive) stage (after 7–8 days or more from the onset of the disease) of diffuse alveolar damage, macroscopically lungs are enlarged, low air, dense, fleshy, can resemble the density of the liver, sometimes, with diffuse whitish layers and areas of different sizes (Fig. 6.1). Microscopically we note siderophages, a relative (in comparison with "swine" influenza) small number of hyaline membranes (Fig. 6.2), fibrin.

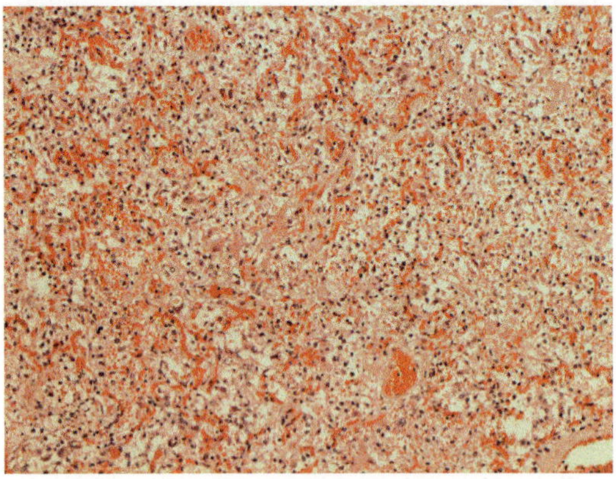

Fig. 6.1 General view of the lung in a deceased from COVID-19. ARDS. H.-E. ×100

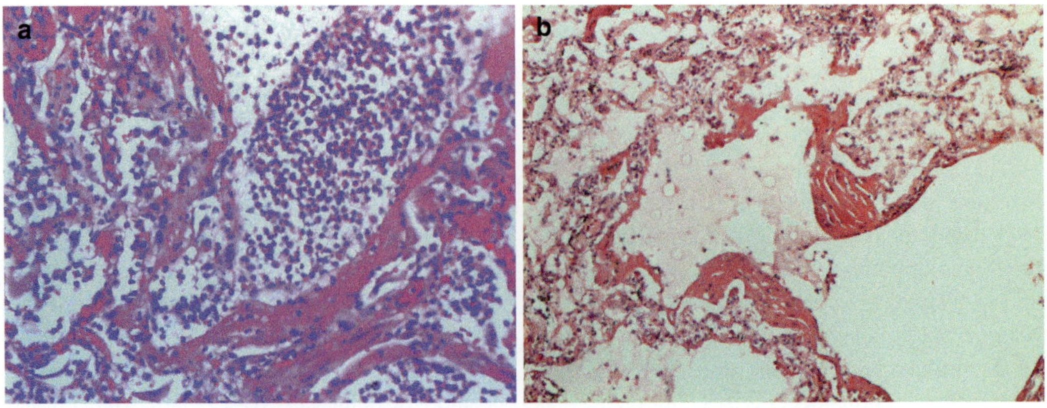

Fig. 6.2 Hyaline membranes in the lung of a deceased from COVID-19. H.-E. ×100. (**a**) Highly expressed with additional neutrophilic infiltration and (**b**) moderately expressed

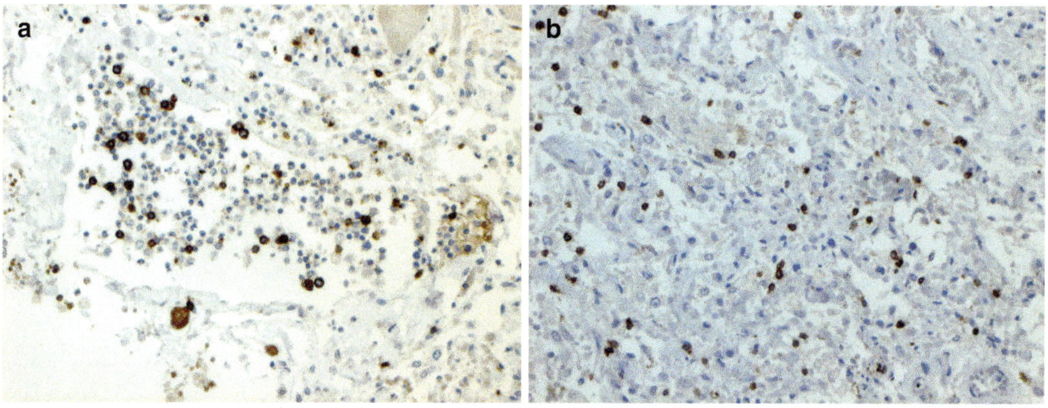

Fig. 6.3 T-lymphocytes in a lung of a deceased from COVID-19. IHC. ×200 (**a**) CD3+ and (**b**) CD8+

Squamous metaplasia of the bronchial, bronchiolar and alveolar epithelium can be detected in the lumens of the alveoli, respiratory and terminal bronchioles. Thickening of the interalveolar septa is noted due to sclerosis, lymphoid (mostly CD3+ and CD 8+) (Fig. 6.3) and macrophageous (Fig. 6.4) infiltration and proliferation of type II alveolocytes. Certain changes we consider to be directly related to virus propagation (Fig. 6.5). The nature of cytoproliferative changes of the epithelium in trachea (Fig. 6.6) and bronchi remains unclear. In the final stage of the disease, sections of fibrous tissue may develop in all parts of the lungs (usually in the lower lobes) (Fig. 6.7), which contributes to the development of chronic respiratory failure. In many vessels, we observe thrombi also in different vessels (Figs. 6.8 and 6.9). The frequency and role of joining a bacterial (mycotic) infection from 4 to 7 days after the onset of the disease remain unclear, which contributes to the development of virus–bacterial pneumonia, which is described mainly in the later stages of the disease. In several cases, we observed lesions with the appearance of PAS-positive extra- and intracellular bodies we regarded as activation of chronic chlamydia infection (Fig. 6.10).

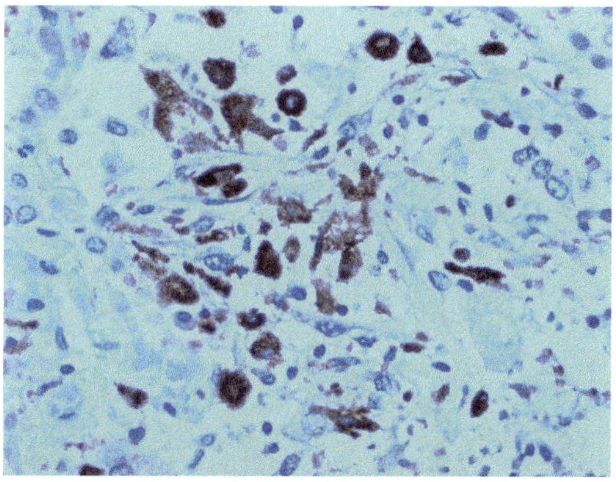

Fig. 6.4 CD68+ macrophages in a lung of a deceased from COVID-19. IHC. ×400

The possibility of developing a generalized infection with damage to other organs is not excluded. In other organs and tissues, alterative and necrotic changes of parenchymal cells, the formation of fibrin thrombi in blood vessels (probably DIC), infiltration by T-lymphocytes, including cytotoxic, as well as pathological changes associated with comorbid chronic diseases that previously existed in the dead, were observed. Many aspects of the pathogenesis of coronavirus infection require further comprehensive study.

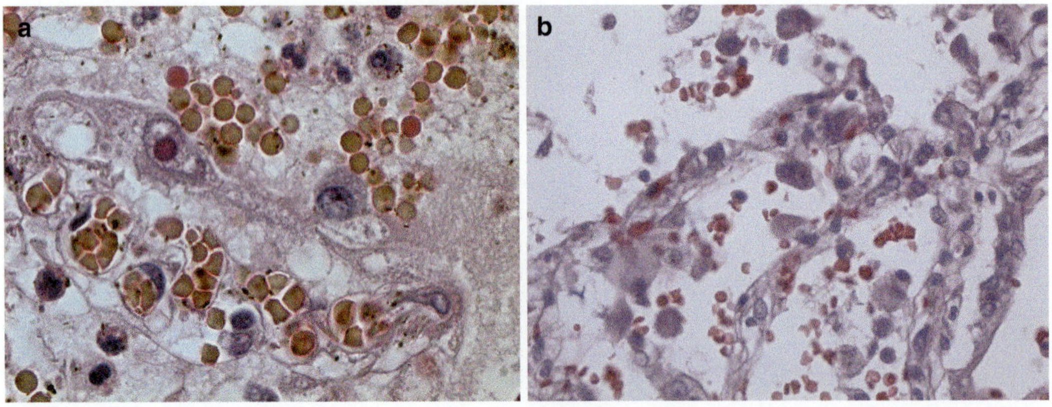

Fig. 6.5 Probably virus-induced changes in the lung of a deceased from COVID-19.H.-E. (**a**) Intranuclear inclusion ×400 and (**b**) alveolocytes and macrophages with irregular form. ×200

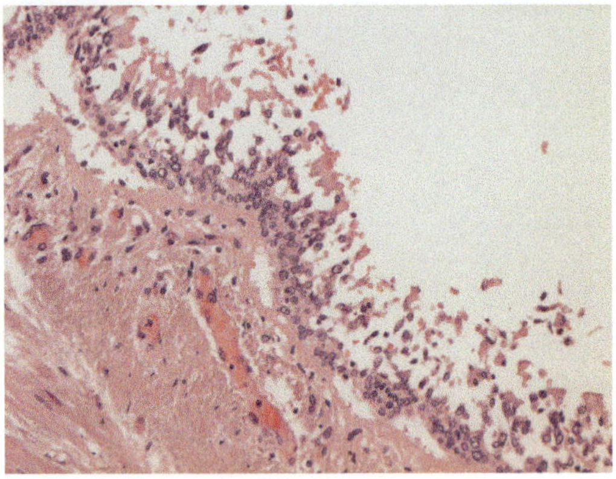

Fig. 6.6 Proliferation of epithelium in a small bronchus. H.-E. ×400

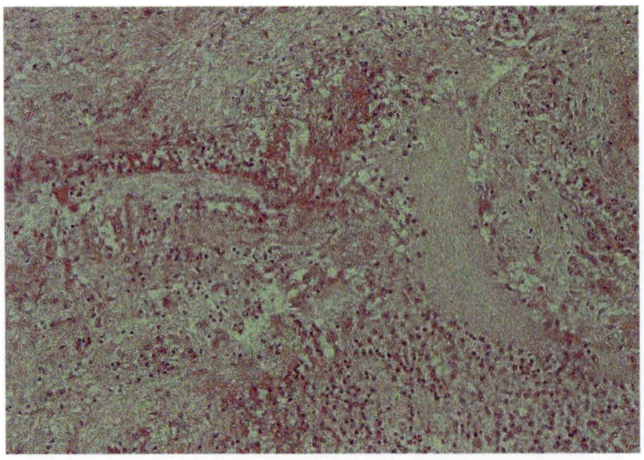

Fig. 6.7 Diffuse fibrosis as an outcome of ARDS in a deceased from COVID-19. H.-E. ×100

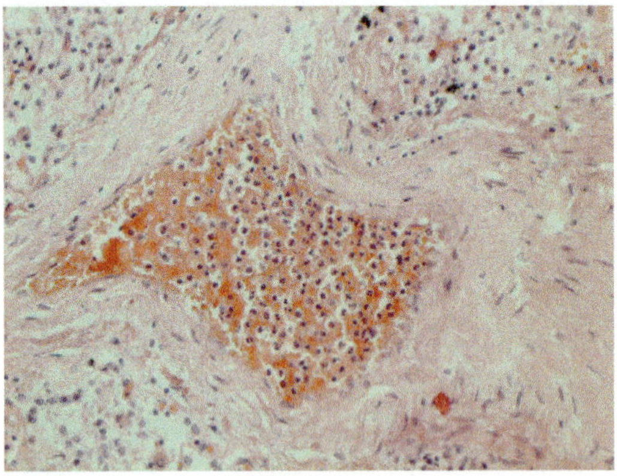

Fig. 6.8 Formation of thrombus in a big artery with disturbance of its wall in the lung of a deceased from COVID-19. H.-E. ×100

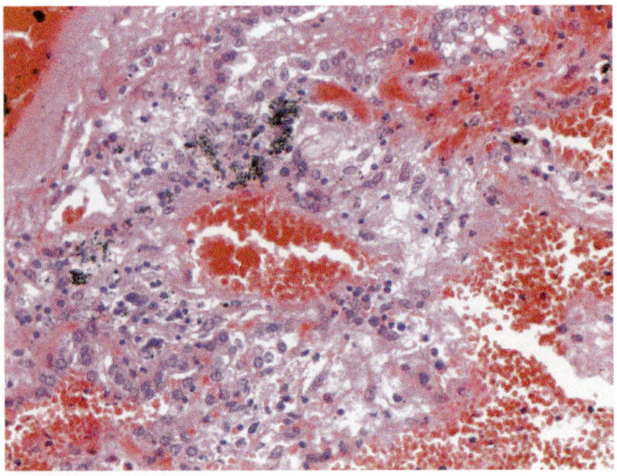

Fig. 6.9 Formation of thrombus in a small branch of an artery with surrounding hemorrhages in the lung of a deceased from COVID-19. H.-E. ×100

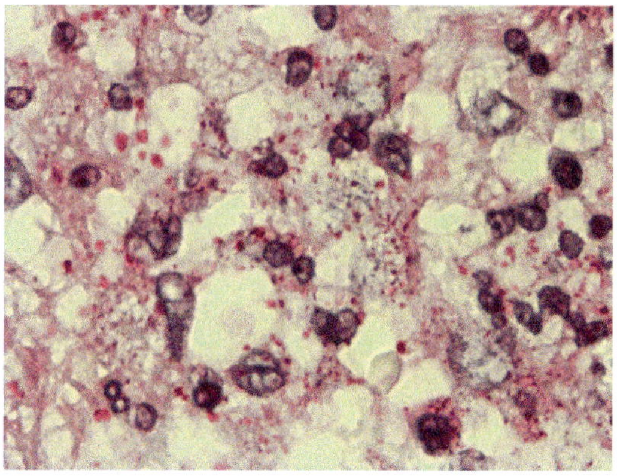

Fig. 6.10 Extra- and intracellular PAS-positive inclusions in the lung of a deceased from COVID-19. PAS ×400

References

1. Ziebuhr J, editor. Coronaviruses. Springer; 2016. 128 p.
2. Cavanagh D, editor. SARS- and other coronaviruses. Springer; 2008. 326 p.
3. Vijay R, editor. MERS-coronavirus. Springer; 2020. 224 p.
4. Bradley BT, Bryan A. Emerging respiratory infections: the infectious disease pathology of SARS, MERS, pandemic influenza and Legionella. Semin Diagn Pathol. 2019;36:152–9. https://doi.org/10.1053/j.semdp.2019.04.06.
5. Shereen MA, Khan S, Kazmi A, Bashir N, Siddique R. COVID-19 infection: origin, transmission, and characteristics of human coronaviruses. J Adv Res. 2020;24:91–8. https://doi.org/10.1016/j.jare.2020.03.005.
6. Skok K, Stelzl E, Trauner M, et al. Post-mortem viral dynamics and tropism in COVID-19 patients in correlation with organ damage. Virchows Arch. 2020. https://doi.org/10.1007/s00428-020-02903-8.
7. Xiao F, Tang M, Zheng X, Liu Y, Li X, Shan H. Evidence for gastrointestinal infection of SARS-CoV-2. Gastroenterology. 2020;158(6):1831–1833.e1833. https://doi.org/10.1053/j.gastro.2020.02.055.
8. Puelles VG, Lutgehetmann M, Lindenmeyer MT, et al. Multiorgan and renal tropism of SARS-CoV-2. N Engl J Med. 2020;383:590–2. https://doi.org/10.1056/NEJMc2011400.
9. Zinserling VA, Semenova NY, Markov AG, et al. Inflammatory infiltration of adrenals in COVID-19 autoimmunity reviews. 2020. https://doi.org/10.1016/j.autrev.2020.102597.

7 Respiratory Infections Due to DNA Viruses

7.1 Adenovirus Infection

Adenoviruses are a family of 49 DNA-containing viruses identified by sequential letters and numbers. In clinical and pathological practice, individual strains are usually not distinguished. Adenoviruses most frequently cause mild infections of the respiratory and digestive systems. After the illness fades away, the virus can persist in the tonsils, adenoids, and other lymph tissue. We have got the data that it may occur also in the brain. Adenovirus does not become latent (like herpes viruses) but instead reproduce constantly and slowly [1]. It is possible to be infected more than once with adenoviruses, because there are many different types.

The transmission may be due to contaminated environment (including swimming pools), medical instruments, crowding. The main transmission way is aerogenic, but also contact, alimentary, and transplacental ways are possible. Although these infections can occur at any time of the year, respiratory tract disease caused by adenovirus is more common in late winter, spring, and early summer.

Adenovirus was first isolated in adenoids in the 50th, but the virus certainly caused respiratory illnesses long before that.

The virus has been studied in detail, but many aspects of the pathogenesis of the disease still remain unclear. Adenovirus is a nonenveloped icosahedral particle. The shell of the virion is made up of two kinds of capsomeres, hexons, and pentons. Hexons have six neighbors and pentons, located at the vertices of the icosahedron, have five neighbors. The predominant protein component of the viral core is an arginine-rich basic protein that presumably aids in the spatial organization of the viral DNA and neutralizes its negative charge. The core protein serves to package the adenoviral DNA. The genome of human adenoviruses is a linear double-stranded DNA molecule of 30,000–36,000 base pairs, depending on serotype. The adenoviral genome has two unusual structural features. First, it possesses inverted terminal repeats: approximately 100 base pairs are repeated in an inverted orientation at each end of the genome. Second, each strand of the genome is covalently attached at its 5′ end to a protein molecule (the terminal protein).

Adenoviruses attach to receptors on the host cell surface through the fiber protein. For the commonly studied adenovirus serotypes 2 and 5, the receptor is a member of the immunoglobulin superfamily of proteins called CAR (coxsackievirus and adenovirus receptor). CAR is present on most human cells and many other vertebrate cell types at up to 10^5 copies per cell. The normal function of CAR is not known. Following attachment, the virus–receptor complex migrates to clathrin-coated pits, which form endosomes that carry the virus particles into the cell. Internalization is dependent on the interaction of a second virion protein (peptone base) with the

V. Zinserling, *Infectious Pathology of the Respiratory Tract*,
https://doi.org/10.1007/978-3-030-66325-4_7

other cell surface proteins. The pH of the endosome falls, inducing the virions to shed their penton capsid proteins and attached fibers. The conformational change in the virions causes the endosome to rupture and releases the partially dissembled virions into the cell cytoplasm. The particles migrate to the nucleus of the infected cell, probably along microtubules, and bind to proteins at the nuclear pore. The viral core then enters the nucleus, leaving behind most of its remaining capsid proteins. The next stages are gene expression, DNA replication, and viral assembly.

Adenoviruses use several mechanisms to evade cell-mediated immune response. Early viral protein blocks the production of MHC class I mRNA in infected cells, thus making them "invisible" for cytotoxic T lymphocytes, and glycoprotein E3 prevents the transport of newly synthesized MHC class I protein to the cell surface. Adenoviruses produce proteins that block the pathways of cell death related to tumor necrosis factor and Fas-ligand. Adenoviruses also break the interferon chain and prevent the inhibition of protein synthesis through the action of small RNA molecules encoded by viral genes.

Adenovirus type 12 was the first DNA-containing virus shown to cause cancer in animals, but there is no clear evidence about their role in carcinogenesis in humans. In recent time, adenoviruses were intensively studied as a possible vector for gene and vaccine transfer. It is estimated that adenoviruses cause about 10% of all respiratory illnesses, but the frequency can significantly vary. Very typical are conjunctivitis and catarrhal tonsillitis. Exact statistics of morbidity and mortality is absent. We can only assume that in different periods of time, the data can vary seriously. There may be single cases and outbreaks.

Adenoviral infection can develop at every age, but generalized forms are diagnosed preferably in infants or immunocompromised adults.

Adenoviruses can cause lesions of many internal organs and brain, but most frequently they are associated with infections of the respiratory tract, eyes, tonsils, and intestines [2].

Acute adenoviral infections are generally self-limiting. However, generalized death threaten forms have also been described especially in infants and immunosuppressed adults.

Structural changes in adenovirus infection have been described by several authors, but the most profound studies were provided by A. Zinserling and his collaborators in the 60th and 70th of the XX century [3, 4].

Macroscopically changes are usually moderate. Catarrhal laryngotracheobronchitis is typical. In lungs with no relation to the duration of the disease are present reddish or dark reddish, seldom gray reddish small sunken foci with the wet cut surface. Such changes can be observed in both lungs usually in the back parts. In front parts of the lungs acute emphysema is typical.

Most important are the changes in the epithelium of the airways. Its nuclei are enlarged and become more basophilic. In some of them, one can observe a basophilic, rich with DNA oval or round inclusion, surrounded with the narrow enlighten zone forming a border from the remaining part of the nucleus. In the cytoplasm and the nuclei of the affected cells can be observed fuchsinophilic inclusions. Not seldom epithelial layer looks to be loosed. At this stage, the cells can desquamate in layers. Under the epithelium can accumulate the serous exudate and with mixture of erythrocytes. Similar changes of the epithelium can be observed in the glands. In the deep layers of the wall of bronchi and trachea can be observed in lymphoid infiltration. In the lumen of the bronchi, one can find the serous exudates with the admixture of macrophages and single leucocytes. At the later stages, epithelial cells undergo karyorrhexis.

The lungs at low power magnification are airless (Fig. 7.1) and in several cases, the radiological changes can be regarded as pneumonia. But a relatively small percentage of neutrophilic leucocytes in the exudate doesn't allow to speak about "common" bacterial pneumonia. Distelectasis (alternation of atelectatic and emphysematic foci) is typical, as well as accumulation of lymphocytes and plasma cells in the interstitial tissue.

In the respiratory parts of the lungs, one can observe the typical changes of the alveolocytes similar to the described in the epithelium of the respiratory tract (Fig. 7.2). The damaged cells are enlarged, predominantly due to the nucleus. The intranuclear inclusions at early stages are oxyphilic, later become basophilic and are rich with DNA. Such giant mononuclear cell later on may desquamate in the alveoli lumen, where at early stages is flocculent protein-rich exudate containing also erythrocytes, macrophages, and not numerous neutrophils (Fig. 7.3). Later on, the exudate undergoes necrosis with the fine-grain appearance. In some infants in lumen of alveoli and small bronchi can be observed hyaline membranes.

In the majority of the deceased are observed also in the lesions of blood vessels. They are plethoric, the walls edematous, in the lumen not seldom thrombi.

Similar changes have been observed in other sites: intestine, brain (Fig. 7.4), liver, kidneys, tonsils, pancreas, and adrenals [5]. Nearby the appearance of increased in seize epithelial and endothelial cells with enlarged nuclei containing basophilic inclusions were noted only nonspecific alterative changes. Inflammatory lymphoid infiltration was expressed moderately. In several observations, adenoviral etiology has been shown in clinical pathology [6].

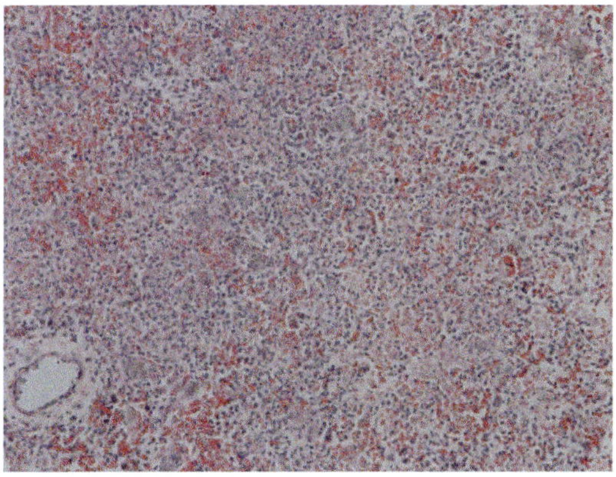

Fig. 7.1 General view of the lung in a child died from a generalized adenovirus infection. H.-E. ×100

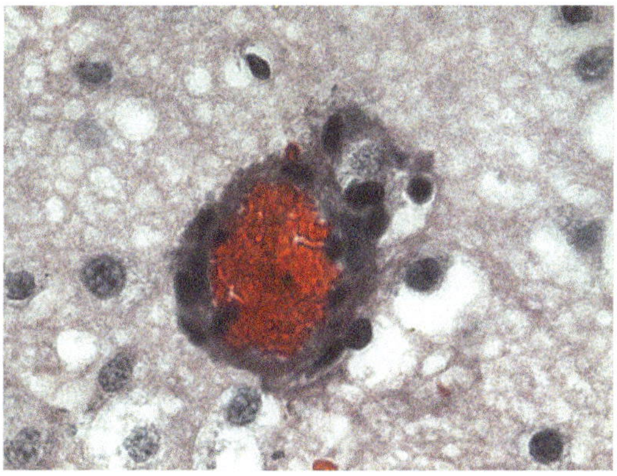

Fig. 7.3 Brain vasculitis with numerous hyperchromic cells in a child died from a generalized adenovirus infection. H.-E. ×200

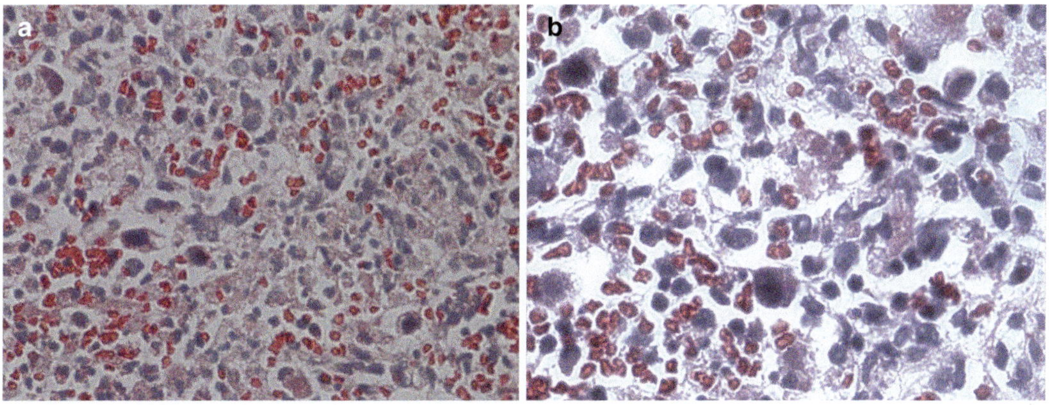

Fig. 7.2 Mixed infiltration in a lung in a child died from a generalized adenovirus infection. Note mononuclear cells with hyperchromic nuclei H.-E. (**a**). ×200. (**b**) Detail of the same picture. Numerous intranuclear basophilic inclusions. ×400

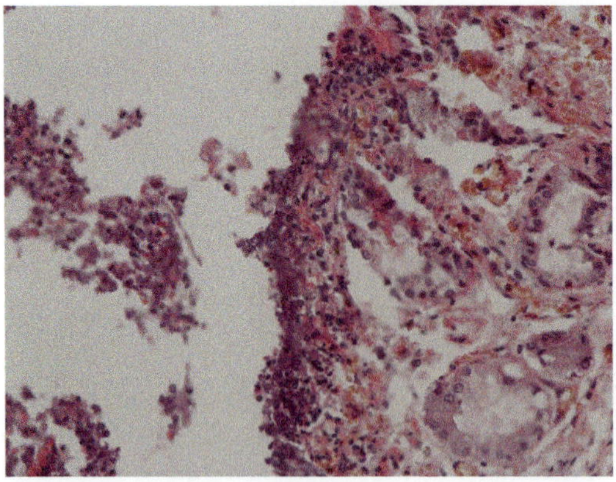

Fig. 7.4 Necrotic bronchitis in a child with herpes simplex infection. H.-E. ×200

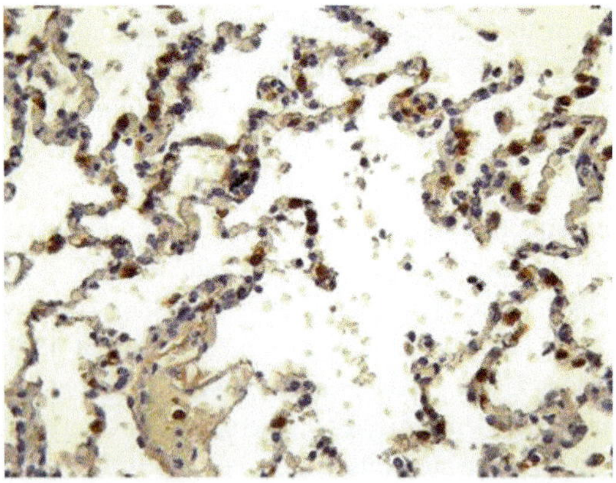

Fig. 7.5 Antigen of herpes symplex type ½ in the lung of a child. IHC. ×200 Courtesy of V.E. Karev

Diagnostic of adenovirus infection can be based upon revealing virus in culture or it's DNA in PCR. Immunofluorescent and IHC diagnostics can be helpful as well. Serological investigation revealing antibodies in blood and CSF can be very informative especially while tested twice in the interval of 5–7 days. In the lethal cases, seroconversion may take place even earlier. For exact diagnostics, IHC has to be used. Histological picture also possesses certain peculiarity and allows at least preliminary diagnosis.

Differential diagnosis. With influenza, other viral and bacterial respiratory infections are based upon the clinical, laboratory, and morphological data. Most problematic is differential diagnosis with generalized herpes simplex infection.

Adenoviral infection can be reproduced in hamsters and guinea pigs [7]. Lesions comparable with those observed in humans can be obtained by pretreatment of animals with corticosteroids.

7.2 Respiratory Herpes

The causative agent of this disease is herpes simplex virus, mainly of type 1. Nowadays it is accepted that both viruses HSV1 and HSV2 can cause similar lesions. The virus is characterized by pantropy and the ability to cause lesions of varying severity. The diseases caused by HSV can occur both as acute and chronic, and periodically with an almost complete absence of clinical manifestations of the disease [8]. At present, it has been proved that apoptosis is the most important pathogenetic factor determining the formation of alterative changes with appearance of small basophilic granules [9].

With any variant of the disease, HSV propagates intracellularly. Affected cells increase in size; inclusions appear in their nuclei [10]. Ions look like small "droplets" in the nuclear mass [10].

There are descriptions of respiratory damage in older children and adults. This includes, in particular, the observation of acute respiratory infections caused by HSV among large groups of the US population [11]. The disease proceeds, like other acute viral infections, with an increase in body temperature. In such patients, pharyngitis and tonsillitis are observed, in about half of ulcerative lesions of the tonsils and posterior pharyngeal wall. According to a serological study, 80% of patients had a primary herpetic infection. In a few publications, respiratory herpes is also considered as a hospital infection [12].

Most often, this disease develops against a background of primary or secondary immunodeficiency. In HIV, in AIDS stage, however, severe herpetic lesions are uncommon. In most of the dead, ulcerations of the mucous membrane of the trachea are revealed, covered with fibrinous films that narrow its lumen (Fig. 7.5). Changes in the lungs have the nature of focal bronchopneumonia with partial necrosis of the interalveolar septa, hemorrhages, the presence in the alveoli of proteinaceous exudate with enlarged alveolar cells with hyperchromic nuclei-containing large eosinophilic inclusions, as well as mononuclear cells and cell debris). In the nuclei of other alveolocytes, perinuclear enlightenments and chromatin margin are visible.

Diagnostics and especially differential diagnostics with other infections due to DNA viruses has to be certainly based upon epidemiological, clinical, and morphological data, but crucial role plays IHC.

There are numerous experimental models in animal experiments [13]; we also succeeded to reproduce generalized infection in new-borne rabbits with the development of typical histological changes in the lungs [14].

Many issues of herpes infection in different localizations, in spite of the fact that its genome has been successfully decrypted, still require profound complex study.

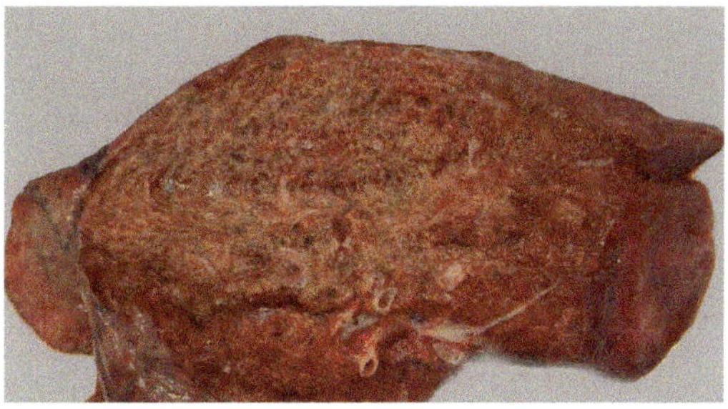

Fig. 7.6 Lung in cytomegalovirus infection. Areas of reduced airiness are yellowish in color; interstitial is well defined in places. Unfixed macropreparation

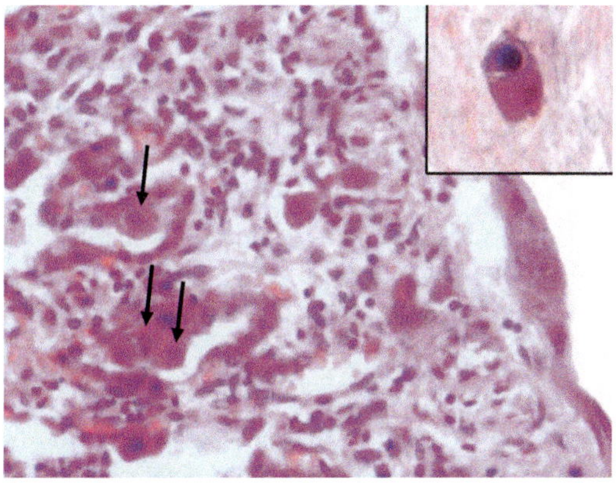

Fig. 7.7 Cytomegalovirus lung damage. Typical "owl's eye" cells (indicated by arrows). Stained with hematoxylin and eosin. ×400 (in the inset ×1000)

7.3 Lung Lesions in Cytomegalovirus in Adults with HIV Infection in AIDS Stage

Cytomegalovirus is ubiquitous pantropic pathogen causing clinically important lesions in patients with T-cell immunodeficiency [15]. Historically, the detailed clinical and morphological characteristics since the early 50th of XX century were made for intrauterine infections [16]. In Sect. 17.6, we are going to present such lesions.

After the outbreak of HIV infection, CMV appeared to be one of its most frequent and clinically important complications able to develop practically in all organs and tissues.

In the late stages of HIV infection, cytomegalovirus infection (CMVI) occurs more often in a severe generalized form. The most commonly affected are the lungs, brain, intestines, and adrenal glands [17].

Macroscopically, the lungs are of a slightly dense consistency; sections in different segments of the lungs showed areas of low-airiness parenchyma of a grayish-yellow color, dryish, sometimes sunken, with a well-noticeable whitish interstitial tissue (Fig. 7.6).

The microscopic manifestations of cytomegalovirus infection are due to the cytopathic effect in the form of a typical cytomegalic giant cell metamorphosis of the alveolar and bronchial epithelium, endotheliocytes. In this case, large intranuclear inclusions are defined that are delimited from the nuclear membrane by a pale rim that does not perceive color, the so-called perinuclear halo. Cells with cytomegalic transformation have a characteristic appearance and are called "owl eye" cells (Fig. 7.7).

During IHC and immunocytochemical studies of histological and cytological preparations, cells infected with the CMV are detected. The value of an IHC study in cytomegalovirus infection is the

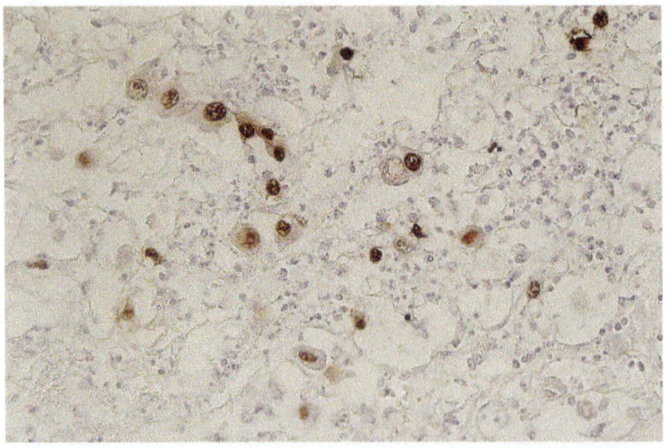

Fig. 7.8 Cytomegalovirus lung damage. Positive immunohistochemical reaction with monoclonal mouse anti-cytomegalovirus. Some of the affected cells are detected before the development of giant cell metamorphosis. ×100

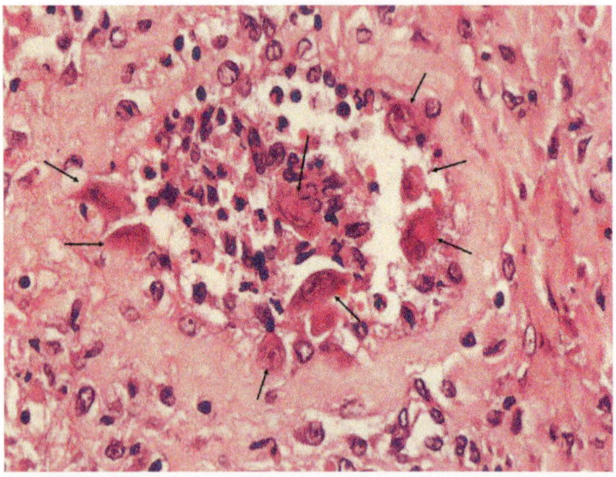

Fig. 7.9 Cytomegalovirus vasculitis–edema and mononuclear infiltration of the vascular wall, cytomegalic transformation of endotheliocytes (indicated by arrows). Stained with hematoxylin and eosin. ×200

possibility of its diagnostics at early stages before the formation of pathognomonic changes of "owl's eye" type, which were not noticeable with overview microscopy (Fig. 7.8).

The lumen of the alveoli contains serous fluid, protein masses, macrophages, a small number of red blood cells, there may be eosinophilic white blood cells. Cellular inflammatory infiltration in the interalveolar septa is usually mild and is represented by small amounts of macrophages, lymphoid, and plasma cells. Squamous metaplasia of the respiratory epithelium of the small bronchi is noted, in the alveoli, the alveolar epithelium can be transformed into cubic.

There are cases with rather pronounced dyscirculatory disorders in interstitial tissue, which are manifested by paretic vasodilation with plethora and stasis of red blood cells, massive hemorrhages in the alveolar septa, and alveolar lumens. The most difficult for morphological diagnosis are cases with severe circulatory disorders in the lung due to cytomegalovirus vasculitis with hemorrhage. The walls of the vessels are thickened due to edema, signs of plasma impregnation, part of the vessels with partial or complete obliteration of the lumen are determined. Endothelial cells with signs of cytomegalic transformation are enlarged, with large nuclei and characteristic perinuclear clearing ("owl eye" cells), with a positive IHC reaction with antibodies to cytomegalovirus (Figs. 7.9 and 7.10). The identification of generalized forms of CMVI in the presence of cytomegalovirus vasculitis, confirmed by IHC, indicates a hematogenous generalization of the process.

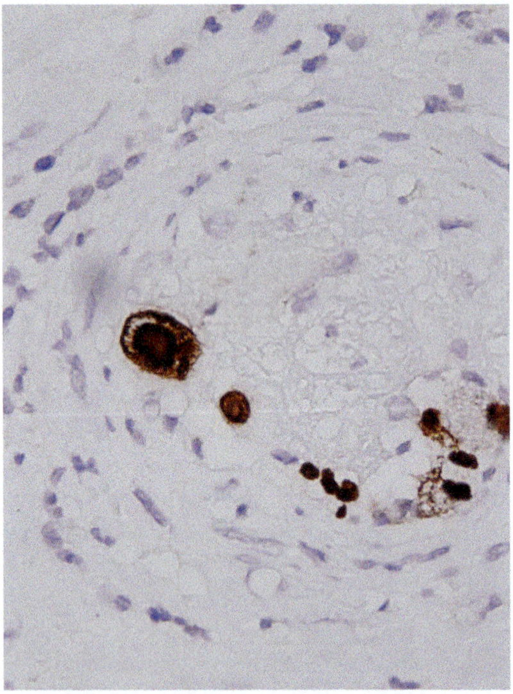

Fig. 7.10 Cytomegalovirus vasculitis, lesions of the endothelial cells. Immunohistochemical reaction with monoclonal mouse anti-cytomegalovirus. ×200

In parallel with cytomegalic metamorphosis, rather early, fibrosis occurs in the interalveolar septa with the cytomegalovirus transformation of the cells of the alveolar epithelium. The morphological picture acquires the features of persistent cytomegalovirus alveolitis with the possible outcome into a “cellular” lung with the development of not only interstitial but also perivascular and peribronchial fibrosis. In the affected areas of the lung, fibrosis of the interalveolar septa with their pronounced deformation is determined. There are areas of pneumosclerosis with diffuse mononuclear infiltration, among the fibers of which there are altered slit-like bronchi and alveoli, sclerosed vessels, micro-islands of the respiratory epithelium with squamous metaplasia.

The fibrotic changes that develop in the outcome of cytomegalovirus pneumonia can be mistaken for post-tuberculous changes, post-pneumonic fibrosis, and the consequences of pneumocystis pneumonia. For cytomegalovirus infection, interstitial fibrosis is more characteristic, in contrast to the focal at the border of the healed foci of caseous necrosis and along the lymphatic vessels typical for tuberculosis.

In some cases, signs of DAD are found in both early and late stages. In cases of pneumosclerosis after cytomegaly, the diagnosis of the late stage of DAD was difficult and only the detection of hyaline membranes in single alveoli allows it to be established. Clinically DAD was not found in any of our observations.

We have not seen any destructive forms with the formation of caverns in cytomegaly. There are publications associating lung decay cavities with CMV infection [18], however, in the presented illustrations, changes typical for tuberculosis, pneumocystosis, and chronic lung abscess in the walls of the cavities were seen. The most likely such cavities developed as a result of a combined pathology, in which CMV was not playing the leading role.

References

1. Jane FS, et al. Human adenoviruses: from villains to vectors. Springer; 2017. p. 416.
2. Ginsberg HS. The adenoviruses. Springer; 2012. p. 605.
3. Zinserling AV. Etiology and pathologic anatomy of acute respiratory infections. L.: Meditsina; 1977. 170 p. (In Russian).
4. Zinserling AV. Peculiarities of lesions in viral and mycoplasma infection of respiratory tract. Virchows Arch A Pathol Pathol Anat. 1973;361:19–30.
5. Zinserling AV, Zinserling VA. Modern infections: pathologic anatomy and issues of pathogenesis: a guide. SPb: Sotis; 2002. 346 p. (In Russian).
6. Lenaerts L, De Clerc E, Naesens L. Clinical features and treatment of adenovirus infections. Rev Med Virol. 2008;18(6):357–74.
7. Davies D, Dungworth D, Mariassy A. Experimental adenovirus infection of lambs. Vet Microbiol. 1981;6(2):113–28.
8. Diefenbach R, Fraefel C. Herpes simplex virus. Springer; 2020. p. 457.
9. Esaki S, Goshima F, Katsumi S, et al. Apoptosis induction after herpes simplex virus infection differs according to cell type in vivo. Arch Virol. 2010;155(8):1235–45. https://doi.org/10.1007/s00705-010-0712-2.
10. Cowdry EV, Nicholson FM. Inclusion bodies in experimental herpetic infection of rabbits. J Exp Med. 1923;37(4):431–56. https://doi.org/10.1084/jem.37.4.431.
11. Ishihara T, Yanagi H, Ozawa H, Takagi A. Severe herpes simplex virus pneumonia in an elderly, immunocompetent patient. BMJ Case Rep. 2018;2018:bcr2017224022. https://doi.org/10.1136/bcr-2017-224022. Published 2018 July 18.
12. Mohan S, Hamid NS, Cunha BA. A cluster of nosocomial herpes simplex virus type 1 pneumonia in a medical intensive care unit. Infect Control Hosp Epidemiol. 2006;27(11):1255–7. https://doi.org/10.1086/508843.
13. Kollias CM, Huneke RB, Wigdahl B, Jennings SR. Animal models of herpes simplex virus immunity and pathogenesis. J Neurovirol. 2015;21(1):8–23. https://doi.org/10.1007/s13365-014-0302.
14. Tsinzerling VA, Popova ED, Baikov VV, et al. Experimental model of generalized herpetic infection in newborns. Arkh Patol. 1993;55(5):28–32. (In Russian).
15. Griffiths P, Baraniak I, Reeves M. The pathogenesis of human cytomegalovirus. J Pathol. 2015;235(2):288–97. https://doi.org/10.1002/path.4437.
16. Halwachs-Baumann, editor. Congenital cytomegalovirus infection. Springer; 2010. p. 350.
17. Kradin RL, editor. Diagnostic pathology of infectious diseases. Elsevier; 2018. 698 p.
18. Parkhomenko YG, Zyuzya YR, Mazus AI Morphological aspects of HIV infection. M.: Literra; 2016. 168 p. (In Russian).

8 Pneumonias. General Aspects

Without dwelling in detail on the discussion of the boundaries of the term "pneumonia," we will, in accordance with modern medical practice, understand by this word the inflammatory process in the respiratory parts of the lungs, characterized by certain radiological symptoms. Thus, usually under this term are understood the lesions of bacterial, mycoplasma, and fungal etiology, frequently with admixture of different viruses. The existence of pure viral pneumonias is disputable. In the previous chapters, we presented results of our studies of respiratory organs lesions due to different viruses, some of them (relative rare) can radiologically be considered as pneumonias as well, but we decided not to include such data in the present chapter.

Pneumonia remains a very common disease, which is both a frequent cause of disability and death. The relevance of this problem is also evidenced by the data of pathological statistics in St. Petersburg, according to which the percentage of unrecognized in lifetime focal and lobar pneumonia among the deceased in hospitals and under the supervision of ambulatory service has been constantly fluctuating for many years within 10–20%. Nowadays increase in mortality due to different forms of pneumonia is noted worldwide [1].

Mortality from acute pneumonia, both primary and secondary, in the pre-antibiotic era was very significant, then after the introduction of a wide range of drugs with antimicrobial activity into medical practice, it significantly decreased. However, in recent years, due to the spread of multiresistant microorganisms, as well as objective and subjective difficulties in diagnosing a disease in socially maladapted individuals, mortality rates are again becoming more alarming.

Despite the crucial importance of this issue, in the world literature of recent decades, there are very few original studies devoted to pathology and clinical and morphological comparisons in pneumonia. The vast majority of textbooks and manuals traditionally quote statements speculatively formed more than a century ago. Thus, we present views upon pneumonia that have developed in the works of V.D. Zinserling (1891–1960) and his numerous collaborators and followers [2–4]. The main evidence of the reliability of these studies, which in many respects, contradicts the generally recognized textbooks, and is their successful verification by medical practice for many decades.

Over the past century, a huge number of different classifications of pneumonia have been proposed, most of which cannot be considered satisfactory due to the lack of strict logical construction, numerous speculative ideas, and incompleteness. Thus, we are proposing our own classification approaches that are logical and based on long-term scientific and practical experience, which, however, do not claim to be ideal.

V. Zinserling, *Infectious Pathology of the Respiratory Tract*,
https://doi.org/10.1007/978-3-030-66325-4_8

1. Etiology
    - Bacterial: pneumococcal, hemophilic, staphylococcal, streptococcal, *Pseudomonas aeruginosa*, klebsiellosis, escherichiosis, chlamydiosis, legionellosis, and others, including those caused by mixed bacterial microflora
    - Mycoplasma
    - Fungal: candidiasis, pneumocystis, aspergillosis, mucorosis, etc.
    - Viral: herpetic, adenoviral, coronavirus and, as an exception, other pathogens
    - Mixed etiology in various combinations, most often viral–bacterial
2. The size of the lesion
    - Lobar
    - Large focal
    - Small focal
    - It is necessary to take into account the frequent simultaneous presence of several foci, possibly of different sizes.
3. According to the topography of the focus with the determination of the localization of the inflammatory process in a certain lobe or segment.
4. By simultaneous involvement in the process of adjacent organs and tissues: pleura, bronchi, bronchioles.
5. By the type of the inflammatory reaction: serous-desquamated, purulent, purulent-necrotic, fibrinous-purulent, as well as with a hemorrhagic component. Proliferative reactions expressed to varying degrees are possible.
6. According to pathogenesis features: aspiration, secondary (e.g., associated with infection with endotracheal anesthesia), on the background of immunodeficiency, in combination with atelectasis and hypostasis.
7. It is also acceptable to divide all pneumonia into community acquired and secondary—hospital acquired, nosocomial. However, it should be noted that in practice, especially in cases of superinfection, such division is difficult and does not have great practical significance.
8. In certain cases, pneumonia is not a separate disease, but one of the manifestations (or specific complications) of certain infections (diphtheria, rickettsiosis, glanders, malaria, typhoid fever, meningococcal infection, etc.). Thus, diphtheria with descending croup can lead to the development of fibrinous pneumonia (Fig. 8.1) [5].

Many types of pneumonia can be determined already macroscopically at the autopsy (Fig. 8.2). However, in some cases, especially in children, the immediate cytological investigation of smears

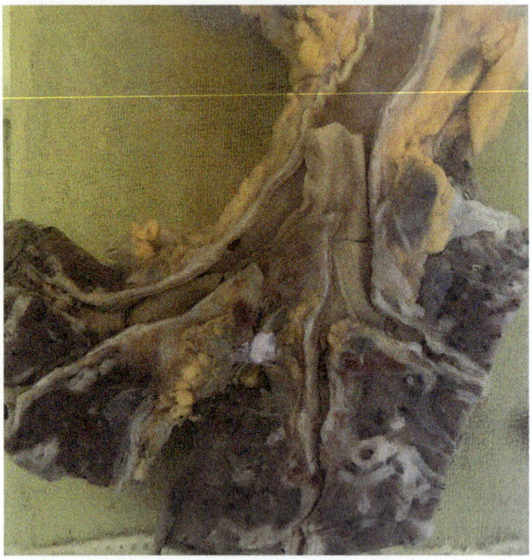

Fig. 8.1 Descendent croup followed by the development of fibrinous pneumonia in an adult deceased from diphtheria in 90th of XX century. Macro-preparation from museum of pathology department of SP Botkin Infectious Hospital, Saint-Petersburg, Russia

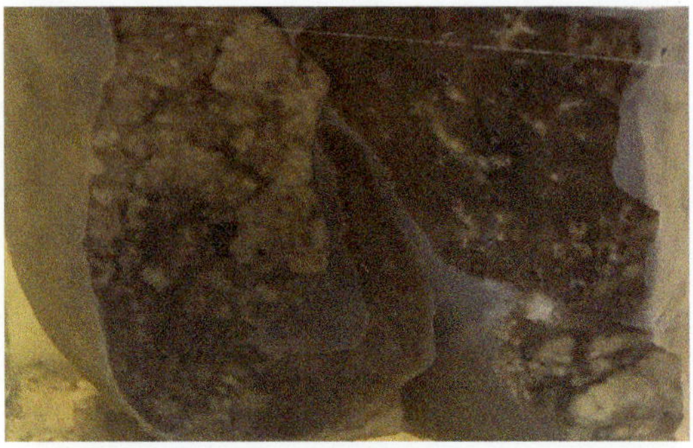

Fig. 8.2 Necrotic pneumonia in a child deceased in 50th of the XX century. Macro-preparation from museum of pathology department of SP Botkin Infectious Hospital, Saint-Petersburg, Russia

from the cut service of the lungs is highly advisable.

Clinical and morphological analysis also allows in many cases with fairly high accuracy to judge the duration of the process, which justifies the judgment of the acute or prolonged course of the disease.

It should be noted that although some researchers started talking about the role of biological pathogens in the etiology of pneumonia in the 19th century (in Russia SP Botkin in 1885) till now they are frequently neglected. This issue is considered to be important only in recent decades due to the appearance on the market of new antibiotics. It is regrettable that the authors of numerous articles and reviews on modern methods of treating pneumonia, discussing their etiology, cite only studies of recent years, often not knowing that they repeated results of V.D. Zinserling and his collaborators with a 50-year delay.

The pathogenesis of different etiologic forms of acute pneumonia is much the same, which allows us to state it in total.

Microorganisms are normally not found in the respiratory parts of the lungs. In the respiratory tract, they are detected relatively often, but there is no obligate microbiota in them. It can be assumed that microorganisms entering the trachea and bronchi are usually destroyed and excreted. Therefore, the flora in them is changing.

The main source of germs entering the respiratory tract is through the oral and nasal cavities. However, microorganisms can appear here as a result of exogenous infection. Numerous studies have shown that microbes penetrate the lungs almost always through the respiratory tract. Initial lesions, as a rule, occur at the level of respiratory bronchioles, which is explained by the sharp expansion of the airway lumen here and the significantly reduced ability to remove microbes due to the lack of ciliary epithelium and less developed muscle tissue.

The most important role in the development of pneumonia is due to the lesions of ciliated epithelium by respiratory viruses. A careful study of the etiology of pneumonias, especially community acquired, shows that viral–bacterial associations can be detected in the vast majority of cases [4].

Of great importance for the occurrence of pneumonia are also violations of the normal functioning of the cleansing mechanisms. This is indicated, first of all, by numerous experimental studies conducted in the middle of the last century [6]. It was shown that such interventions as narrowing or closing the lumen of the bronchi, the introduction of foreign bodies into the lumen of the trachea and bronchi, or various injuries of their mucous membranes, with different frequencies, can lead to the development of pneumonia. There are also observations on clinical material, according to which, in patients with brain damage, respiratory disturbances contribute to aspiration and then the development of pneumonia. The occurrence of pneumonia is also, of course, facilitated by disorders of the innervation of the bronchial tree, for example, transection of the vagus nerve in the experiment. Intra- and antenatal asphyxia also leads to aspiration of amniotic fluid [4].

Estimating the importance of aspiration, of course, one cannot think that the particles themselves that can appear in the lungs (plant, squamous epithelium, dust, meconium bodies, lanugo) cause pneumonia. Pneumonia is caused by germs that enter the respiratory tract along with aspirated particles. The presence of the latter only contributes to the delay of pathogens. Findings in the respiratory organs during microscopic examination of foreign particles are an important indicator of the disorder in protective function and help to understand the pathogenesis of pneumonia.

V.D. Zinserling and his collaborators convincingly proved that the inflammatory process in the lungs cannot develop only on the basis of hemorrhage, edema, or hypostasis. The so-called hypostatic pneumonia does not occur due to vascular disorders, but because in poorly ventilated parts of the lungs, the evacuation function of the bronchi is sharply impaired. In addition, in patients with such changes, the risk of infection with hospital strains of microorganisms is sharply increased.

Often, an important role in the pathogenesis of pneumonia is noted previous pulmonary atelectasis, which serves as a reason for the radiologists and clinicians to identify "atelectatic" pneumonia. This, usually focal, pneumonia is observed mainly in the lower lobes of the lungs, as a rule, in the presence of previous inflammatory changes in the bronchi. In the vast majority of patients, it is more correct to talk about the development of pneumonia not on the background of atelectasis, but in parallel with it because of the same reason—violations of the drainage function of the bronchial tree.

Of particular importance for the topography of inflammatory changes are the structural features of segmental bronchi—the level and angle of their departure from the lobar bronchi, as well as their course, length, and width [7, 8]. So, it is known that the sixth upper basal segmental bronchus departs from the lower lobar bronchus at a right angle higher than the seventh, eighth, ninth, and tenth bronchi, and goes immediately posteriorly; it is relatively long and wide. The functional and anatomical isolation of this bronchus and the worst drainage conditions are especially clearly manifested by the most frequent development in this segment of pneumonia in children of the first months of life. In the case of a similar discharge of adjacent segmental bronchi, the inflammatory process often develops in two segments simultaneously, as is usually the case in 9 and 10, as well as 1 and 2 segments.

The virulence of the pathogen, which is determined by the specific properties of the microorganism and the degree of their expression in a particular strain, is also of great importance.

An extremely important role in the implementation of pneumonia is played by the state of the host. At present, one can speak of the importance of primary and secondary immunodeficiency of various nature as well as various defects of local resistance of the respiratory tract. Thus, at least 24 different genes have been found to result in neutropenia when mutated and these patients have an increased risk of infections including pneumonia [9]. It should be noted that in clinical practice, among the factors that suppress the human defense mechanisms, cooling and intoxication are especially relevant, especially those acting in combination. There are no reliable data in literature or our own long-term experience in favor of the significance in the pathogenesis of pneumonia, including croupous, immunopathological (allergic) factors. In contrast to croupous pneumonia, the pathogenic mechanisms of focal bacterial pneumonia are relatively well understood. We can talk about the possibility of developing community-acquired focal pneumonia, most often caused by pneumococci and hemophilic bacillus, and secondary focal pneumonia, mainly caused by a variety of nosocomial microbiota. The basis of their pathogenesis is a violation of the protective functions of the respiratory system of various kinds, which contributes to the free penetration of microbiota into the lower parts of the respiratory tract and ensures the onset of the disease. Such situation is typical for postoperative period, with prolonged mechanical ventilation and in patients with acute cerebral vascular disorders. These are the so-called pathogenetic determined pneumonia, uncharacteristic in morphology, caused, as a rule, by a low-virulent and often mixed microbiota. Unlike croupous pneumonia, they are characterized by a primary lesion of the bronchi with a further spread of the process along the airways, that is, the primary lesion develops in the acinus. They have no specificity in morphological manifestations, and clinically, as a rule, they are not accompanied by collapse, however, developing in severe and weakened patients are often the cause of death.

In some cases, hospital pneumonia can also be caused by highly virulent strains of pathogens. In these cases, we can talk about pneumonia with a morphological feature typical for Staphylococcus, *Pseudomonas aeruginosa*, and Klebsiella.

The youngest children and older adults have a much higher frequency of pneumonia than do older children and young adults. The mechanisms of this phenomenon are becoming elucidated [10].

In modern literature, it has been demonstrated that pneumonia of different bacterial etiology is characterized by different influences upon the mechanisms of programmed cell death [11]. The biological mechanisms responsible for making some individuals more susceptible to pneumonia need to be better defined. Variations in the inflammatory response are a major component of interindividual variability in pneumonia risk [12].

Many issues of the etiology, pathogenesis, clinic, and pathology of pneumonia need further comprehensive study.

References

1. Torres A, Chalmers JD, Dela Cruz CS, et al. Challenges in severe community-acquired pneumonia: a point-of-view review. Intensive Care Med. 2019;45(2):159–71. https://doi.org/10.1007/s00134-019-05519-y.
2. Zinserling VD. Several questions of pathogenesis of croupous pneumonia in the light of new morphological investigations. Clin Med. 1939;9–10:3–12. (In Russian).
3. Zinserling VD, Zinserling AV. Pathological anatomy of acute pneumonia of different etiology. Gos Izd Med Lit. Leningrad; 1963. 175 p. (In Russian).
4. Zinserling AV, Zinserling VA. Modern infections: pathologic anatomy and issues of pathogenesis: a guide. SPb: Sotis; 2002. 346 p. (In Russian).
5. Zinserling AV, Kadyrova SN, Zinserling VA. Lesions of respiratory organs in diphtheria in adults. Pulmonologia. (1):71–75. (In Russian).
6. Anichkov NN, Zakharyevskaya MA. Experimental studies on autogenic infectious processes in lungs. Vest Khir. 1954;113(5):19–25. (In Russian).
7. Minnich DJ, Mathisen DJ. Anatomy of the trachea, carina, and bronchi. Thorac Surg Clin. 2007;17:571–85.
8. Leslie KO, Wick MR, editor. Practical pulmonary pathology. A diagnostic approach. 2nd ed. 2011. 828 p.
9. Donadieu J, Beaupain B, Fenneteau O, Bellanne-Chantelot C. Congenital neutropenia in the era of genomics: classification, diagnosis, and natural history. Br J Haematol. 2017;179(4):557–74.
10. Quinton LJ, Walkey AJ, Mizgerd JP. Integrative physiology of pneumonia. Physiol Rev. 2018;98(3):1417–64. https://doi.org/10.1152/physrev.00032.2017.
11. FitzGerald ES, Luz NF, Jamieson AM. Competitive cell death interactions in pulmonary infection: host modulation versus pathogen manipulation. Front Immunol. 2020;11:814. https://doi.org/10.3389/fimmu.20.00814.
12. Mizgerd JP. Inflammation and pneumonia: why are some more susceptible than others. Clin Chest Med. 2018;39(4):669–76. https://doi.org/10.1016/j/ccm.2018.07.002.

9 Atypical Pneumonias Due to Chlamydia and Mycoplasma

9.1 Respiratory Chlamydiosis

Chlamydia is a large family of Chlamydiaceae, capable of causing, on the one hand, various, often chronic, lesions of almost all organs and tissues in numerous animals and plants, and on the other hand, initiating autoimmune lesions. The in vitro cycle of their development includes extracellular (reticular) and intracellular (initial) particles [1]. Currently, it has been shown that under adverse conditions for the pathogen (e.g., antibiotic therapy), the formation of intracellular persistent forms occurs. Recently it has been demonstrated that Chlamydia interacts with different cells of innate immunity, toll-like receptors, different pattern recognition receptors, interferon signaling, inflammatory responses, factors regulating apoptosis, macrophages, dendritic cells, masts cells, eosinophils, and neutrophils [2]. It is postulated that so quite different variants of chlamydia infection can be explained by them. This question has not been studied enough.

Respiratory chlamydia is usually subdivided into ornithosis/psittacosis (parrot disease) caused by *Chlamydia psittaci* and the disease proceeding by manifestations associated with *Chlamydia pneumoniae*.

Information about the frequency of respiratory chlamydia in humans is very controversial. Some authors give them up to 20% of all etiological forms of pneumonia, while others do not even mention respiratory chlamydiosis. At the same time, there is a very extensive literature on chlamydia of various localizations, including those with damage to the respiratory system, in a wide variety of animals.

Clinical symptoms can vary from extremely severe, life-threatening, then mild with a primary lesion of the upper respiratory tract. As the most characteristic symptom, a prolonged cough is indicated. According to some reports, respiratory chlamydiosis is identical to interstitial pertussis-like eosinophilic pneumonia [3].

Structural changes in the respiratory system in humans are described as very incompletely. The possibility of both focal and lobar lesions is indicated. Microscopic examination noted serous-fibrinous exudate with an admixture of monocytes, macrophages, and desquamated alveolocytes (Figs. 9.1 and 9.2). In cells, elementary and extracellular (rarely) larger reticular bodies can be determined.

Here are the changes typical for respiratory chlamydia in a man who died in the outcome of the disease "swine flu."

A 31-year-old male patient I.V. with obesity got ill acutely, with fever up to 39 °C. Three days later, he was hospitalized to the intensive care unit with severe respiratory insufficiency. Intubation and, later on, tracheostomy were performed. The clinical diagnosis of "swine influenza" was supported by RT PCR and serology (increase of antibody level 0–640). In spite of

V. Zinserling, *Infectious Pathology of the Respiratory Tract*,
https://doi.org/10.1007/978-3-030-66325-4_9

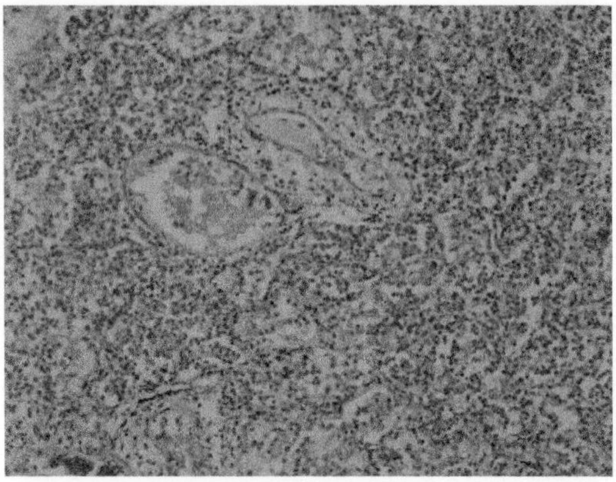

Fig. 9.1 General view of lung in a child deceased from respiratory chlamydiosis. H.-E. ×100

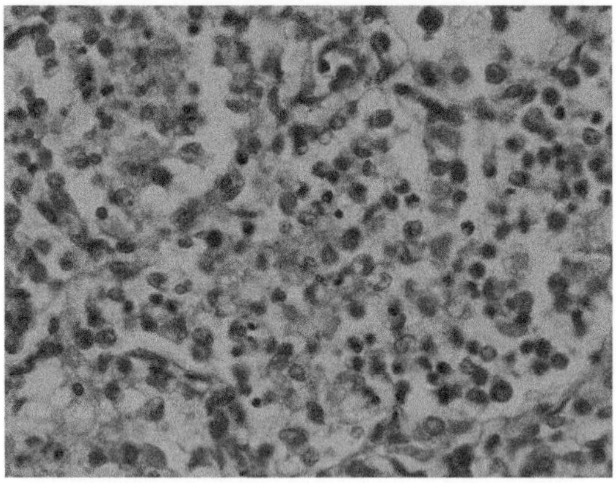

Fig. 9.2 Detail of a previous slice. Note macrophages with vacuolated cytoplasm. ×400

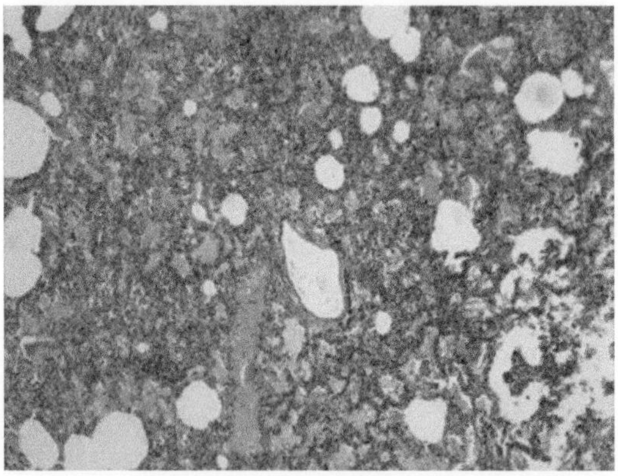

Fig. 9.3 General view of lung of an adult with the activation of respiratory chlamydiosis in a late stage of influenza. H.-E. ×100

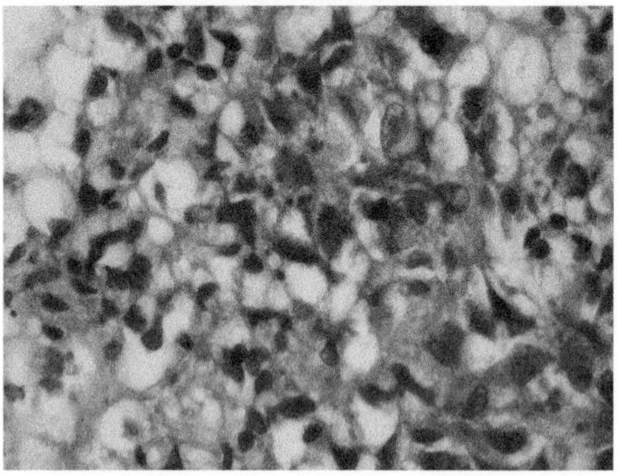

Fig. 9.4 Detail of a previous slice. Note macrophages with vacuolated cytoplasm. ×400

intensive treatment including antibiotics and antiviral drugs, patient died on the 35th day of the illness.

Macroscopic changes. At the autopsy, remarkable changes were found only in the lungs: necrotic post-tracheostomic tracheitis, large abscesses in the lower lobes of the lungs in the stage of organization, bilateral fibrinous pleuritis. The rest of the lung tissue was dark red, firm.

Microscopic changes. During the histological examination in the lungs, changes typical for rather old abscesses, late stages of respiratory distress syndrome were noted (Fig. 9.3). The changes that we consider to be typical for influenza (virus-induced transformation of epithelial cells) were expressed only in the moderate number of the cells. We notified numerous intra-alveolar macrophages, partly with vacuolated cytoplasm (Fig. 9.4), and PAS-positive inclusions. Some cells had slightly enlarged hyperchromic nuclei. Similar changes were noted in other organs as well.

Postmortem laboratory investigation. Postmortem RT-PCR of lung and spleen specimens for influenza A/H1N1sw was negative. During the bacteriological investigation of lung specimens cultures of *Escherichia coli*, non-pathogenic *Corynebacteria*, *Enterococcus*, *Streptococcus Viridans,* and *Staphylococcus epidermidis* were isolated.

Immunohistochemical investigation. In the lungs, strong positive reaction with serum against *Chlamydia spp.* (Fig. 9.5), moderate against

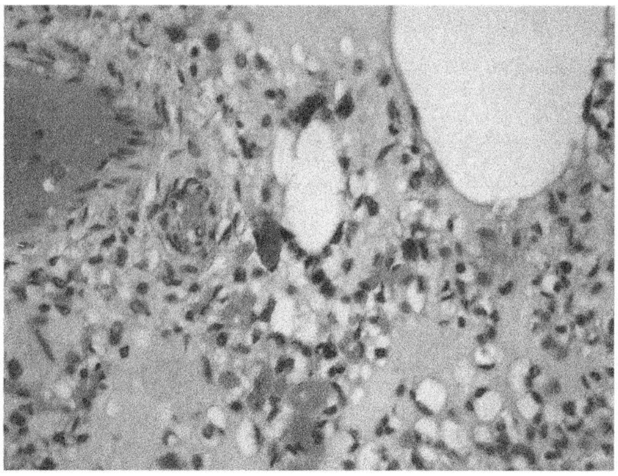

Fig. 9.5 Antigen of *Chlamydia trachomatis* in lungs of the same case. IHC ×200

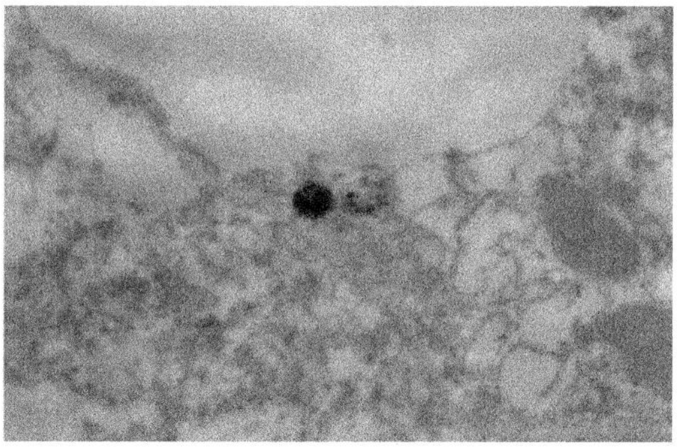

Fig. 9.6 Elementary and reticular bodies in the lung of the same patient. EM. ×20,000

Adenovirus and weak against influenza H1N1 were obtained. The reactions with sera against HSV1/2, CMV, EBV, RS, entero-, and parvoviruses, as well as *Mycoplasma pneumoniae* were negative.

Electron microscopy was performed as follows. Samples were fixated in glutaraldehyde 4 h after death then treated with osmium oxide; uranyl acetate was used for contrast enhancement. Dehydration and embedding were performed using conventional techniques. Sections were analyzed on electron microscope JEM-100S.

During the electron microscopic investigation of lungs, we succeeded to evaluate numerous elementary and reticular bodies of *Chlamydia* (Fig. 9.6), in brain only reticular bodies, predominantly in cytoplasm of endothelial cells. In their nuclei, several PML–nuclear bodies (small intranucleolar inclusions containing promyelocytic leukemia protein) were found (Fig. 9.7).

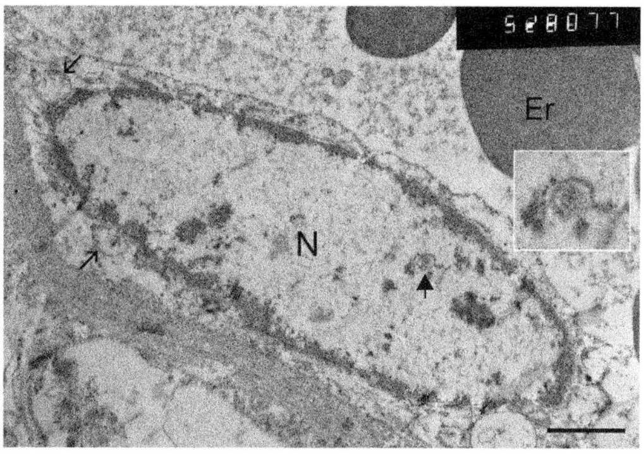

Fig. 9.7 Reticular body (on thin arrows) and PLM particle (thick arrow and insertion) in endothelial cell of the brain vessel in the same case. EM ×30,000

Conclusion. Death of a young healthy man occurred on the 35th day of illness clinically regarded as influenza with bacterial superinfection. The results of postmortem morphological and laboratory investigation proved that clinically diagnosed infections were expressed rather weakly, but provoked the activation and severe course of respiratory chlamydiosis (with probable generalization) and adenoviral infection.

9.2 Respiratory Mycoplasmosis

9.2.1 Microbiology

The causative agent of human respiratory mycoplasmosis is *M. pneumoniae*. The modern term appeared in 1962 when R. Channock, L. Hayflick first isolated the pure culture of Agent Eaton on a cell-free environment and, after a detailed study of it, established mycoplasma affiliation [4].

The frequency of respiratory mycoplasmosis in the structure of acute respiratory infections and pneumonia, according to various authors, varies quite significantly in different periods of time and age groups, but the figure of 20% of all pneumonia is quite realistic. According to long-term data, respiratory mycoplasmosis takes 4–6 places among the causative agents of acute respiratory infections [5]. It is worth recalling that for

ARI and pneumonia account for 50–60% of the total morbidity of the working population.

M. pneumonia cultivated on amino acid-rich media (these are tryptic digests of the beef hearts, etc.), as well as in various cell cultures and chicken embryos. *M. pneumonia* on dense media grows in the form of spherical granular colonies without peripheral zones, less often in the form of two-phase colonies of 10–100 μm in size, which are clearly visible with an increase of 20–60 times. Typical colonies look like fried eggs—with a dense center and a transparent narrow periphery. *M. pneumonia* ferments carbohydrates: glucose, xylose, maltose, mannose, starch, etc. *M. pneumonia* is movable. This differs from other types of mycoplasmas in its ability to adsorb on the surface of red blood cells, to produce hemolysin, which is hydrogen peroxide. *M. pneumonia* sensitive to pH, the optimum for its growth is 6.5–7.5, a change in pH leads to the death of the pathogen. *M. pneumonia* is very sensitive to moisture, and therefore they are grown in desiccators with water [6].

Among the properties of *M. pneumonia*, tropism to the basal membrane of the cells of the ciliated epithelium lining the airways, as well as some other cells of the internal organs and the brain, is important. Avirulent strains lose their ability to hemadsorption and adsorption on the surface of epithelial cells, while their complementary adhesin—protein P1—remains. Probably, the virulence of the strains is largely due to the genetically determined antigenic characteristics of the P1 protein. Recently other adhesins (P30, HMW) were detected [7]. Gene *M. pneumoniae* almost completely studied and mapped. The binding of certain sequences in the genome of *M. pneumonia* is shown. Antigenic structure of *M. pneumonia* is more studied and more stable than other mycoplasmas. There are two groups of antigens—membrane and intracellular.

Membrane glycolipid antigen is related to similar antigens in the lung, liver, and brain tissue, which creates the prerequisites for the cross reaction of antibodies.

The glycoprotein fraction stimulates antibody production and is considered as the most important criteria characterizing pathogenicity of the strain M. pneumonia (in vitro assessment) on cell cultures [7].

1. The presence of adhesive properties
2. The ability to cause the cytopathogenic changes
3. The ability to multiply and persist in cells

Respiratory mycoplasmosis is registered everywhere, more often in countries with a temperate climate. People of any age are ill, but most often the disease is described in children aged 5–15, especially when forming groups in school and kindergarten. Very high morbidity (up to 45%) in closed military collectives is also very characteristic. With an interval of 4–8 years, epidemic outbreaks are recorded. The peak incidence is observed in late summer and the first autumn months. The main transmission is airborne. The source of infection is humans.

In the development of the disease, the individual properties of the pathogen play an important role. It is believed that hemolysin of *M. pneumonia* contributes to the development of DIC syndrome in patients, which in the most severe course can be manifested by skin hemorrhages, as well as focal hemorrhages in the lung tissue and pleura. The fundamental ability of mycoplasmas to cross over the blood–brain barrier has been proved [8].

9.2.2 Clinical Picture

The incubation period is 1–12 days. Among the first clinical manifestations, pharyngitis and tracheobronchitis occurring at normal or subfebrile temperature are described [5]. In addition, much less often the disease can manifest in the form of conjunctivitis, eustachitis, and otitis media. Pneumonia often develops gradually; the leading clinical symptom is a dry cough. In most cases, the so-called atypical course of pneumonia is noted, which patients often carry on their feet. However, the literature describes a fairly wide range of severe complications etiologically associated with *M. pneumonia*—meningitis and meningoencephalitis, myocarditis, arthritis. With generalized forms, especially in children, deaths are described [9].

Relation of *M. pneumonia* to antibiotics is determined by their lack of a cell wall. Naturally, they are resistant to all drugs that inhibit biosynthetic processes in the cell wall and are sensitive to drugs that affect intracellular processes. *M. pnweumonia* is sensitive to such drugs as to the action of tetracycline's, macrolides, aminoglycosides. However, to date, cases of *M. pneumonia* resistance have been described. It is important that it was not possible to prove the ability of the strains to inherit it.

Other types of mycoplasmas can also inhabit the human respiratory tract. Their role in respiratory pathology is not entirely clear. So, many researchers detected in the respiratory tract *Mycoplasma hominis* (in 1–3% in healthy individuals and 8% in patients with chronic acute respiratory infections), cases of its isolation in acute pharyngitis, pneumonia, and pleural fluid have been described [9]. There are a large number of publications on mixed infections of *M. pneum.* + *M. hominis* + a variety of respiratory viruses. A number of researchers point to the necessity of study to the role of *M. orale* and *M. salivarium* [6]. However, there are no data allowing to exactly determine their importance in human pathology.

9.2.3 Laboratory Diagnostics

The diagnosis of respiratory mycoplasmosis can be made on the basis of:

1. Isolation of the pathogen
2. PCR
3. Fourfold increase in antibody titers in the dynamics of the disease.

Bacteriological culture material: swabs from the pharynx, sputum (better morning portion), pleural fluid, fluid in bronchioalveolar lavage, biopsy specimens of the bronchi, lung tissue (surgical or autopsy material), other fluids (e.g., CSF), and tissues in cases of suspected generalization of infection. In practice, the most commonly examined are the swabs from the back of the throat.

9.2.3.1 Serological Methods

These methods are usually used in the study of paired sera.

1. CBR (complement binding reaction) is characterized by 100% sensitivity. A number of companies produce glycolipid diagnostic for *M. pneumonia*. Maximum titers are observed in 90% of patients starting from the 14th day from the onset of the disease and persist for 3–7 weeks; the antibodies completely disappear by the 12th month. If there is only one sample, then the diagnostic titer is considered to be 1:64 and higher. In paired sera, the diagnostic criterion is a fourfold increase in titer.
2. ELISA Enzyme-linked immunosorbent assay systems for the differentiated determination of IgG and IgM to *M. pneumonia* antigens have only limited use.
3. PCR diagnostics allows identification of *M. pneumonia* nucleotide sequences of the genome in blood, sputum, swabs from the nasopharynx, lavage fluid, and other materials.

In conclusion, it can be noted that the diagnosis of respiratory mycoplasmosis in routine practice is advisable to carry out by serological methods: RBC and ELISA. The cultural method is very laborious, and the frequency of positive results is very low. The use of immunofluorescence diagnostics, along with the well-known subjectivity of the method and the possibility of cross-reactions, is also limited by the absence of certified commercial diagnostic sera.

9.2.4 Pathology

In the world literature, the pathology of human respiratory mycoplasmosis is not described, with the exception of a number of studies conducted in past decades in Russia on pediatric autopsy material [9].

The respiratory tract of children with respiratory mycoplasmosis usually seems almost unchanged. It is possible to note only moderate focal hyperemia of the mucous membrane of the trachea and large bronchi. In the lumen of the respiratory tract is a little relatively viscous grayish, less often bloody mucus. The lungs with respiratory mycoplasmosis, which was not combined with other infections or other lesions, are moderately firm, mainly in the posterior sections, on a cut of a dark red color with a bluish edema. When pressed, a little bloody liquid-containing gas bubbles flow from the cut surface. It should also be noted that typical arer also numerous small hemorrhages both in the respiratory organs and outside them, which can be explained by the action of β-hemolysin, secreted by *M. pneumonia* and its hemagglutinating properties. It seems impossible to describe macroscopic changes in adults since they are always combined with other pathology.

In the respiratory tract, especially in children, changes are noted primarily at the mucosal epithelium, where pronounced alterative changes are observed, leading to desquamation of individual cells of the ciliated epithelium or even its entire layers. Mycoplasmas are found in the cytoplasm of such epithelial cells, which, under light microscopy, look like very small bodies stained with azure, thionine, orcein, and by PAS reaction. Around the agent, focal enlightenments of the cytoplasm or, less commonly, the nucleus are detected. Affected cells can be slightly enlarged, as if swollen. Such changes are best seen not in sections, but in smears. It should be noted that, unlike viral infections, in mycoplasmosis fuchsinophilic inclusions are absent. Along with changes in cells in the respiratory tract, there is a marked swelling of the submucosa and its slight lymphohistiocytic infiltration and plethora of the entire wall. The lumen of the respiratory tract, especially its lower sections, along with desquamated epithelium contains a little serous fluid, macrophages, as well as granular leukocytes and erythrocytes (Figs. 9.8 and 9.9). Among the exudate, one can also find, usually in small quantities, mycoplasmas lying freely and located in the cytoplasm of cells. In the respiratory parts of the

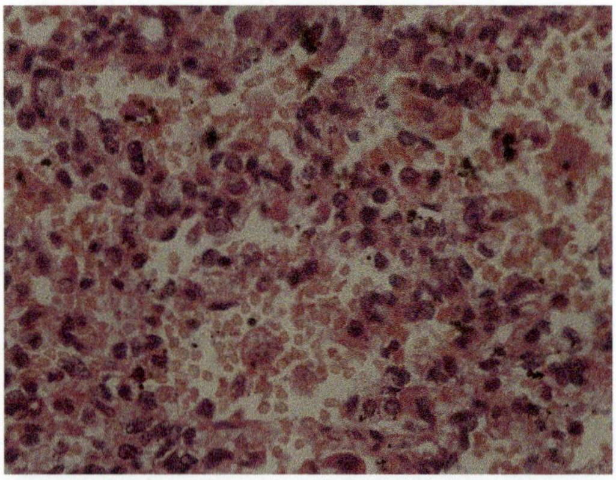

Fig. 9.8 Lung of a child with respiratory mycoplasmosis. Note macrophages with vacuolated cytoplasm. H.-E. ×400

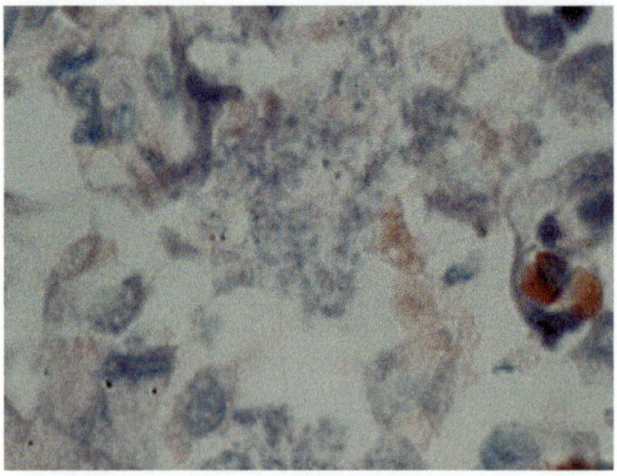

Fig. 9.9 Similar case. Note azure-positive inclusions in vacuolated cytoplasm. Stained by azure–eosin ×400

lungs in many areas, a peculiar change of alveolocytes attracts attention. In the cytoplasm of such cells, and sometimes in their nuclei, mycoplasmas are found in the form of single small bodies or their groups. They, as in the ciliated epithelium, are surrounded at the beginning by indefinite, then very clearly defined enlightenments. Such cells are significantly increased in size. At earlier stages of the process, they retain a connection with the wall, later they are desquamated and lysed. At this stage, the agent is not detected in them, and the cytoplasm and nucleus acquire a foamy appearance. Fuchsinophilic inclusions in the cytoplasm are not available. Alveolar lumens, along with the changes described above, contain serous fluid and usually numerous red blood cells, as well as macrophages and single granular leukocytes. Some children also have hyaline membranes. The volume of many alveoli in areas with acute inflammatory changes is reduced, which, apparently, is associated with a violation of the formation of surfactant by the affected alveolocytes. In areas with changes that are older in time of development, moderate fibrosis of the interalveolar septa and focal peribronchial and perivascular infiltrates are detected. They consist mainly of lymphocytes, to which histiocytes, plasmocytes, and single eosinophilic leukocytes can be added. Development of plethora of vessels of various calibers, especially small ones, is possible, there are small hemorrhages. The walls of the blood vessels of the lungs are often swollen, mycoplasmas are found in some endothelium cells. Separate vessels contain small fibrin thrombi, weakly connected to their wall.

Often, respiratory mycoplasmosis was combined with other viral and bacterial respiratory infections.

In children, it was often possible to identify signs of generalization of respiratory mycoplasmosis with the development of typical lesions in the kidneys, liver, intestines, central nervous system, and lymph nodes [9].

9.2.5 Experimental Models

Experimental studies with *M. pneumoniae* began in 1944 with the work of M.D. Eaton. The literature provides numerous data on the results of modeling respiratory mycoplasmosis using various animal species and mycoplasmas. These works were carried out most intensively in the 1960–1970s of the 20th century and were summarized in the most complete form by I.G. Shroyt et al. [9]. The most commonly used model was the challenge of Syrian hamsters with *M. pneumoniae*. In these works, almost exclusive attention was paid to changes in the respiratory system.

In subsequent years, experimental work on experimental respiratory mycoplasmosis was carried out only to a very limited extent. Thus, we present the results of our experimental work (V.A. Zinserling, 1980), which had never before been published in the press.

A study was conducted on 163 Syrian hamsters at the age of 3 weeks infected with *M. pneumoniae* (strain N13) in four series of experiments.

In the first series of experiments, 45 intact animals were used, which were challenged intranasal with 0.1 suspension of mycoplasmas at a concentration of 108 CFU/mL. Animals were sacrificed on days 1, 3, 5, 10, 15, 20, 25 after infection. Specimens from all major organs were taken for a detailed histological examination using HE, azure-eosin, PAS reaction and thionine according Nissl on paraffin sections prepared according standard methods. IF studies on cryostat sections were provided as well. In parallel to other, but simultaneously infected animals, a microbiologist using a special nutrient medium isolated quantitatively mycoplasmas from the lungs on the 5th, 10th, 15th, and 20th days, and detected neutralizing antibodies in the blood of animals on the 5th, 10th, 15th, 20th, and 25th days. As control, we used both intact animals and hamsters to which the growing medium mycoplasmas were introduced intranasally.

In these series of experiments, it was possible to reproduce a generalized mycoplasma infection and to follow up its development. After an early, probably hematogenous dissemination in the body, which was histobacterioscopically recorded already for the first day, later occurred lesions of various internal organs. The morphological picture observed in the lungs (Fig. 9.10), kidneys, and liver was similar to that described with human mycoplasmosis. The results of a microbiological study of the lungs of infected animals showed that the intensity of reproduction of mycoplasmas increased with each day of infection, reaching a maximum at 15th days, which correlated with the most severe lesions in the lungs. The results of serological studies were consistent with microbiological data. The increase in the level of neutralizing antibodies following the number of mycoplasmas in the lungs of infected animals. The maximum level of neutralizing antibodies (1:16) was determined on

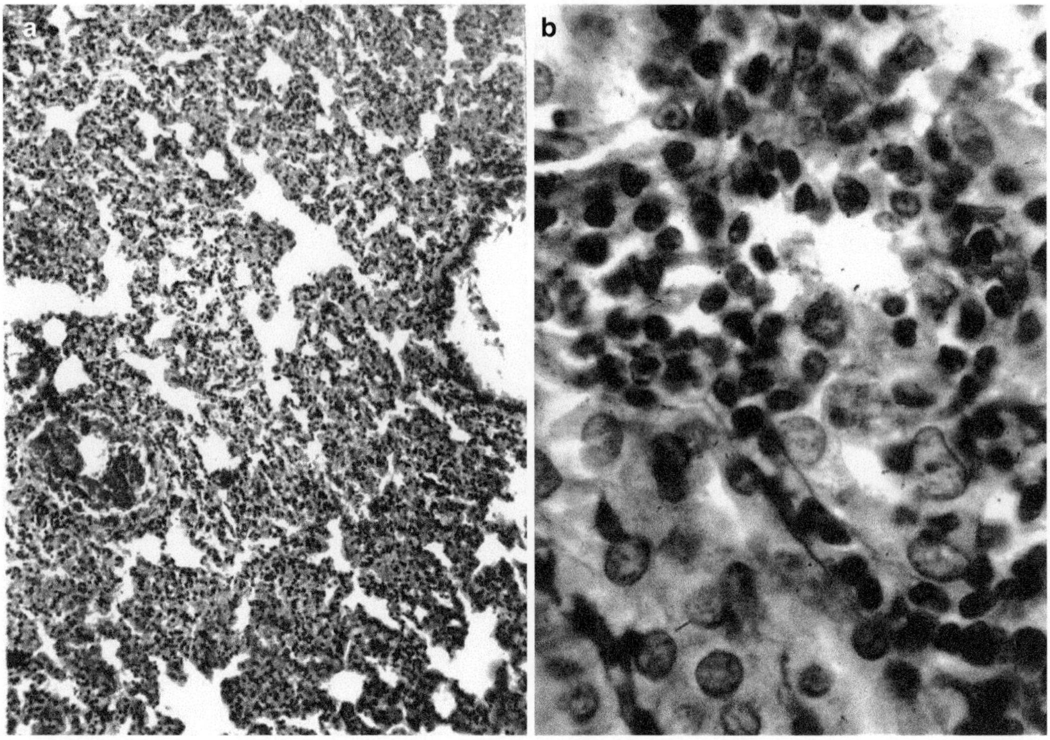

Fig. 9.10 Pneumonia in a Syrian hamster on the third day after intranasal challenge with high virulent strain of *Mycoplasma pneumoniae*. H.-E. (**a**) General view ×100. (**b**) Macrophages with vacuolated cytoplasm in the lung of the same animal ×400

the 20th day of infection and remained during the subsequent development of the pathological process.

In the second series of experiment 35 animals have undergone radiobiological and IF study. The culture of *M. pneumoniae* strain N13 was grown on standard nutrient medium supplemented with 2 μg/ml H3 thymidine. The first group of animals was infected intranasal at the same dose as in the first series of experiments. In the second group, animals were challenged by inactivated pathogen. In group 3, live culture at the same dose was administered intraperitoneal. Animals were examined at 1, 3, 7, 14 days after infection. For radiological research, the lower lobe of the right lung, the cerebral cortex of one of the hemispheres, and the hypothalamic region with the medulla oblongata were taken. A hydrolysate was prepared from tissue specimens according to standard methods, to which scintillation fluid was added and pulse counting was performed on a MARK-II counter. To obtain reliable results, the counter readings were correlated with 1/10 of the organ sample. The results were subjected to statistical processing (Table 9.1). The control was organs of uninfected animals. In parallel, histological and IF studies were performed.

The results of a comprehensive study of materials from animals of the first subgroup demonstrate a clear multiplication of mycoplasmas in the lungs. However, unlike other series of experiments, a large number of pathogens were not located intracellularly, but lay freely or were adsorbed on the surface of bronchial or alveolocytes (Fig. 9.11). In most animals, pronounced structural changes associated with exposure to mycoplasmas were absent, only on the 14th day in a number of animals a moderate histiocytic infiltration and thrombosis of small vessels were noted. Radiobiological, IF, and histological studies proved the ability of mycoplasmas in this

Table 9.1 Results of radiobiologic investigation of Syrian hamsters (in impulses)

Group	Object of investigation	Days of experiment			
		1	3	7	14
Intranasal challenge with viable pathogen	Lungs	117.3 ± 37	20.1 ± 4.0	59.8 ± 6.6	47.8 ± 1.9
	Big hemispheres of brain	9.0 ± 2.0	2.5 ± 0.3	19.0 ± 7.0	14.2 ± 2.4
Intranasal challenge with inactivated pathogen	Lungs	23.2 ± 3.1	9.4 ± 1.1	5.0 ± 0.8	3.9 ± 0.8
	Big hemispheres of brain	3.5 ± 0.6	1.8 ± 0.3	2.7 ± 0.5	3.0 ± 0.2
Intraperitoneal challenge with viable pathogen	Lungs	4.4 ± 0.4	10.5 ± 3.5	36.5 ± 6.8	66.3 ± 17.0
	Big hemispheres of brain	3.1 ± 0.9	7.5 ± 0.9	18.4 ± 8.0	29.5 ± 4.0
Control animals	Lungs	4.1 ± 0.4			
	Big hemispheres of brain	2.6 ± 0.4			

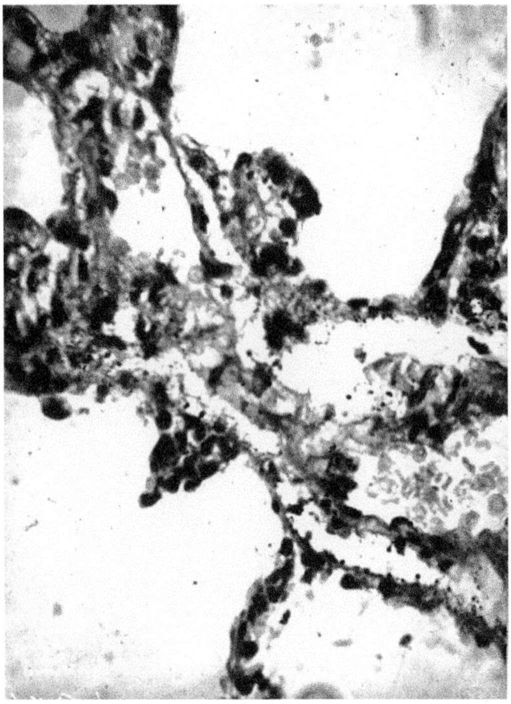

Fig. 9.11 Mycoplasma on the surface bronchial cells in lung of a Syrian hamster on the third day after intranasal challenge with non-virulent strain of *Mycoplasma pneumoniae*. PAS ×400

experiment to hematogenous dissemination to the brain, where they were located mainly on the surface and, rarely, in the cytoplasm of the vascular plexus ependymocytes, as well as extracellularly in perivascular spaces.

The results of the study of the second group indicate that inactivated mycoplasmas do not penetrate in the animal's body beyond the lumen of the bronchi and lose their ability to adsorb on the surface of cells. The absence of mycoplasmas in the brain confirms that with intranasal infection, hematogenous dissemination of only a viable pathogen is possible. The results of a comprehensive study of materials from animals of the third group indicate a significantly pronounced hematogenous dissemination of the pathogen during its intraperitoneal administration. It can be assumed that the transfer of mycoplasmas contributes to their ability to adsorb on blood cells. Marked penetration of the pathogen into the lungs and brain occurred, starting from 3 days after infection, and reached a maximum of 14 days.

In the third series of experiments, infection of 43 animals was carried out, as in the first series of experiments, but the strain passed additional passages and lyophilization. Animals were euthanized on 3, 6, 9, 12, 15, 18, 21, 24, 27, and 30 days after infection. Histologically and microbiologically (6 and 12 s), the lungs and brain were examined.

The data obtained in the third series of experiments showed that the *M. pneumoniae* strain used for infection underwent significant changes in its properties during its one-and-a-half-year storage. It was not possible to give a clear microbiological explanation for this phenomenon. In this series of experiment during morphological and microbiological studies, it was shown that the pathogen as a result of intranasal infection in a significant amount was in the lungs, where it multiplied and, despite partial elimination, continued to be seen till the end of observation (30 days). The localization of the pathogen was fundamentally different from that described in the first series of experiments. In the present study, almost exclusively the extracellular location of the pathogen was noted, mainly around the bronchi, blood vessels, as well as in the lumens of the alveoli. Intracellular mycoplasmas were determined only in a small amount on 12–15 days after infection, when they were observed in the cytoplasm of macrophages located in the zone of moderate macrophage–histiocytic infiltration. On the 15th day after infection, signs of intravascular hemolysis, swelling of endotheliocytes, and increased permeability of the vascular wall and hemorrhage into the lumen of the alveoli were also noted. The almost complete absence of brain damage, both according to morphological and microbiological data, suggests that the culture of the strain used in this study, along with the ability to penetrate into cells and cause pronounced inflammatory changes in the lungs, also lost the ability to penetrate into blood vessels and other organs, in particular to the brain, and cause a generalized infection.

In the fourth series of experiments, delivered simultaneously with a similar technique, the animals before infection were once (for 3 weeks) or twice (for 4 and 3 weeks) intramuscularly vaccinated with an inactivated by ultrasound culture. Forty animals of this series of experiments were investigated on the 5th, 10th, 15th, 20th, and 25th day after infection using histological, morphometric, microbiological, and serological methods.

In this series of experiments, it was shown that although vaccination initially inhibits the reproduction of pathogens, later they nevertheless undergo a fairly significant reproduction, along with which there was an increase in the area of airless foci in the lung. At the same time, an increase in the area of perivascular lymphoplasmacytic infiltrates and the average thickness of the vascular wall, which can be considered as indirect signs of the development of immunopathological processes, is noted.

Beginning at 10th day moderate, and from 15 days, distinct morphological signs of a generalization of the process with damage to the kidneys, liver, and brain were revealed, the nature of the changes in which corresponded in principle with those described in the first series of experiments. Signs of fibrinoid swelling were revealed in the walls of the vessels of all organs.

The data obtained in this experiment indicate that the course of respiratory mycoplasmosis, including generalization with brain damage, depends not only on the severity of the inflammatory process and the level of specific antibodies. Immunopathological reactions are also of great importance, among the morphological manifestations of which we were able to evaluate peribronchial and peribronchial infiltrates from lymphoid cells, which literature data allow us to associate with T-cell cytotoxicity. It should be noted that changes of this kind are considered characteristic of mycoplasmosis, for which the intracellular location of the pathogen is characteristic. Intracellular localization of Mycoplasma was confirmed by EM as well (Fig. 9.12).

Thus, in our experimental studies, using various methods the ability of mycoplasmas to cause severe lesions of lungs and other organs was proved. The dissemination of pathogens occurs only when used cultures are able to adsorb on the surface of the cells. The penetration properties of mycoplasmas are clearly related to their ability to cause pronounced structural changes in both the lungs and other internal organs, including the brain. The development of extrapulmonary lesions is delayed in the presence of antibodies in animals, but they do not protect hamsters from the enhancement of the process after reducing their titer. The sensitization of animals after their unsuccessful vaccination leads to the development of immunopathological processes in the lungs, probably of the type of delayed-type hypersensitivity and pathological immune complexes leading to fibrinoid swelling of the vascular wall and impaired permeability, which contributes to the late generalization of the process.

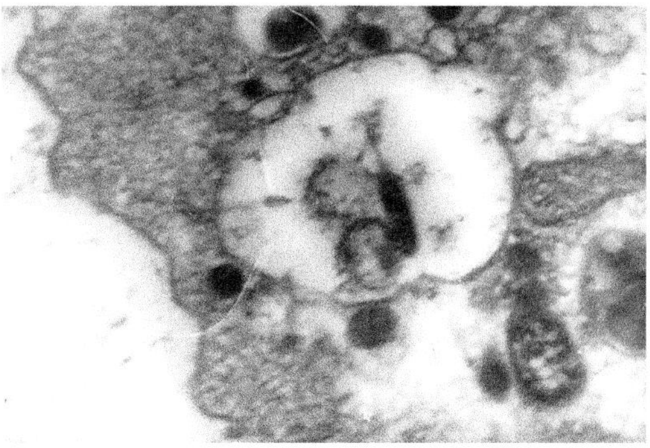

Fig. 9.12 Dividing mycoplasma in the cytoplasm of alveolar macrophage of a hamster with experimental infection. EM ×40,000. Courtesy of A.S. Kozlyuk

References

1. Bayramova F, Jacqquuir N, Greub G. Insight in the biology of Chlamydia-related bacteria. Microbes Infect. 2018;20(7–8):432–40. https://doi.org/10.1016/j.micinf.2017.11.008.
2. Chen H, Wen Y, Li Z. Clear victory for Chlamydia: the subversion of host innate immunity. Front Vicrobiol. 2019;10:1412. https://doi.org/10.3389/fmicb.2019.01412.
3. Shaad UB, Rossi E. Infantile chlamydial pneumonia—a review based on 115 cases. Eur J Pediatr. 1982;138(2):105–9. https://doi.org/10.1007/BF00441148.
4. Chanock RM. Mycoplasma infections of man. N Engl J Med. 1965;273(23):1257–64. https://doi.org/10.1056/NEJM196512022732307.

5. Waites KB, Xiao L, Liu Y, Balish MF, Atkinson TP. Mycoplasma pneumoniae from the respiratory tract and beyond. Clin Microbiol Rev. 2017;30(3):747–809. https://doi.org/10.1128/CMR.00114-16.
6. Blanchard A, Browning G, editors. Mycoplasmas. Springer; 2005. p. 600.
7. Chaubdhry R, Ghosh A, Chandolia A. Pathogenesis of mycoplasma pneumonia: an update. Indian J Med Microbiol. 2016;34(1):7–16.
8. Zinserling VA, Chukhlovina ML. Infectious lesions of nervous system. Issues of etiology, pathogenesis and diagnostics. Saint-Petersburg, ElbiSPb; 2011. 583 p. (In Russian).
9. Shroyt IG, Kozlyuk AS, Zinserling AV, et al. Comparative pathology of mycoplasmosis in respiratory organs. Kishinev, "Shtiinza"; 1977. 119 p. (In Russian).

10 Lobar Pneumonia

10.1 General Characteristics

Pneumonia remains a very important cause of morbidity and mortality in the world. We assume that these data include quite different etiological and pathogenical variants of the disease. But it is widely accepted that the main causative agent of "community acquired" pneumonia is pneumococcus (*Streptococcus pneumoniae*). In the manual of Engelberg, we can find the estimation that about 500,000 cases of pneumococcal pneumonia occur each year in the United States [1]. Pneumococcal infection causes approximately two million deaths globally and costs hundreds of billions of dollars per annum [2], making it one of the leading infectious causes of mortality, it allowed Sir William Osler to call *S. pneumoniae* "the captain of the men of death" [3].

Previously it was commonly accepted that clinicopathological data allow to divide pneumonia into lobar (croupous) and focal (bronchopneumonia), such division remains in the pathology textbooks all over the world. It was accepted that croupous pneumonia is characterized by acute development and quick involvement in the inflammatory process of the whole lobe. The main morphological sign at the upper point of the disease is the so-called hepatization, histologically characterized as dense fibrinous-neutrophilic infiltration. On the contrary, the development of focal pneumonia is much slower. Only croupous pneumonia can be regarded as an immediate cause of death, at least in adults.

Pneumococcus was first isolated from patients with croupous pneumonia in 1886. The paired arrangement of bacteria determined its historical name—the Fränkel–Weichselbaum diplococcus—by the names of the authors who isolated it in pure culture and began its study as a pathogen for humans (A. Fränkel 1848–1916, A. Weichselbaum 1845–1920), although the first to isolate pneumococcus were G. Sternberg, L. Pasteur (1881). However, they did not attribute it to the causative agents of pneumonia since similar microbes were sown by them in healthy people as well. Until now, not all microbiologists share the legitimacy of including pneumococcus in the genus Streptococcus according to a number of phenotypic characteristics, including those that determine its relationship with the human body. In the classical descriptions, the form of pneumococcus is compared with the flame of a candle or lancet, hence the lanceolate diplococcus. Due to the differences in the polysaccharide capsule, at least 92 serotypes of pneumococcus are known to date [2]. The tendency of pneumococcus to autolysis under the influence of autolysin can undoubtedly have pathogenetic significance since pneumolysin (autolysin) has a high membranolytic activity and is capable of damaging the endothelium. This ensures the speed and severity of vascular reactions, pro-

V. Zinserling, *Infectious Pathology of the Respiratory Tract*,
https://doi.org/10.1007/978-3-030-66325-4_10

motes hemorrhage and abundant exudation into the alveolar spaces. In addition, it contributes to the self-destruction of pneumococcus and the release of inflammatory mediators, while repeated contact with pneumococcus is not accompanied by sensitization, it is quickly recognized and captured. Pneumolysin causes a sharp increase in the permeability of the pulmonary vessels, and its effect does not depend on the participation of resident or migrating phagocytic cells. In addition, pneumolysin promotes the taxis of neutrophils and monocytes into the lumen of the alveoli. The main autolysin of LitA is an essential virulence factor. Pneumococcus tolerates the oxygen environment, which ensures its existence in the respiratory tract.

It is widely believed that pneumococcus is present in the nasopharynx of the majority of healthy people. Pneumococcus is completely dependent from the host and quickly perishes in the environment without necessary nutrient media. The constant presence of pneumococcus supports the human immune system in tension.

Pneumococci are differentiated by antigenic characteristics of capsular polysaccharides. The so-called C-polysaccharide has unique properties. Due to its properties, it can bind to acute-phase serum proteins called the C-reactive protein.

It is believed that in the vast majority of cases we are talking about endogenous infection. However, in some cases, it was noted that the serotypes of the strains from the nasopharynx and isolated from the patient during the illness and after it did not coincide. Nosocomial outbreaks of pneumococcal pneumonia were also described. Thus, the possibility of exogenous infection exists. However, the interaction of pneumococcus with the human body is highly individual, and only in exceptional cases leads to the development of the disease. The nature of such a paradoxical contradiction has not yet been disclosed. According to most authors, elderly people are more likely to get a pneumococcal infection, in this regard, pneumococcus received the ironic nickname "old friend," although pneumococcal infections are found in all age groups. In addition to pulmonary lesions, pneumococcal meningitis and otitis media are widespread. According to N.G. Engleberg [1] to date, about 10% of adults are colonized by pneumococcus, approximately 40% of otitis media are also caused by it. Carriage of pneumococcus in children of 2 months was 53.9%, and in children of 6 months—70.2% [4].

The nature of pneumococcus virulence factors requires further study. The high invasiveness of the pathogen is associated with its unique capsule, which allows to resist phagocytes and complements at the beginning of the infection process. Among the pneumococcal enzymes, hyaluronidase and neuraminidase are known to be able to destroy the basic substance of connective tissue. However, many authors note that the pathogenetic significance of these enzymes needs further study. The causes of the toxic effects of pneumococcus on the human body are also not entirely clear. Hemolysin and leucocidin available in pneumococcus do not have toxin properties. The capsule material is also nontoxic. An essential morphological characteristic of pneumococcus is its ability to cause fibrinous (croupous) inflammation, due to damage of the endothelium, which begins to miss fibrinogen and red blood cells. Substances that can violate the integrity of the endothelium were found in the products of pneumococcus autolysis, primarily peptidoglycan derivatives. The second component capable of exerting a membranolytic effect on alveolocytes and vascular endothelium is hydrogen peroxide, which in the absence of the catalase enzyme is produced by pneumococcus in large quantities; in addition, it inhibits other microorganisms and prevents their adhesion. Pneumococcus can be considered as a low-virulent bacterium. However, the existence of its more virulent strains is very likely. Most types of pneumonia are associated with pneumococci of types 1–4, 6–8, 14, 18, and 19. It was revealed that type 3 is the most dangerous in this regard. This serovar produces the largest amount of capsular substance; therefore, it is more reliably protected from phagocytosis. Molecular biological studies conducted with pneumococcal infections indicate that the human body has a number of factors affecting the severity of their course. So, in the works of F.F. Yuan and coworkers [5], it was shown that the genetic variability of the

TLR2, TLR3, CD14, Fc-gamma RIIA genes increases the risk of developing an invasive disease in infected patients. A pronounced protective effect against pneumococcus I11-beta is shown. Galectin-3, which is produced by alveolar macrophages, has a significant effect on the course of the disease [6]. Thus, the conducted molecular biological studies indicate the role of genetic mechanisms associated with the inability of alveolar macrophages to resist pneumococcus and affect the onset and development of the disease. These mechanisms explain the relatively small number of patients with croupous pneumonia with a high number of bacteria.

Bacteria are associated with the ability of pneumococcus to transfer the oxygen environment, which ensures its existence in the respiratory tract, and due to the ability of pneumococcus in the absence of the catalase enzyme to produce hydrogen peroxide, it can inhibit the adhesion and reproduction of other bacteria.

The onset of the disease is associated with the penetration of pneumococci into the alveoli, due to the action of resolving factors, among which defects in the immune system associated with malnutrition, alcohol abuse, and hypothermia are more often mentioned. Among the most common causes, acute respiratory viral infections and influenza are mentioned as factors contributing to the violation of the barrier properties of the epithelium of the respiratory tract, preventing the subsidence of the flora, due to sedentary macrophages [7]. It is noted that in people who are intoxicated, the cough reflex decreases sharply, which contributes to the penetration and adhesion of the flora in the deep parts of the respiratory tract. The high invasiveness of pneumococcus is associated with a unique polysaccharide capsule that can withstand phagocytes and complement until specific antibodies appear. The greatest number of capsular factors is in pneumococcus type 3, and therefore, it has the greatest virulence [2]. When pneumococcus enters the alveoli, under conditions of weakened phagocytic activity of alveolocytes due to genetic defects, it is destroyed with the release of a large number of enzymes and inflammatory mediators. With repeated contact with pneumococcus, sensitization does not occur, but its rapid recognition and phagocytosis occur. Hyaluronidase and neuraminidase, capable of destroying the main substance of the connective tissue, provide adhesion and colonization of pneumococcus in the initial stages. In modern studies, it has been demonstrated that *S. pneumoniae* induces intrinsic apoptosis, necroptosis, and pyroptosis of different cell lines [8]. The pneumococcal capsule itself is non-toxic, but toxic are products of its autolysis. Among them are derivatives of peptidoglycan, which have a membranolytic effect and damage the capillary endothelium. The second component with the same damaging effect is hydrogen peroxide. The third, important factor that has a membranolytic and damaging effect on the capillary endothelium is pneumolysin. It is under the influence of these three components that vascular reactions are triggered with the release of serous fluid, red blood cells, and fibrin into the alveolar spaces, the morphological equivalent of which is the so-called microbial edema. Pneumolysin, among other things, has a pronounced chemotactic effect against neutrophils and monocytes, resulting in their active migration into the alveoli and induces their necroptosis. This fact explains the reason that in one case, in the microscopic picture, circulatory disorders associated with the action of peptidoglycans and hydrogen peroxide will prevail, in the other, accumulations of leukocytes and fibrin will appear and prevail. Similar mechanisms explain the speed and brightness of not only the clinical but also morphological manifestations in croupous pneumonia. The morphological pattern found in the lungs upon microscopic examination depends on the predominant effect of peptidoglycans, hydrogen peroxide, pneumolysin, and its chemotactic properties. The action of these factors explains the mechanisms of exudation and the principles of the formation of microbial edema, its rapid spread over the lung with the capture of large spaces in a short time. These mechanisms suggest that the diversity of morphological manifestations in the lungs should not be considered as stages, but as morphological variants or types of changes associated with the virulence of pneumococcus and the state of the protective mechanisms of the human body. This position confirms the views of V.D. Zinserling expressed about 80 years ago [9]. The key factor underlying the allergic theory of the pathogenesis of croupous pneumonia was the speed and prevalence of the process. At the same time, in the available literature, we were not able to find works in which adequate evidence was provided from the standpoint of modern immunology and allergology of this theory. From the point of view of modern ideas about the pathogenic properties of pneumococcus, the rapid spread of the process in croupous pneumonia with damage to the entire lobe can be easily explained. The inability to withstand pneumococcal invasion can be explained by the weakening of the phagocytic function of alveolocytes due to genetic mechanisms. Important for understanding the clinical and epidemiological data from practical point of view is recently demonstrated fact that alcohol exposure is associated with reduced granulopoiesis and enhanced growth of *S. pneumoniae* in the lungs [10]. In addition, to date, it is impossible to deny the possibility of exogenous infection with the subsequent development of the disease.

After pneumonia, immunity is type specific in nature. The duration of the protective effect is 6–12 months. This stimulated the elaboration of the vaccine.

10.2 Views Upon Pathology in a Historical Aspect

The first studies of croupous pneumonia apparently belong to C. Rokitansky (1842) and were based on a small number of cases [11]. He was the first to describe the stages of the disease, distinguishing inflammatory tide, hepatization, and purulent infiltration. Moreover, a description of the stages of the disease was made on isolated examples. The first stage is very similar to the usual stasis and swelling. In the second stage, the lung is dense, the cut surface is fine-grained. Later on, the lung turns pale, its surface becomes gray. During this period of the disease, the lesion may be called gray hepatization. Further, the stage of purulent infiltration occurs. The lung becomes yellowish, the graininess disappears from the surface, a large amount of sticky, pus-like liquid with an unpleasant odor flows from it. C. Rokitansky proposed the terms "red," "gray," and "yellow" hepatization. Later, during recovery, pus is released with sputum or its resorption. C. Rokitansky emphasized that very often all stages are observed in one lung at the same time, and death, as well as recovery, can occur with any of them.

Subsequently, in a number of manuals, substantial changes were introduced into the concept of C. Rokitansky. They began to claim, with reference to his authority, that croupous pneumonia is always lobar or strictly lobar in nature. "Hepatization" was divided into red and gray with a strict temporal pattern of their replacement. The purulent infiltration phase has been called the resolution phase.

N. Loeschke [12] introduced changes in the concept of the course of the disease. He postulated that the inflammatory process in the lungs spreads due to the spreading of the serous fluid containing a large number of pneumococci. Then fibrin falls out and colonization of granular leukocytes phagocytic pneumococci occurs.

Subsequently, the possibility of hematogenous ingestion of the pathogen into the lungs was unproven postulated, leading to the rapid development of the pathological process with hyperergic reactions. There were speculative representations of a consistent sequential change in a number of stages. According to them, hyperemia is observed in the tidal stage; serous fluid, red blood cells, and fibrin accumulate in the alveoli. After 2–3 days, the tide stage is replaced by the second stage—the stage of red hepatization. The proportion is increased in size, red–brown, and granular due to fibrin corks. In addition to alveoli, fibrin falls in the blood and lymph vessels. Subsequently, with the accumulation of exudate in the alveoli, on the fourth–sixth day, the changes enter the next, third stage—the stage of gray hepatization. It is based on the absence of hyperemia, the disappearance of red blood cells from the exudate with a progressive accumulation of leukocytes. The lung becomes gray, granular, and later gray–yellow. With a favorable course in the stage of gray hepatization, a "disease crisis" occurs, with a critical drop in temperature. There comes the fourth stage of the disease—the resolution stage, which in fact is a favorable outcome of croupous pneumonia. The exudate gradually dissolves; the pulmonary parenchyma is restored.

Subsequently, all the description of the pathology of croupous pneumonia remained practically the same in all textbooks all over the world, differing only in details, without reference to the own primary data [12, 13].

The most complete study of croupous pneumonia was conducted by V.D. Zinserling and his collaborators. In numerous publications of V.D. Zinserling and representatives of his school examined the etiology, pathogenesis, morphological manifestations, and clinical symptoms of the disease [9, 14, 15]. A detailed description of pulmonary complications was given, as well as information about extrapulmonary complications. The relationship between morphological changes in the lungs and the virulence of various strains of pneumococci was emphasized. It was shown that strains 1–3 are especially pathogenic for humans. The disease begins with the penetration of pneumococcus directly into the alveoli. It was proved that with croupous pneumonia at the onset of the disease, a small focus of serous inflammation occurs in the posterior, posterior–lateral, or central parts of the lungs, which then spreads out like an "oil stain." Initially, the focus of inflammation is represented by serous exudate, containing a large number of multiplying pneumococci, which quickly spreads through the Kohn pores throughout the lobe. In this regard, the most acute changes are found in the peripheral parts of the lungs. With the further course of the disease, fibrin falls out, the number of leukocytes increases, and more or less red blood cells are found in the exudate. In this phase of the disease, macroscopic changes in the lungs in different people can vary: in some of they correspond to the "red hepatization", due to the pronounced hyperemia of the alveolar septa and the prevalence of red blood cells in the exudate, in others to the "gray hepatization" option. At the same time, hyperemia subsides, and the exudate in the alveoli is predominantly leukocyte in nature. The amount of fibrin decreases, or it disappears altogether. In the future, the exudate is resorbed, and the lesser the fibrin in the exudate, the faster it dissolves. The third variant of the course may be a mucous variant, which is similar to the second, but the exudate acquires a mucous character. The processes occurring in the lungs with croupous pneumonia cannot be considered as stages of the disease with their strict and consistent replacement. We can evaluate the variants of the disease, which directly depend on the virulence of the pneumococcus strain and the state of the host. Detection of various stages of the process in the lung of the same patient is usual in the practice of pathologists.

Along with lesions in the lungs with croupous pneumonia, changes occur in other organs, which are of great importance in the clinical picture. First of all, this applies to the kidneys, liver, myocardium, brain, and spleen. Among the complications of croupous pneumonia pulmonary and extrapulmonary have to be distinguished. Pulmonary complications include carnification, abscessing, and lung gangrene. In cases where the resorption of fibrin does not occur, the processes of its organization begin. At the same time, overgrowth of the connective tissue is visible in the lumen of the alveoli, some of the alveoli fall off, and the interalveolar septa look thickened, which is denoted by the term carnification (from Latin caro, carnis—meat). With the addition of pyogenic and putrefactive flora, abscesses or gangrene can develop. Of extrapulmonary complications, the most significant are complications associated with lymphogenous (pleurisy, pericarditis, mediastinitis, peritonitis) or hematogenous pathways of spread: meningitis, endocarditis, arthritis, etc. Similar information is provided by other researchers.

V.D. Zinserling provides statistics on the complications of croupous pneumonia. So, meningitis, as the most severe complication, occurs in 6% of cases. Initially, it proceeds as serous, then acquires a fibrinous-purulent or purulent character.

In approximately 4–5% of cases, the disease can be complicated by pneumococcal endocarditis, more often in patients with rheumatic defects. In some cases, the course of the disease may be complicated by sepsis.

In the works of the V.D. Zinserling's scientific school croupous pneumonia is considered as one of the manifestations of pneumococcal infection. The author was the first to distinguish sublobar croupous pneumonia. His work also gives a comparative description of croupous and focal pneumococcal pneumonia, which is practically not discussed by other authors.

10.3 Clinical Manifestations

Pneumococcal croupous pneumonia in many cases has a fairly typical course. A person usually gets sick acutely. In cases with the prodromal period, the onset of weakness is noted at first: headache, loss of appetite. In socially maladaptive persons entering a hospital in serious condition, the anamnesis is often absent.

The classical temperature curve fluctuates around 40° with morning remissions, followed by a critical drop at 5–10 days. However, there are remittent and intermittent temperature curves. In about half of those affected, a rise in temperature is accompanied by chills.

Often there is a cough, but in some people, especially the elderly, it is absent. Most patients have a characteristic appearance for this disease: a reddened face, herpetic eruptions on the lips, nose wings are involved in breathing. Pain in the affected part of the chest is typical. They have a prickling character, intensified with a deep breath, cough, and movement. Other changes include tachycardia, leukocytosis, toxic granularity of leukocytes, and a shift in the leukocyte count to the left, albuminuria, and hyaline cylinders in the urine.

Sputum is typical: usually, it is viscous with a rusty tint, appearing on the second to third day of illness in different quantities.

Mortality in croupous pneumonia before the introduction of modern treatment methods was great. According to various authors, it ranged quite significantly from 8 to 43%.

10.3.1 Own Results

Taking into consideration high morbidity and mortality due to croupous pneumonia at least in Russia and leak of fundamental investigations during the last 50 years we provided our own research in Irkutsk (Eastern Siberia, Russia).

Among 152 cases from Irkutsk 117 deceased (77%) were males, out of which 108 (71.1%) were people younger than 60 years. The majority (72.4%) belonged to the group with a lower level of income, in another 11.8% the social status remained unknown. In 44.7% of cases, alcoholism was mentioned in medical records, these data corresponded well with liver steatosis, which was revealed in 78% of the deceased. The majority of cases occurred in spring and summer (61.8%), which could probably be explained by overcooling while bathing in the cold water of Baikal lake.

Eighty-four (55.3%) died on the first day after hospitalization, 36 (23.7%)—during the next 2 days. The final clinical diagnosis was wrong in 22.4% of cases. Among the false diagnoses, the most frequent were myocardial infarction, septicemia, shock of unclear origin, and lung tuberculosis.

The most important clinical signs were immediate outset (in 63.8%), febrile fewer (documented in 62.5%), and the manifestations of vascular insufficiency (in 87.5% cases). In 67.8% cases, blood was noted leukocytosis (more than 7×10^9), but in 11.2%—leucopenia (less than 4×10^9).

In 110 cases, we succeeded to get the information about the duration of the disease. In 93.6%, the duration of the disease was less than 2 weeks, the median 7.1 ± 0.39. In 21.8%, it was less than 3 days.

10.4 Pathology. Own Data

Macroscopically changes at the autopsy allowed to speak in 84,9% of cases about lobar involvement (Fig. 10.1) and 15.1% of sublobar (mostly in the patients over 70 years with the injury appreciatively of two-third of the lobe) (Fig. 10.2).

Fibrinous pleuritis was extremely typical and was diagnosed in all cases. One side lesion was noted in 61.2% (77.4% among them in the right lung), both sides were involved in 38.8% of cases. One lobe was injured in 16.4% of cases, 2—in 30.3%, 3—in 30.3%, 4—in 9.2%, and total lesions of all five lobes were noted in 13.8%.

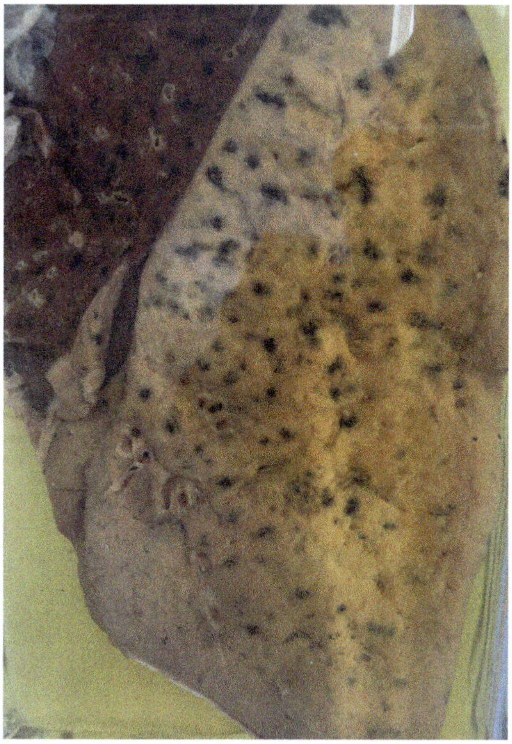

Fig. 10.1 Lobar pneumonia. Macro-preparation from the museum of pathology department of SP Botkin Infectious Hospital, Saint-Petersburg, Russia

Bacterioscopically, in the smears from the cut surface of the lung typical lancet-shaped diplococci were found in all the cases both by bacteriologist and pathologist. In paraffin slices stained with azur-eosine, the typical diplococci were seen in 86.2% of cases, including 25.9% with the mixed microbiota. The culture *S. pneumoniae* was obtained in 24% of cases investigated bacteriologically.

During the histological investigation of lung lesions, we distinguished six variants: microbeous edema—ME (Fig. 10.3), "red hepatization"—RH (Fig. 10.4), "gray hepatization" with equal quantity of neutrophils, and fibrin—GH (Fig. 10.5), "gray hepatization" with a predominance of leucocytes—GHPL (Fig. 10.6), "gray hepatization" with a predominance of fibrin—GHPF (Fig. 10.7), "gray hepatization" with a

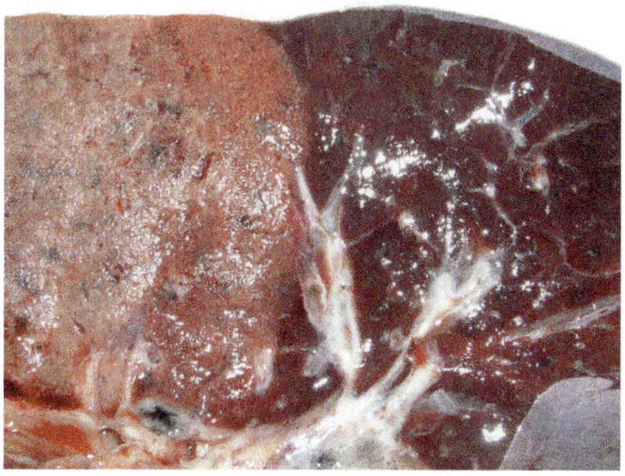

Fig. 10.2 Sublobar pneumonia. Unfixed lung

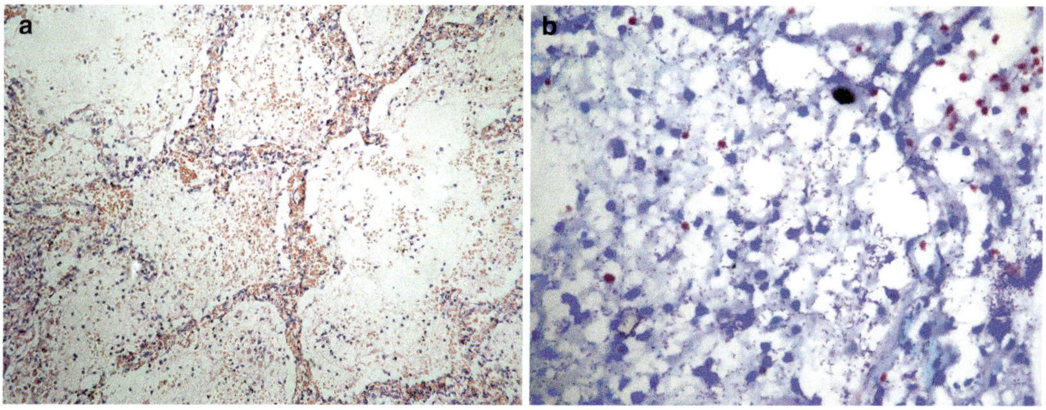

Fig. 10.3 "Microbious edema" in lobar (croupose) pneumonia (**a**) H.-E. ×400, (**b**) Azur-eosin staining ×1000

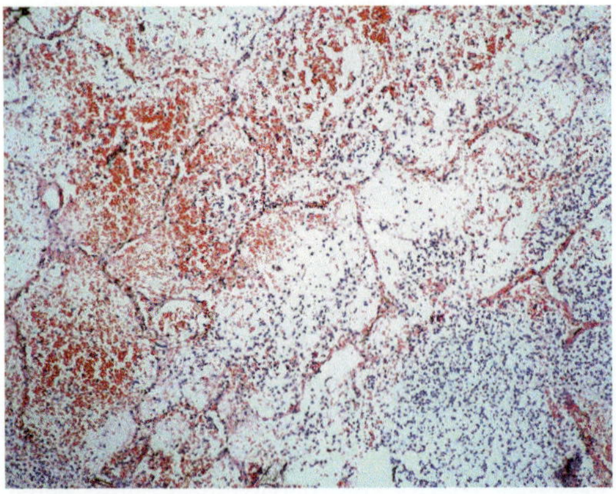

Fig. 10.4 "Red hepatization" in lobar (croupose) pneumonia H.-E. ×100

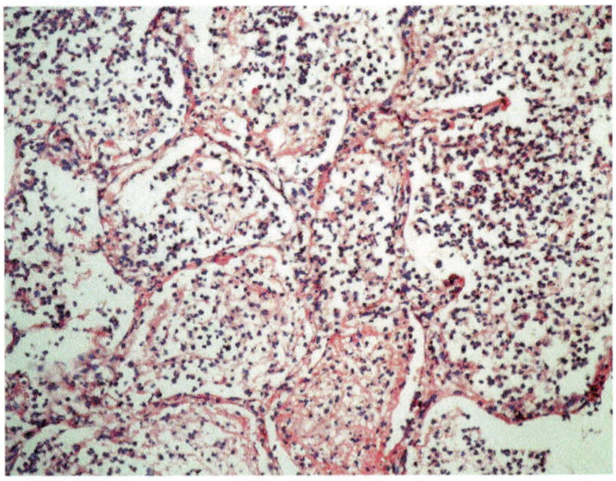

Fig. 10.5 "Gray hepatization" with equal number leukocytes and fibrin in lobar (croupose) pneumonia H.-E. ×100

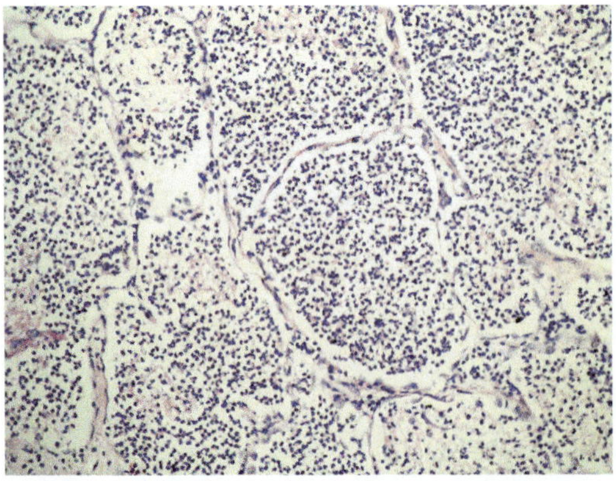

Fig. 10.6 "Gray hepatization" with a predominance of leukocytes in lobar (croupose) pneumonia H.-E. ×100

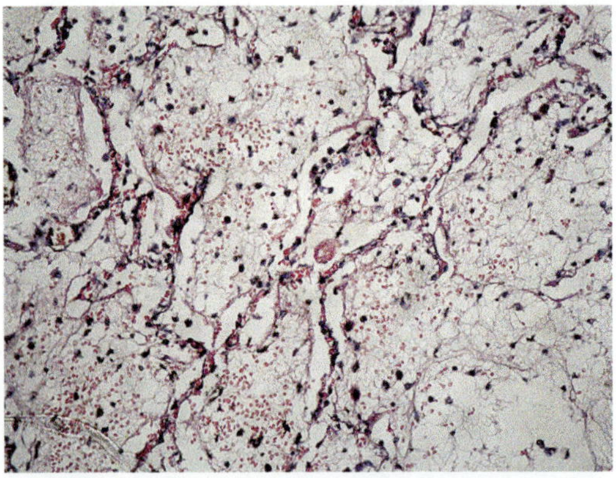

Fig. 10.7 "Gray hepatization" with a predominance of fibrin in lobar (croupose) pneumonia H.-E. ×100

predominance of fibrin and macrophages—GHPFM. The types of histological changes at different days of the disease are shown in Table 10.1.

We have to note that in each deceased, usually, several types of morphological changes were found. So, in 110 cases, we met 417 variant of changes—with the mean 3, 8 variants per case.

The most frequent lung complications were exudative pleuritis (19.1%) and carnification (7.9%). We regarded the formation of microabscesses (in 30.9%) and phlebitis (in 21.1%) important, and in many cases, they were present simultaneously. Based upon the results of bacteriologic and bacterioscopic studies, we connect their development with superinfection along with staphylococci.

Among the extrapulmonary complications, we have to note purulent meningitis (11.2%), in more than half of the cases, with the involvement of brain matter and ventricles. Pericarditis was diagnosed in 3.3% of cases and hemorrhages in adrenal in 4.6%. In 46% of the cases, notable changes in myocardium were seen. In 12.5% of the cases, they were regarded as "disturbances of blood flow," in 25.6% as the microscopical equivalent of acute heart failure (Fig. 10.8), and in 7.9% as early myocardium infarction.

In 21.1% of cases, oliguria and azotemia were noted clinically, which corresponded with the morphological picture of acute renal failure with

Table 10.1 The timing of the occurrence of different histological variants of lobar (croupose) pneumonia

	Terms from the start of acute clinical symptomatic (in days)									
Type of inflammatory reaction	1	2	3	4–5	6–7	8–9	10–11	12–14	>14	all
ME	1	4	9	12	16	6	2	8	3	***61***
RH	1	4	11	8	20	8	–	9	2	***63***
GH	1	5	13	21	22	7	3	10	4	***86***
GHL	1	4	11	18	20	6	3	9	5	***77***
GHF	–	4	9	18	16	5	2	8	3	***65***
GHFM	–	3	12	17	18	4	1	7	3	***65***
Total	***4***	***24***	***65***	***94***	***112***	***36***	***11***	***51***	***20***	***417***

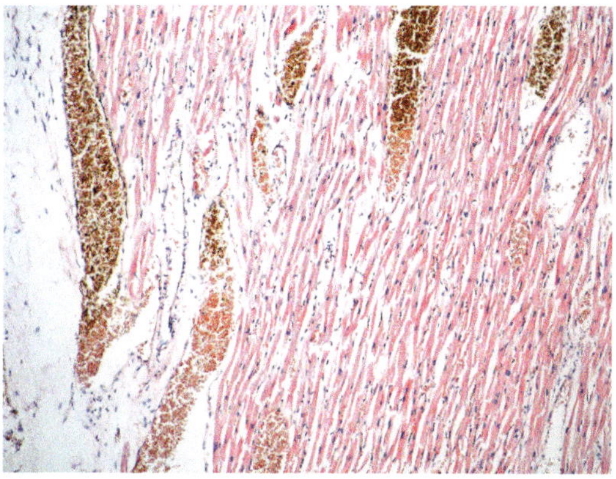

Fig. 10.8 Acute coronary insufficiency in lobar (croupose) pneumonia H.-E. ×100

anemia of the cortex and expressed alteration (till necrosis) of the nephrothelium.

In the pathological department of SP Botkin Clinical Infectious Hospital (Saint-Petersburg) during the period 1993–2007 269 autopsies were provided with the main pathological diagnosis being croupous pneumonia. The number of autopsies with this diagnosis strongly varied from 7 cases (in 1996) till 33 (in 1993). The deceased were dominated by males (77.3%). The information on alcohol abuse was present in 84.4% of clinical records. In half of the cases, the patients died during the first day after hospitalization.

During the postmortem bacteriological investigation, the growth of *S. pneumoniae* was obtained in 33.8% of cases, *Klebsiella* spp. in 13%, but we do not possess the information about the frequency among these cases of the typical Fridländer pneumonias. In 13.4% cases, the serological or histological signs in favor of acute viral respiratory infections were noted, their frequency varied significantly in different years. HIV infection at early stages was detected in eight cases in recent time. Purulent meningitis and meningoencephalitis were diagnosed in 25.3% of all cases.

10.5 Conclusion

The similarity of croupous pneumonia in different Russian cities located in different parts of the country allows verifying the clinical and pathological data as being typical for the whole of Russia. We can also assume that they may be actual true for the other countries with a high level of mortality from pneumonia.

- Croupous pneumonia is a clear separate nosology, playing a very important role in morbidity and mortality in many countries, caused by pneumococcus.
- Certain properties of the pathogen, environmental, and social factors influence the course and outcomes of the disease.
- We have to regard low social status, alcohol abuse, and cooling as the main factors for the development of the disease.
- In the clinical course, the acute onset with febrile temperature is very typical. In many cases, the final clinical diagnosis was wrong predominantly due to the short time of surveillance.
- The morphological changes are comparable with the classical descriptions, but we have to speak about clinico-morphological variants of the disease and not timely restricted stages.

Our data support the views of V.D. Zinserling, first published on the 30th of XX century.

- Our data allows to distinguish 6 histological variants of changes (microbeous edema, "red hepatization", "gray hepatization" with equal quantity of neutrophils and fibrin, "gray hepatization" with predominance of leucocytes, "gray hepatization" with predominance of fibrin, "gray hepatization" with predominance of fibrin and macrophages).
- We have to notify the frequency and importance of extrapulmonary complications—purulent meningitis (11.2—25%), severe heart (46%), and kidney (42.8%) lesions.
- Many questions concerning the mechanism of the disease are still to be investigated.

One of the debate issues regarding the etiology of croupous pneumonia is the reliability of its determination according to the results of cytological and histobacterioscopic studies in the absence of pneumococcus seeding during in vivo and postmortem bacteriological studies. It should be remembered that pneumococcus is very demanding on cultivation conditions and bacterial cultures can never be obtained in all cases of lesions caused by this pathogen. The consequence is widespread views on the polyetiology of croupous pneumonia. We on limited material compared the results of bacteriological, PCR, and histobacterioscopic studies. An almost complete coincidence of the results of PCR and histobacterioscopy was shown, and pneumococcal etiology of community-acquired pneumonia was confirmed in most cases (11 positive PCR results with one positive seeding).

We have analyzed and compared the materials in detail from Irkutsk with the data from St. Petersburg, and literature, primarily the publications of V.D. Zinserling and his schools allow us to conclude that the clinical and morphological manifestations of modern croupous pneumonia are similar in different regions of Russia (and probably in the world) and have not changed significantly over the past half-century.

References

1. Engleberg NC, Di Rita V, Dermodi TS. Shaechter's mechanisms of microbial disease. Philadelphia: Lippincott Williams &Wilkins; 2007.
2. Mackenzie G. The definition and classification of pneumonia. Pneumonia. 2016;8:14. https://doi.org/10.1186/s41479-016-0012.
3. Dockrell DH, Whyte MKB, Mitchel TJ. Pneumococcal pneumonia. Mechanisms of infection and resolution. Chest. 2012;142(2):482–91.
4. Bogaert D, De Groot R, Hermans PW. Streptococcus pneumoniae colonisation: the key to pneumococcal disease. Lancet Infect Dis. 2004;4(3):144–54. https://doi.org/10.1016/S1473-3099(04)00938-7.
5. Yuan FF, Marks K, Wong M, et al. Clinical relevance of TLR2, TLR3, CD14 and Fc gamma RIIA gene polymorphisms in Streptococcus pneumonia infection. Immunol Cell Biol. 2008;86(3):268–70.
6. Farnworth SL, Henderson SL, MacKinnon AC, et al. Galectin 3 reduces the severity of pneumococcal pneumonias by augmenting neutrophil function. Am J Pathol. 2008;172(2):395–405.
7. Garcia-Vidal C, Fernàndez-Sabe N, Carratalà J, et al. Early mortality in patients with community acquired pneumonia: causes and risk factors. Eur Respir J. 2008;32:733–9.
8. FitzGerald ES, Luz NF, Jamieson AM. Competitive cell death interactions in pulmonary infection: host modulation versus pathogen manipulation. Front Immunol. 2020;11:814. https://doi.org/10.3389/fimmu.20.00814.
9. Zinserling VD. Several questions of pathogenesis of croupous pneumonia in the light of new morphological investigations. Clin Med. 1939;3–12:9–10. (In Russian).
10. Siggins RW, Melvan JN, Welsh DA, et al. Alcohol suppresses the granulopoietic response to pulmonary Streptococcus pneumonia infection with enhancement of STAT3 signalling. J Immunol. 2011;186:4306–13. https://doi.org/10.4049/j/immunol.10002885.
11. Rokitansky C. Handbuch der speziellen pathologischen Anatomie, II, Wien; 1842.
12. Cotran R, Kumar V, Collins T. Robbins pathologic basis of disease. 8th ed. Philadelphia: W.B. Saunders Company; 1999.
13. Paltsev MA, Anichkov NM. Pathologic anatomy. Vol. 2. Moscow, "Meditsina"; 2001. p. 433–41. (In Russian).
14. Zinserling VD, Zinserling AV. Pathologic anatomy of acute pneumonias of different etiology (Rus), Leningrad, Medgiz; 1963.
15. Zinserling A. Pathologische Anatomie der wichtigsten Formen bakteriellen Pneumonien. Zbl Allg Path path Anat. 1990;136:3–13.

11 Other Community-Acquired Pneumonia

11.1 Focal Pneumococcal Pneumonia

Focal pneumococcal pneumonia occurs most often among primary pneumonia in all age groups, both according to long-term pathological studies [1, 2] and modern clinical data [3]. On the autopsy material, focal pneumococcal pneumonia as the main disease is found either in young children (in recent years, at least in St. Petersburg, it is extremely rare) or in the elderly. Most often, pathologists meet with them as complications of other very diverse diseases. Obviously, timely adequate antibiotic therapy plays a decisive role in reducing mortality. With a virological and qualified histological examination, the vast majority of observations reveal viral–bacterial associations.

Reliable data on the causes of the development in most cases of a meeting of pneumococcus with a host in the respiratory parts the lungs focal, and not lobar pneumonia, are absent in the literature. It can be assumed that this is due to the lower virulence of the infecting strains, which, in the case of the normal human resistance, more often causes a relatively mild, nonlife-threatening disease. In other observations, when the patient is weakened, or due to age, various intercurrent diseases, even a moderately virulent pathogen can lead to death.

Focal pneumococcal pneumonia in most cases does not have a course typical for croupous pneumonia. However, sometimes even relatively small foci of inflammation are able to give a vivid clinical picture similar to that described with croupous. In most cases, this disease is typically lighter with a gradual development of symptoms.

Pathological anatomy. With focal pneumococcal pneumonia, changes in the lungs most often develop in the lower lobes, less often in the upper ones. A typical predominant lesion of the posterior portions of the lungs is where the first changes occur, which can then spread anteriorly. Isolated lesions of the anterior parts of the lungs are very rare.

In the absence of specific treatment in the lungs, scattered small foci of inflammation are formed, which often merge into larger areas, sometimes capturing most or almost the entire lobe of the lung (confluent, pseudo-lobar pneumonia). They are easily detected while touching during the autopsy. The cut surface has the appearance of reddish, gray, sometimes dark red, airless patches, several protruding above the surrounding lung tissue.

In some atypical cases of focal pneumococcal pneumonia, microbial edema, both during the onset and during the development of the process, is very weakly expressed. With such pneumonia without typical features, pneumococci are found in little amounts, often they are not determined at all. Sometimes accumulations of pneumococci are found only in scanty serous fluid on the walls of respiratory bronchioles and alveoli. Later, as a

V. Zinserling, *Infectious Pathology of the Respiratory Tract*,
https://doi.org/10.1007/978-3-030-66325-4_11

result of the release of neutrophils, on the walls of the alveolar passages and alveoli, a half-moon infiltration is formed. Such foci of inflammation can be so small that they are not macroscopically detected. With the progression of the infectious process in the lung in such cases, only the bronchogenic spread matters. This nature of pneumonia was described with a maximum weakening of the host (e.g., alimentary dystrophy during the siege of Leningrad 1941–1944) and was probably associated with a low-virulent pathogen.

Focal pneumococcal pneumonia cannot be sharply distinguished from croupous. Between them, there are transitional forms—large-focal and confluent pneumonia, in which foci increase in size due to a sufficiently pronounced microbial edema. Morphologically, they differ from croupous pneumonia in that their serous exudation is less pronounced, the zone of microbial edema is narrower, the spread of the process is slower, and there is no clear staging.

With the progression of the inflammation, the involvement of new parts of the lung occurs in two ways: (1) by capturing the lung tissue surrounding the focus by contact spread using a serous fluid spreading through the interalveolar pores containing pneumococci and (2) by transferring them through the bronchi to the new lung sections. Unlike croupous pneumonia, with a focal second path usually becomes leading.

On the autopsy material, it is often possible to observe focal pneumococcal pneumonia in the remission stage. Such lesions are usually found in patients who received antibiotic treatment and died not from pneumonia. In such observations, the peripheral zone of edema is absent in the foci of inflammation, and pneumococci (both bacteriologically and bacterioscopically) are not detected at all or in extremely small quantities. Later, exudate resorption with a complete restoration of the lung structure was observed.

Numerous experimental works were conducted mainly in the first half of the last century, when various animals were infected with pneumococcus focal or lobar pneumonia arose, similar in structure to that described in humans [4]. Various experimental models are used contemporarily, usually to check the efficacy of the vaccine and new antimicrobic drugs.

Thus, the characteristic features of pneumococcal pneumonia are: (1) the absence of necrosis, (2) the spread of pneumococci in the edematous fluid as an "oil stain," and (3) a large amount of fibrin in a purulent inflammatory exudate. These signs are most pronounced in diseases, probably caused by more virulent (stronger expressing their pathogenicity factors) strains of pneumococcus.

11.2 Pneumonia Caused by a Hemophilic Bacillus (Hist. Afanasyev–Pfeifer Rod)

Pneumonia of this etiology is quite important among primary pneumonia; however, certain difficulties in the bacteriological diagnosis of their pathogen and the extreme rarity of the associated fatal outcomes, especially in recent decades, lead to the extreme scarcity of their clinical and morphological descriptions in the literature. Nowadays hemophilic bacillus is most often reported in adults with chronic obstructive pulmonary disease [1–3, 5].

It is very important to remember that during bacterioscopy examination, this pathogen can look not only like a thin tender rod, but (under unfavorable conditions for the pathogen) as a polymorphic rather large coccus. In addition, it is necessary to keep in mind the high exactingness of this pathogen to nutrient media, as well as the possibility of suppressing its growth by other microorganisms in case of mixed infection. All of the above leads to a frequent underestimation of the etiological role of the hemophilic bacillus; in some institutions, they are almost never diagnosed. According to V.D. Zinserling and A.V. Zinserling [1] on autopsy material such pneumonia was revealed in about 1% observation.

The clinical picture has no characteristic features. This etiology can be supposed if focal pneumonia with a relatively mild course is combined with severe purulent bronchitis. In addition, it should be remembered that this pathogen plays a very important role in the etiology of purulent otitis and sinusitis, which can be diagnosed simultaneously with pneumonia, espe-

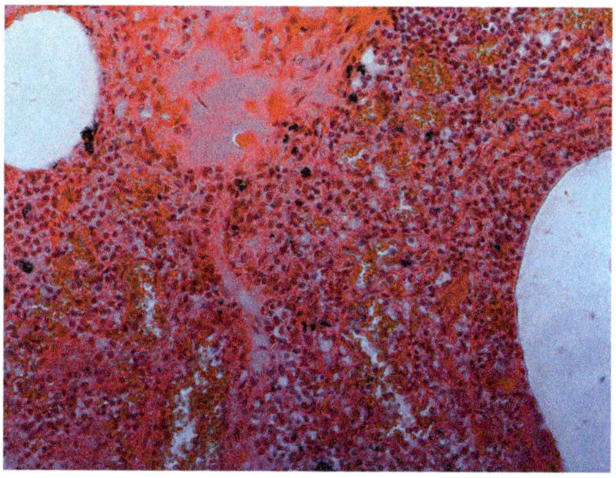

Fig. 11.1 Pneumonia due to *Haemophilus influenza*. H.-E. ×100

cially in young children. Virus–bacterial and viral–bacterial–bacterial associations are frequent.

Pathological anatomy. Damage to the lungs can be focal and less often large focal. Localization of lesions and their appearance are similar to the focal pneumococcal pneumonia (Fig. 11.1). With focal hemophilic pneumonia, there is also a zone of serous inflammation along the periphery with a large number of freely lying rods. Furthermore, toward the center in the alveoli, leukocytes phagocyting microbes are found. The central parts of the foci are predominantly occupied by leukocyte exudate that does not contain rods. With large-focus pneumonia, the swelling zone is wider. Here, pneumococci are sometimes detected as well. Pulmonary necrosis is not observed with this form of pneumonia.

11.3 Pneumonia Caused by Klebsiella (Hist. Fridländer Pneumonia)

Pneumonia caused by *Klebsiella pneumoniae*, whose capsule strains have long been called Friedländer's bacillus, have been known since the late 19th century, but have always been regarded as a rare form that can occur in different age groups [1, 5].

It is important to note that in recent years, significant heterogeneity of various strains has been shown, including those due to different plasmid profiles.

Klebsiella (Friedlander) pneumonia was described as a relatively rare primary disease, but most often acts as a complication of other diseases, including a proven hospital infection (see Sect. 12.2).

According to some authors of the early 20th century, the disease begins acutely, often with chills, cough, and chest pains. Unlike pneumococcal croupous pneumonia, herpes is often absent. The temperature curve is not characteristic, more often it is high, wavy; in severe condition of the patient, it is often low. On average, after 9 days (from 2 to 48 days), a critical or lytic drop in temperature occurs. Sputum is very characteristic. Usually, it is bloody, viscous, and has the smell of burnt meat. During its cytological examination, a significant number of gram-negative rods surrounded by a mucous capsule can be detected.

According to reports of researchers working in the pre-antibiotic era, mortality in Friedländer pneumonia ranged between 30 and 50%. In cases of combination with bacteremia, it reached 80%.

According to A.V. Zinserling frequency of this etiological form on the autopsy material, depending on the treatment ranged from 2 to 5% [1].

Pathological anatomy. Changes in the lungs with Friedländer's pneumonia were studied by a number of authors, starting with A.I. Moiseev (1900), but it is described in detail in the works of A.V. Zinserling. Lesions have the appearance of large, rounded foci, located mainly in the posterior parts of the lobes. They often cover almost the entire lobe or even several lobes of the lung. In addition, in other lobes of the lungs, as a rule, focal lesions of the same etiology are found. The lung tissue in the lesions is sharply densified, grayish-pink, or gray. Dark red hemorrhages are often visible of various sizes. The cut surface is slightly grainy or smooth. A very characteristic macroscopic feature of pneumonia of this etiology is the separation from the cut surface of a more or less thick, mucus-rich pus-like pink fluid that stretches for a knife up to half a meter (Fig. 11.2). A peculiar smell from the lung tissue often resembles the smell of burnt meat.

During microscopic examination (Fig. 11.3), the foci of consolidation do not have a homogeneous structure throughout. In terminal bronchi-

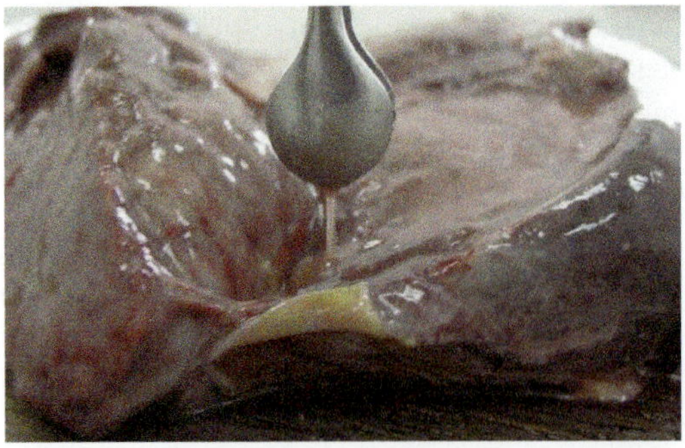

Fig. 11.2 Pneumonia due to *Klebsiella pneumonia* (Fridländer type). Lung at the autopsy

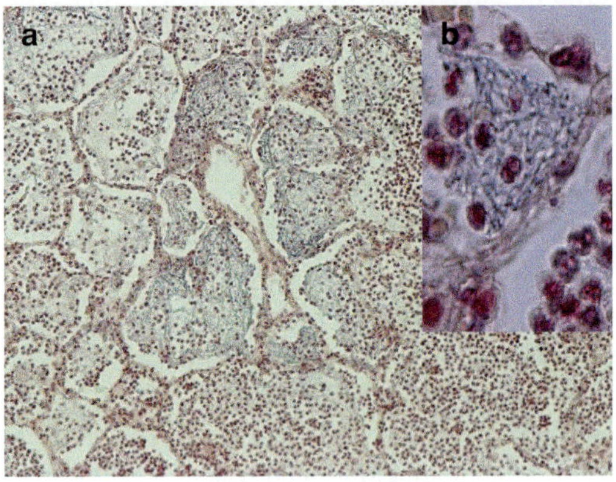

Fig. 11.3 General view upon Fridländer pneumonia. Gram stain ×100. (**a**) ×100; (**b**) numerous rods × 1000

oles, alveolar passages, and alveoli, poor neutrophilic exudate is detected. Fibrin fibers are thin and not numerous and are located mainly in the peripheral regions. A large number of bacteria are found in the exudate. In the central parts of the foci, almost all rods are phagocytosed by neutrophils. Closer to the periphery, they lie mostly freely, sometimes making up the bulk of the contents of the alveoli. On the periphery of the pneumonic foci, there is either a narrower or wider zone of alveoli filled with serous exudate. It also contains rods, usually in smaller numbers, sometimes in the form of rings. With a longer course of the process, a large number of macrophages are found in the exudate, which also phagocytizes microorganisms. With a relapse of the process, a significant amount of neutrophilic white blood cells may again appear. In most of the deceased, in areas with older changes pronounced lymphangitis and lymphadenitis can be found. In dilated lymphatic vessels, neutrophilic leukocytes and microbes are detected.

Some patients have extensive infarctions, occupying up to one-third of the lung lobe. From the surrounding lung tissue, the area of necrosis is clearly delimited by the leukocyte shaft. Many blood vessels in the lungs, including arteries, are thrombosed.

The spread of the inflammatory process in the lungs can occur both by contact and bronchogenic.

In observations of previous years, foci of the generalization of the process with the development of extrapulmonary lesions, as a rule, were not described, and epidemiology was not analyzed. However, it cannot be ruled out that in A.V. Zinserling's observation with the development of severe Friedländer's pneumonia on the fifth to sixth day after abdominal surgery, it is a hospital infection.

In numerous experimental studies conducted in the mid-20th century, it was possible to reproduce a large focal, often pseudo-lobar lung lesion with a predominantly bronchogenic, less often vague distribution of the process, serous-leukocyte nature of the exudate with a huge number of rods, and the frequent addition of pleurisy and pericarditis, moreover, infarctions were often observed as well.

Thus, despite a number of similarities between lobar pneumococcal and *K. pneumoniae*, a number of significant features do not allow us to say that croupous pneumonia is polyetiological and can be caused by both pneumococcus and Klebsiella.

In recent years, classic forms of Friedländer pneumonia are extremely rare.

11.4 Streptococcal Pneumonia

Streptococcal pneumonia was observed relatively often (1–10%) on autopsy material in the pre-antibiotic era either as an independent primary disease or as a complication of scarlet fever. Currently, such lesions are extremely rare.

The hemolytic streptococcus of group A acts as the main pathogen.

The clinical picture according to the descriptions of a number of the older authors was characterized by gradual onset with rare chills. Cough, high fever with large swings in temperature, and difficulty in breathing were noted. Sputum is not very characteristic: scanty, mucopurulent, and sometimes with an admixture of blood.

The morphological manifestations of streptococcal pneumonia were most thoroughly studied in the school of V.D. Zinserling [1, 5, 6].

The most severe are focal necrotic lung lesions, which in a typical form occur with scarlet fever as primary foci or bronchogenic metastases in the early days of the disease. They immediately cause a serious general condition of the patient, not corresponding to the volume of local lesions.

A microscopic examination reveals a huge number of streptococci in the necrotic tissue of the lung (Fig. 11.4). In the early stages, the lung tissue in these places still retains its general structure, although the cell nuclei are already absent; later it is destroyed. Along the periphery, such focal necrosis is surrounded by zones of lung tissue containing fibrinous effusion, and further from the center is serous exudate. In these areas, streptococci are absent. At the same time, a shaft is formed on the border of necrosis, consisting initially of individual white blood cells, and then of a significant number of them. At this stage, leukocyte phagocytosis of streptococci is clearly visible.

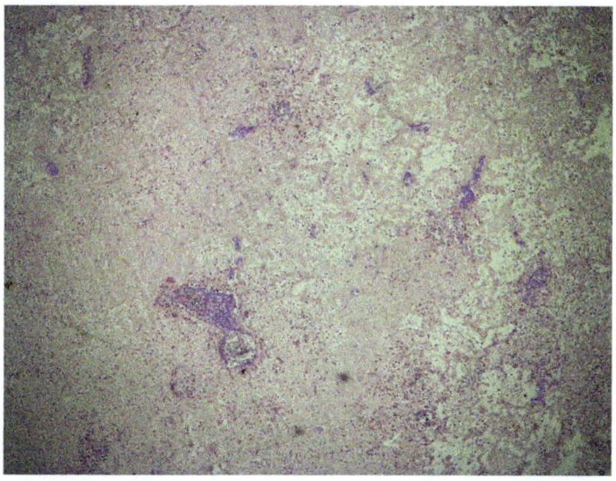

Fig. 11.4 Necrotic streptococcal pneumonia. Stained according to Gram. ×100

Macroscopically, these are, as a rule, single irregularly shaped foci 1–2 cm across, less often large, located subpleural, somewhat more often in the lower lobes. Their center is occupied by one or more sites of necrosis. These focuses in the early stages are unclearly outlined, grayish red in color, flabby. At later stages, areas of necrosis become gray or whitish; they are clearly delimited from the surrounding inflammatory-altered lung tissue. Usually, corresponding to the lesion in the lung, pleura is also necrotic, which quickly leads first to serous and then serous-purulent pleurisy and pyopneumothorax. In the pleura and interlayers of connective tissue, lymphangitis easily develops, spreading from the focus toward the root, which is accompanied by damage to the regional lymph nodes. In the early stages of the disease, toxic (fibrin prolapse in the marginal sinuses) and hyperplastic, and later necrotic and purulent changes are observed in them. Mediastinal phlegmon may also occur. The process captures the veins in which septic thrombophlebitis is observed, often spreading to larger veins outside the focus.

Another variant was pneumonia with the absence of necrotic changes, but a more pronounced lesion of the bronchi. In such bronchi, the wall can be necrotic throughout the entire thickness; the bronchus takes the form of a channel with pus surrounded by inflamed lung tissue with alveoli containing fibrinous and serous exudate, but not microbes.

Streptococcal bronchopneumonia and bronchitis with even more mild necrotic changes can be considered as the third variant. With such pneumonia, neutrophilic exudate is contained in the bronchi and the corresponding alveoli. Its cells are often devoid of nuclei, due to which it turns into a mass without structure. Perifocal toxic changes may be absent.

11.5 Staphylococcal Pneumonia

The frequency of staphylococcal pneumonia according to reports of various authors ranges from 1 to 7% among all their etiological forms. They can develop under different circumstances as a complication of influenza, as complications of staphylococcal tonsillitis, laryngotracheitis, and also as a hospital infection [1, 3]. Primary development of pneumonia of this etiology seems rare. It is important to note that the frequency of staphylococcal pneumonia, as well as lesions of other organs of the same etiology, can undergo very significant fluctuations upon time.

As a causative agent, *Staphylococcus aureus* usually acts, although there is evidence of the importance of *S. epidermidis*. Astonishingly, modern literature distinguished both extra- and intracellular forms [7], although we have never met the latter. Among the pathogenic mechanism are noted induction of apoptosis, necroptosis, and pyroptosis [8].

One of the most pressing clinical problems is the widespread occurrence of staphylococcus strains resistant to many antibiotics.

The clinical course. Staphylococcal pneumonia develops gradually, but, as a rule, within a few hours the patient's condition becomes severe; acute onset of the disease is rarely observed. Clinical manifestations are dyspnea, cyanosis, cough, vomiting, and less chest pain. The temperature curve is irregular, with a reminder temperature prevailing. Often there is severe sweating. High leukocytosis with a severe toxic granularity of neutrophils is noted in the blood. Purulent sputum, often with bloody insertions, is usually excreted in a small amount. It reveals many gram-positive cocci lying in heaps. As a peculiarity of staphylococcal pneumonia, many authors note early abscess formation, early and frequent lesions of the pleura. Many researchers consider the presence of air cavities in a radiological examination as typical for staphylococcal pneumonia in children. They do not manifest themselves or almost do not manifest clinically, do not contain pus, do not have a capsule, and change relatively quickly in both quantity and size. The formation of these cavities is not entirely clear. According to one version, we are talking about a site of necrosis, the cavity of which, due to the elasticity and retractability of the lung, soon exceeds its original size. According to another opinion, with the development of a peribronchial abscess, a valve mechanism appears in the wall of the bronchus, leading to a rapid inflating of the lung tissue.

Mortality from staphylococcal pneumonia in the pre-antibiotic era exceeded 50%. We do not have reliable modern statistics.

Changes in the lungs with staphylococcal infections are different. A special place is occupied by a rare form of staphylococcal infection with severe intoxication, resembling scarlet fever. With this form, brain swelling and a scarlet-like rash on the skin are noted.

In the lungs, single, fairly large, up to 6 cm, foci of necrosis are found, located subpleural, usually in the posterior parts of the lungs or multiple foci of necrotic pneumonia. Such foci usually develop as a complication of necrotic tonsillitis or damage to the respiratory tract. Larger single foci are heterogeneous in the cut section: against the background of dark red densified lung tissue, gray areas of necrosis with blurry contours are visible. Multiple lesions of the lungs are more uniform: red or dark red with small grayish-yellow patches in the center. With such pneumonia, the lesions of the bronchi often come to the fore. In their place, abscesses of an elongated form are formed.

A histological examination in necrotic tissues and the central zones of purulent foci always determines a significant number of staphylococci (Fig. 11.5). The sites of lung tissue necrosis with huge accumulations of staphylococci in the alveoli sometimes have a peculiar appearance: the

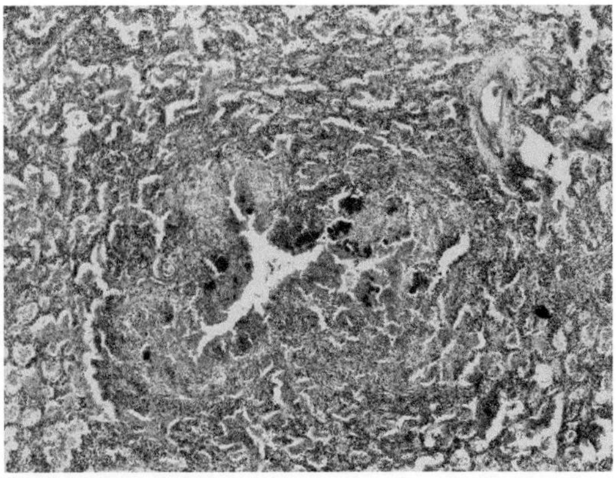

Fig. 11.5 Necrotic staphylococcal bronchopneumonia. H.-E. ×200

alveolar septa are devoid of nuclei the alveolar cavities contain only microbes. In the circumference of the focus of necrosis is a more or less pronounced shaft of granular leukocytes that phagocytize staphylococci. In the initial stages of the process in the bronchi, as well as in the respiratory tissue, clusters of staphylococci are found in serous or hemorrhagic exudate, initially with a small admixture of leukocytes. The presence of such changes with a large number of microbes indicates the progression of the disease.

Staphylococcal pneumonia without scarlet fever intoxication often also occurs violently. Morphological changes in the lungs are similar to those described earlier.

With milder staphylococcal lung lesions, necrotic and perifocal toxic changes in the form of serous or fibrinous effusion are less pronounced and may be absent. In the central parts of such foci, a small number of often phagocytized staphylococci are found.

Thus, staphylococcal pneumonia in morphological manifestations (the presence of necrosis and perifocal toxic changes) is close to streptococcal. The differences between these two forms of pneumonia are that with staphylococcal pneumonia there is a great tendency to the formation of abscesses, the process often has a hemorrhagic character, and there is no systematic involvement of lymphatic vessels and nodes.

11.6 Legionellosis of the Lungs (Syn. Disease of Legionnaires)

The causative agents of this disease are Legionella, primarily Legionella pneumophila. These are sticks with sizes of 0.5–0.7 × 2–3 μm, but they can also have large sizes. They are well stained with aniline dyes according to Gimenez and impregnated with silver. Most bacteria have fat vacuoles detected by black Sudan. Some species have relative acid resistance [3]. In the modern literature the pathogen is considered to be intracellular and characterized by inducing parthanatos, payroptosis, and autophagy, but depressing apoptosis of different cell lines [8].

Infection occurs by airborne droplets. The causative agent can exist in the external environment and enter the human body with dust, water, air conditioning, as evidenced by epidemiological studies conducted in the United States in the early 1980s of the 20th century.

The disease is most often described in the United States, but can be determined almost everywhere, where there are necessary diagnostic capabilities. There is evidence that legionellosis accounts for up to 8% pneumonia of unknown etiology. Extensive serological studies conducted in many countries have proven the high prevalence of legionellosis, which can occur easily, and not only with almost constant lethal outcomes, as was initially assumed.

Legionella spp. produces pulmonary infections ranging in severity from a mild respiratory illness to life-threatening pneumonia [3].

Macroscopically, pneumonia has the nature of focal or lobar. The cut surface of the lung is grayish-red or grayish, with a rusty tint; abscessing is often noted. Very often, serous or serous-fibrinous pleurisy develops.

Microscopic examination in the alveoli is characterized by the accumulation of exudate from neutrophilic leukocytes and macrophages mixed with red blood cells, fibrin, and serous fluid. There are also hyaline membranes, indicating a sharp violation of vascular permeability. In the central parts of the foci, leukocytes prevail, which undergo a decay with karyorrhexis, which is very typical for this disease (Figs. 11.6 and 11.7). Thrombosis of small blood vessels, especially veins, often occurs. Along with this, damage to the distal airways occurs. In all areas of the foci of inflammation, the presence of legionella is described, lying both freely and intracellularly, in particular, in macrophages and leukocytes. Legionella is gram-negative coccobacillus, can be weakly stained with gram stains, by Z-N and silver impregnation. The greatest number of them is found in areas with pronounced alterative changes in leukocytes. They were also found in hyaline membranes, in the vessels of the microvasculature, and pleural exudate. Among serous and serous-hemorrhagic exudate along the periphery of the foci of legionella are detected less often.

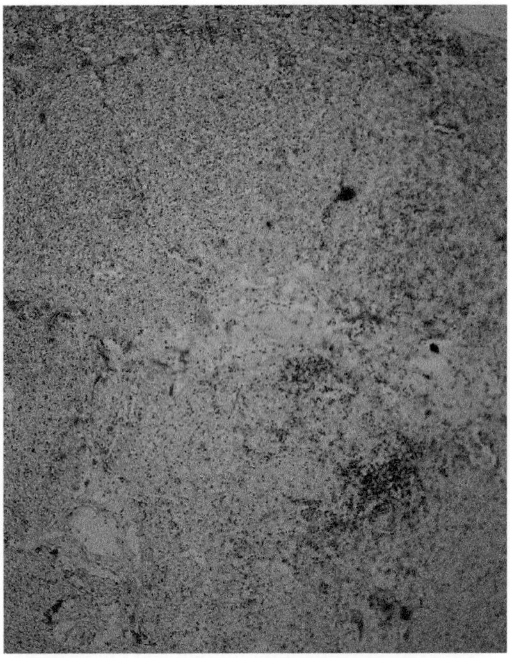

Fig. 11.6 Necrotic focus in pneumonia due to Legionella. H.-E. ×40. Courtesy of V.V. Svistunov

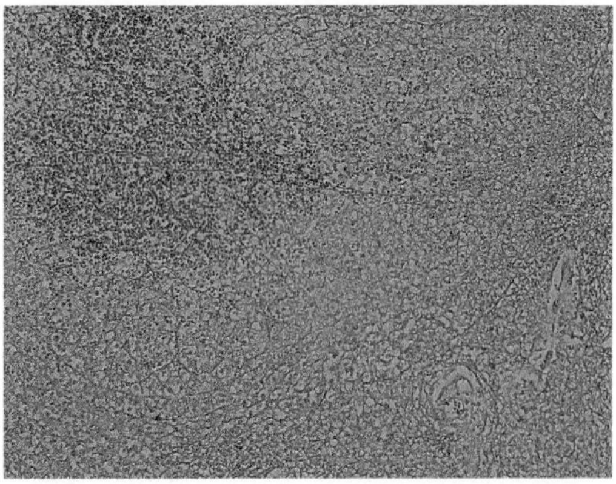

Fig. 11.7 Necrotic focus and hemorrhage in the same case. H.-E. ×200

There is evidence in favor of the possibility of both lymphogenous and hematogenous dissemination of the pathogen with the development of lesions of the lymphatic vessels, heart, kidneys, and appendix.

Other current forms of legionellosis are described, in particular, Pontiac fever (a respiratory disease without pneumonia) caused by the same type of pathogen. Possible lung damage caused by other types of legionella. Their clinical and morphological manifestations are largely similar to those described earlier.

We do not have complete information about the thoroughly studied deaths from legionellosis in Russia.

11.7 Plague

The causative agent of this acute infectious disease from the group of anthropozoonosis is Yersinia pestis [3]. The disease occurs in people of different ages, sometimes sporadically, usually in the form of outbreaks and epidemics. Although in recent years this disease has been recorded extremely rarely in the world, there is no discussion about its complete eradication. Infection occurs in various ways, most often from wild rodents (rats, ground squirrels, etc.) through bloodsucking insects, mainly fleas. Less commonly—in the midst of an epidemic—aerosol contamination from people suffering from plague pneumonia is possible. Among the pathogenic mechanisms nowadays are distinguished activation of anoikis and necrosis, meanwhile, pyroptosis is suppressed [8].

In the works of previous years, various clinical and morphological forms of the disease (skin, bubonic, septic, and pulmonary) were distinguished. Respiratory injuries are typical of the latter two. Autopsy of dead from the plague or with reasonable suspicion of this diagnosis requires special precautions.

Macroscopically, foci have various sizes—from a few centimeters across to lobar lesions. In the early stages of the development of plague pneumonia, the lungs in the affected areas are enlarged in volume, in the section of a dark red color, with a smooth surface with which red fluid flows. In the later stages of the disease, the lungs acquire a gray–red color.

With a microscopic examination, the main characteristic is the development of serous-hemorrhagic inflammation, associated with the rapid multiplication of plague bacteria (Figs. 11.8 and 11.9). In the early stages of the disease, only a few macrophages and white blood cells are

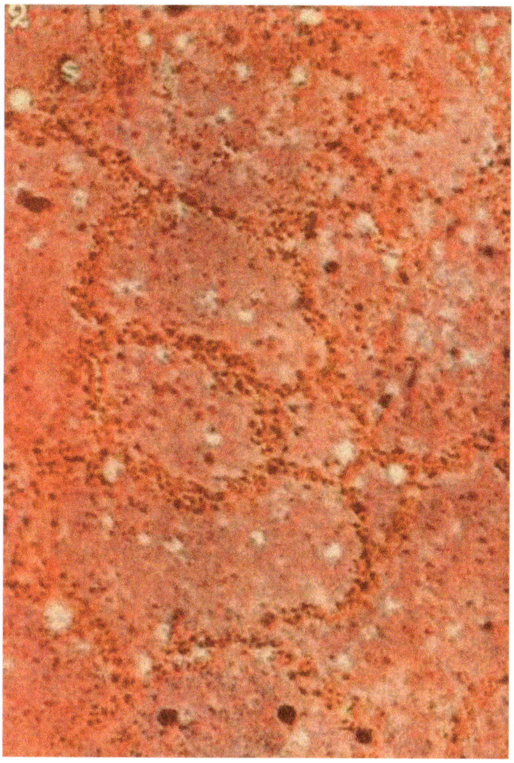

Fig. 11.8 Lung tissue of the deceased from lung plague. Hemorrhagic pneumonia. Stained by Methylenblau-Eosin. ×200. From "Lung Plague in Manchuria in 1910-11." Report of Russian scientific expedition. Ed. Prof. D.K. Zabolotny Vol. II, Petrograd 1915 (in Russ)

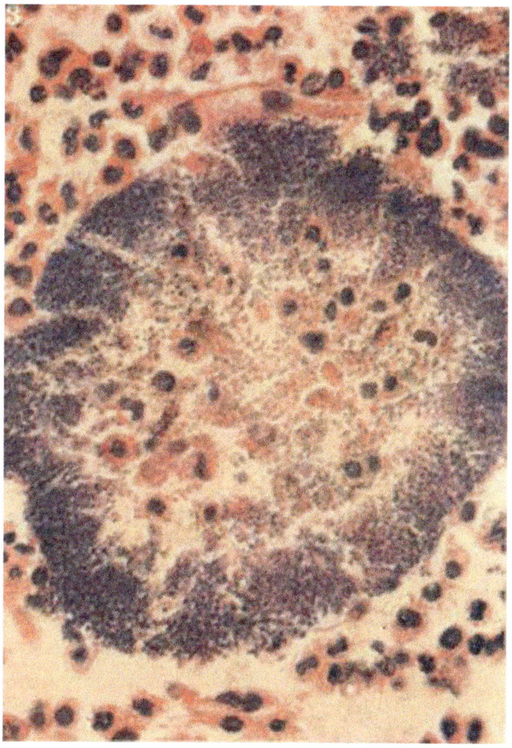

Fig. 11.9 Colonies of plague bacteria in the lymph node sinus. Stained by Methylenblau-Eosin. ×800. ibidum

found in the pneumatic foci. Under the influence of bacterial enzymes, necrosis of exudate cells and even organ tissue often occurs. With the progression of the disease, plague bacilli spread in all possible ways—in extent, bronchogenic, lymphogenous, and hematogenous, especially in the lung, and then beyond. With a longer duration of pneumonia in the alveoli, as well as in the bronchi, an increasing number of white blood cells appear, and the exudate becomes purulent. It is generally accepted that plague pneumonia is characterized by 100% mortality.

11.8 Anthrax

The causative agent of this acute anthropozoonosis is Bacillus anthracis—sizes 1.0–1.2 × 3–5 μm with rounded ends, located in pairs or short chains. People of any age are ill. Infection is possible from sick animals, mainly domestic ones (large and small horned honeycombs, horses, and deer), and occurs most often through the skin. Spores, which were also considered as biological weapons, very often act as infectious material. In Russia, an outbreak of anthrax with aerogenic infection and a significant number of deaths in 1979 was described [9]. In this case, serous hemorrhagic pneumonia with areas of necrosis was noted.

11.9 Actinomycosis

The causative agents are several representatives of the genus Actinomyces, which was previously attributed to fungi. In tissues, the pathogen usually consists of closely interwoven filaments 0.4–0.7 nm thick with side branches. On the periphery of a drusa the filaments are swollen. This accumulation of bacteria is called drusen (Fig. 11.10).

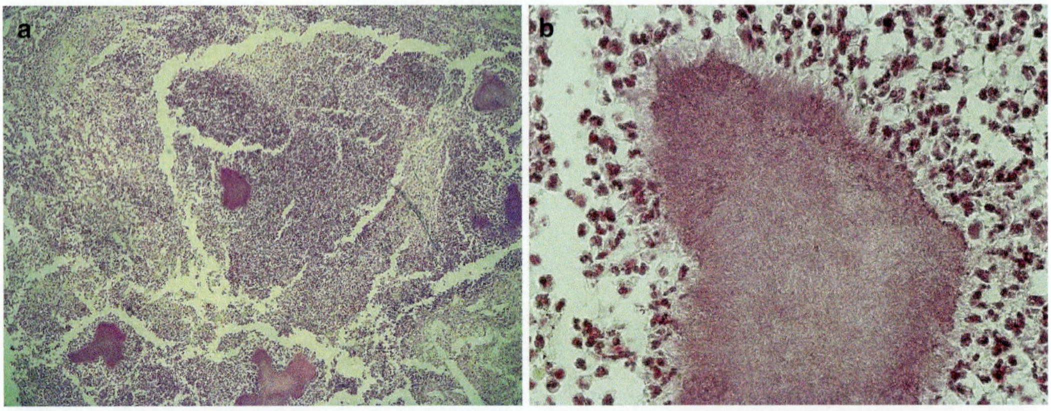

Fig. 11.10 Lung lesions in actinomycosis. (**a**) General view. H.-E. ×40. (**b**) Detail of the previous preparation ×400

The causative agent is gram-positive, well stained with hematoxylin, and according to Z-N. Bacteria are widespread throughout the world. Epidemiological features are not well understood. With actinomycosis, almost all organs and tissues can be affected, clinical diagnosis is extremely difficult. Among the affected organs, lungs are also noted. Around even a long druse existing for a long time, neutrophilic infiltration is characteristic. In the later stages of the disease, fibrosis without characteristic features is noted.

11.10 Whooping Cough

The causative agent is Bordetella pertussis—gram-negative bipolar bacilli 0.2–0.3 × 1-, 0–5 nm in size. They are located singly or in pairs, very rarely in short chains.

Pertussis usually affects children under 5 years, most often in the form of small outbreaks. The disease is contagious and almost all people are susceptible to it. Due to the widespread vaccination, the incidence worldwide has sharply decreased, and deaths are almost not recorded.

The pathological anatomy of whooping cough was studied in detail in the middle of the last century in Russia [1]. Propagation of bacteria occurs in the respiratory system. The characteristic clinical picture with paroxysmal cough is associated with the effect on the centers of the medulla oblongata produced by the pathogen exotoxin.

Macroscopically, a moderate plethora of the respiratory tract with a mild semifluid overlay on the mucous membrane was noted. Light swollen, in the anterior sections they are pale, grayish pink in color, often with manifestations of bullous emphysema. In the posterior sections, the lungs are gray–red, often with punctate hemorrhages. In the section, individual protruding small gray or gray–red foci of densification and smaller sunken dark red areas are visible.

Microscopic examination of part of the bronchi managed to see rods located in the form of a thin strip on the surface of the epithelium. Later, alterative changes in the epithelium with its desquamation and signs of catarrhal inflammation were detected. Serum exudate with a small admixture of leukocytes and macrophages was contained in the lumens of such bronchi; it contained free or phagocytic pertussis bacilli. In the walls of the bronchi—small lymphocytic infiltrates. In some children, the spread of the inflammatory process to the respiratory departments with the development of small focal pneumonia with serous–macrophage–leukocyte exudate and mainly free-lying microbes was noted. When children died in the late stages of whooping cough, only changes due to secondary microbiota were detected.

References

1. Zinserling VD, Zinserling AV. Pathological anatomy of acute pneumonia of different etiology. Gos Izd Med Lit. Leningrad; 1963. 175 p. (In Russian).
2. Zinserling AV, Zinserling VA. Modern infections: pathologic anatomy and issues of pathogenesis: a guide. SPb: Sotis; 2002. 346 p. (In Russian).
3. Leslie KO, Wick MR, editors. Practical pulmonary pathology. A diagnostic approach. 2nd ed. 2011. 828 p.
4. Borsa N, Di Pasquuale M. Restrepo M.I animal models of pneumococcal pneumonia. Int J Mol Sci. 2019;20:4220. https://doi.org/10.3390/ijms20174220.
5. Zinserling AV. Pathologische Anatomie der wichtigsten Formen bakterieller Pneumonien. Zbl Allg Path Pathol Anatomie. 1990;136:S3–13.
6. Zinserling AV, Ioakimova KG. Streptococcal infections: forms and morphological appearance. Arkh Pathol. 1987;(5):3–11. (In Russian).
7. FitzGerald ES, Luz NF, Jamieson AM. Competitive cell death interactions in pulmonary infection: host modulation versus pathogen manipulation. Front Immunol. 2020;11:814. https://doi.org/10.3389/fimmu.20.00814.
8. Bradley BT, Bryan A. Emerging respiratory infections: the infectious disease pathology of SARS, MERS, pandemic influenza and Legionella. Semin Diagn Pathol. 2019;36:152–9. https://doi.org/10.1053/j.semdp.2019.04.06.
9. Abramova FA, Grinberg LM, Yampolskaya OV, Walker DH. Pathology of inhalational antrax in 42 cases from Sverdlovsk outbreak in 1979. Proc Natl Acad Sci U S A. 1993;90(6):2291–4. https://doi.org/10.1073/pnas.90.6/2291.

12 Nosocomial Pneumonias

12.1 Pseudomonas Pneumonia

The causative agent is *Pseudomonas aeruginosa* [1]. Its colonies often emit a smell of trimethylamine, reminiscent of the smell of jasmine. The same smell can come from inflammatory foci of the same etiology. These rods emit various pigments, of which the most characteristic is blue–green. The formation of pigments of brown, red, and greenish-yellow is also possible, the latter glows in ultraviolet rays. Some strains can have no pigment.

P. aeruginosa is resistant to various influences, including many disinfectants and antibiotics. In addition, the possibility of the formation of hospital strains has been proved, which can be judged using intraspecific typing methods, including immuno-, piocyne-, and phagotyping. Various strains of *P. aeruginosa* vary significantly in pathogenicity factors, among which exotoxin A, isoenzyme S, and proteases are currently considered to be the main ones. All this determines the possibility of widespread *P. aeruginosa* in medical institutions. The source of infection can be sick people with various forms of pseudomonosis, items, including medical equipment, bedding, sinks, and toilets.

According to new data, *P. aeruginosa* induces mechanism of cell death such as apoptosis, ferroptosis, pyroptosis, and autophagy [2].

Pneumonia is one of the most important manifestations of *P. aeruginosa*.

It should be noted that, depending on the epidemiological situation, the frequency of *Pseudomonas pneumonia* can fluctuate quite significantly. Most often, their outbreaks are described in burns, postoperative departments, departments for premature babies.

Macroscopic manifestations of the disease can be divided into two options: (1) fuzzy hemorrhagic seals, sometimes with grayish-yellow patches of necrotic parenchyma in the center; (2) dense dark gray or brown necrotic areas with moderately elevated edges, surrounded by a narrow rim of dark red color [3]. The foci of pneumonia have fuzzy borders, various sizes, and shapes. At autopsy, half of the dead in the pleural cavities show a serous or serous-hemorrhagic effusion, and some patients develop fibrinous-purulent pleurisy.

Microscopic examination at the early stages of the disease in the lumens of the alveoli and distal airways reveals a sharp plethora of the interstitial tissue, the accumulation of leukocytes in the capillaries. In the alveoli, there is a little serous fluid with a significant admixture of red blood cells and with single leukocytes.

At a later date, the process is characterized by the appearance of large foci of pulmonary parenchyma necrosis with more massive clusters of rods in necrotic tissues (Fig. 12.1). Destructive changes in these places also undergo blood vessels and bronchi. The inflammatory reaction around necrotic tissues and microbial colonies is

V. Zinserling, *Infectious Pathology of the Respiratory Tract*,
https://doi.org/10.1007/978-3-030-66325-4_12

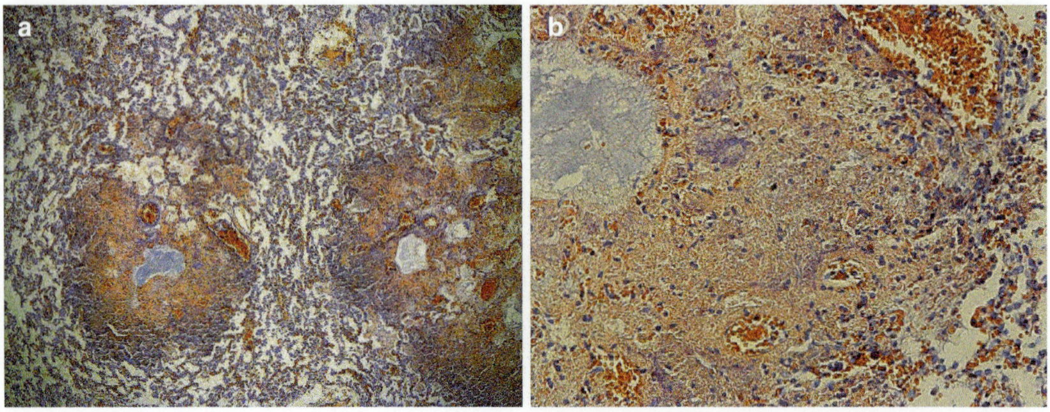

Fig. 12.1 Necrotic pneumonia due to *Pseudomonas aeruginosa*. Stained by azur–eosin. (**a**) General vue ×40 and (**b**) Detail of the previous preparation. ×400

poorly expressed, although necrotic masses often contain fragmented leukocyte nuclei, as well as a few lymphocytes and monocytes. The foci of necrosis are surrounded by a zone of hemorrhages, the vessels are dilated, the lumen of the alveoli contains serous-leukocyte exudate with numerous bacteria. Further to the periphery, the alveoli are made by macrophages, leukocytes, microbes are visible here, some of which are phagocytized, sometimes fibrin can be detected in the alveoli.

P. pneumonia can be reproduced experimentally, including with intratracheal infection of rats. The nature of the structural changes revealed in this case is similar to that observed in humans.

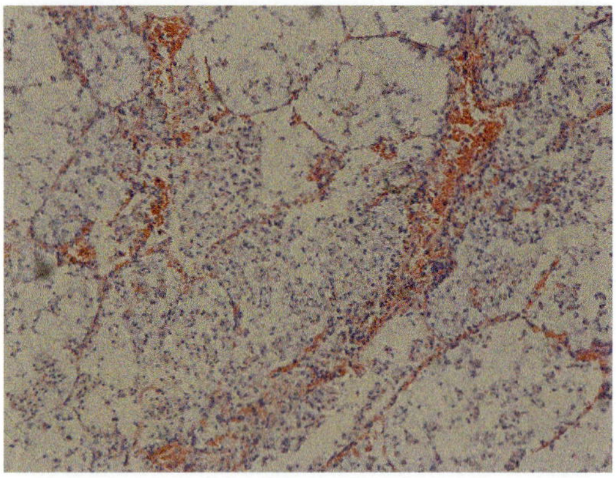

Fig. 12.2 Lung lesion in nosocomial generalized infection due to *Klebsiella pneumoniae*. Stained by azur–eosin × 100

12.2 Hospital Pneumonia Due to Klebsiella

It remains unclear why several decades ago we started to meet nearby Fridländer pneumonia (see Sect. 11.3) a new clinicopathological entity—nosocomial pneumonia. We have also to consider that in reports of postmortem bacteriological investigations are not seldom revealing strains of Klebsiella, to which we are unable to ascribe any pathogenic role. In modern reviews, Klebsiella is astonishingly considered as obligate intracellular pathogen [2], while we see it quite clearly extracellular.

Klebsiella often becomes causative agents of severe hospital infections, most often occurring in the form of pneumonia [4–7]. At the same time, massive reproduction of the rods in various tissues is noted with a minimally expressed predominantly macrophage reaction (Fig. 12.2). In some observations, there were generalized lesions of many organs (hospital sepsis) with a very significant number of pathogens detected with minimal tissue reaction (Fig. 12.2). Performed by L.A. Berezina study under the co-guidance of V.A. Zinserling study showed that significant differences in the clinical and morphological manifestations of klebsiellosis in different observations may depend on the cytotoxicity and adhesion of the strains caused by in-hospital 40 MD and 55 MD plasmids [5].

12.3 Proteus Pneumonia

The disease is caused by various species of the genus Proteus (*P. rettgeri*, *P. mirabilis*). These are usually straight rods, which can take on a cocciform or filiform shape, are mobile due to peritrichous flagella.

Proteosis is rarely diagnosed, although apparently its value is underestimated. There are practically no detailed descriptions of structural changes in this disease. The most complete descriptions were made by A.V. Zinserling [5].

Macroscopically, lung proteosis has the character of small focal pneumonia. Its foci are of moderate density, with a smooth cut surface, grayish-red in the center and red along the periphery.

Microscopically, at the very early stages of the development of such pneumonia in the distal airways and alveoli, serous hemorrhagic exudate with an admixture of gradually accumulating leukocytes and macrophages is detected (Fig. 12.3). This exudate contains a significant amount of rather polymorphic rods, some of which are phagocytosed by leukocytes and macrophages. Sometimes among this exudate, individual fibrin strands are detected. It is typical that both exudate cells and the lung tissue itself undergo necrosis by the type of lysis (Fig. 12.4).

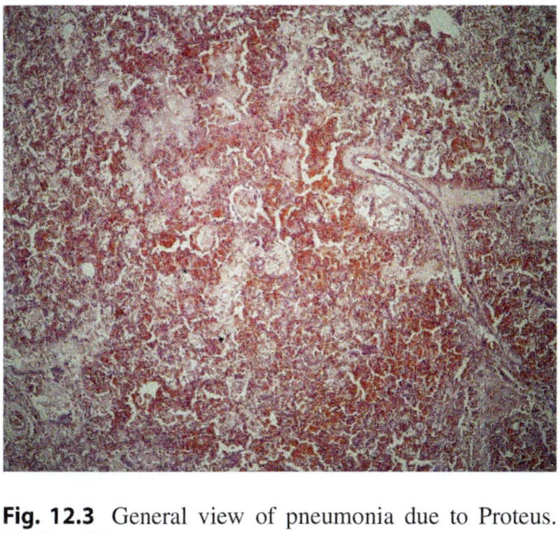

Fig. 12.3 General view of pneumonia due to Proteus. H.-E. ×100

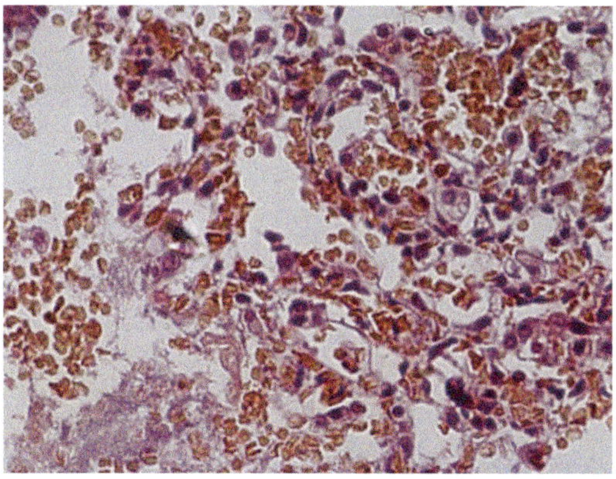

Fig. 12.4 Detail of the same preparation. ×400

12.4 Pneumonia Caused by Pathogenic Escherichia

They are mainly observed as a complication of intestinal coli infection in newborns due to intracanalicular generalization during vomiting. In recent decades, deaths from this form of pneumonia have not been observed. The materials of previous years are most fully observed by A.V. Zinserling [5].

Macroscopically, lung damage has the character of small pneumonic foci, mainly gray–red in color, with a smooth, moist cut surface. They are more often located in the posterior parts of the lungs and are not clearly distinguished from the surrounding air lung tissue.

Microscopic examination at the very early stages of development has only massive contamination of the respiratory organs with microbes, among which there is a sharp predominance of Escherichia. In the trachea and bronchi, there is a violation of the connection between the cells of the epithelium and its desquamation. In about 1/4 of the observations, single Escherichia is determined in the cytoplasm of individual cells. In the bronchi, and often in the alveoli, there are individual cells or layers of desquamated cylindrical, and sometimes flat epithelium, as well as plant particles. This clearly shows the importance of aspiration in this form of pneumonia. Later, serous exudate with an admixture of individual macrophages and neutrophils is gradually sweated to the locations of microbes.

Subsequently, an accumulation of neutrophilic white blood cells occurs in the lungs. At this stage of the development of the process, a relatively homogeneous leukocyte exudate with an admixture of single macrophages predominates. Its distinguishing feature is its "friability." Necrosis of neither exudate cells nor lung tissue associated with exposure to Escherichia is observed. Sometimes in these foci, there is a small amount of serous fluid. In the cytoplasm of neutrophils and macrophages, phagocytosis rods are detected.

With a longer course of pneumonia, areas with rarefied exudate and a predominance of macrophages were found in it, free microbes no longer existed.

The character of structural changes in the lungs of children was in principle consistent with the description of the lesions that developed in the lungs of experimental mice when they were infected with pathogenic *Escherichia coli* [5].

12.5 Lung Gangrene

This disease is characterized by the breakdown of organ tissue as a result of the action of putrefactive bacteria, primarily spirochetes. Under the influence of these bacteria, protein substances are cleaved to form peptones, biogenic amines, phenol, skatol, and other toxic substances.

The main predisposing factor for the development of gangrene is a change in reactivity, associated primarily with hypovitaminosis C. With a sharp deterioration in the living conditions of the population during wars, periods of significant increase in diseases of fusospirochetal gangrene were observed. So, according to autopsy materials, their frequency in 1919 was 10%, while until 1914 it was only 0.5% [8].

However, it should be noted that in sieged Leningrad, the frequency of lung gangrene on autopsy material remained low [9].

For all gangrenous processes, regardless of their localization according to V.D. Zinserling, certain macro- and microscopic features are characteristic, allowing to distinguish three variants of fusospirochetosis: (1) progressive; (2) fibrinous necrotic, and (3) transitional.

The first of them is the most typical and characterizes the entire group of infectious gangrene. This form is characterized by a tendency to a progressive, sometimes uncontrollable course with a blackish, ragged, often extensive decay or fusion of tissue with a very strong specific gangrene odor. Tissue necrosis is detected, often without signs of reaction along its periphery: the border of healthy tissue is indicated only by the appearance of the color of the nuclei. In other cases, a more or less pronounced lymphocytic leukocyte shaft is detected. The tissue is flooded with huge masses of various bacteria, among which the main place is spirochete, which accumulates in large quantities in the marginal parts of necrosis and penetrates deeply, as a rule in pure culture, into the edematous tissue surrounding the necrosis. In second place is a spindle-shaped rod, accumulating in large quantities on the border of necrosis. Further, filamentous bacteria and various uncharacteristic forms, which occupy the first place in the surface layers of necrosis, join the indicated two microbial forms. Similar very progressive forms of gangrene, in addition to their typical and well-known representatives in the form of gangrenous stomatitis such as noma (from the Greek nome—spread around the circumference, erosion) and lung gangrene, were also observed in the ear, intestines, and genitals.

From the described progressive form of infectious gangrene to two other variants, there are gradual transitions, characterized primarily by a lesser spread of necrosis, the presence of a pronounced reactive lymphocytic—leukocyte shaft and the emergence of *Bacillus fusiformis* and other bacteria in the foreground.

With the expressed second variant of fusospirochetosis, the process can even lose its gangrenous character, expressed only in the form of fibrinous inflammation with a sharp reaction from the underlying tissues, while characteristic necrosis may be completely absent, like spirochete, which is generally found in these forms of the process in much smaller quantities. Similar forms are characteristic of the mucous membranes in the oral cavity and pharynx. Transitional forms are usually in the form of ulcerative lesions, with a more or less pronounced dirty appearance, smelly, sometimes typical ragged, decay at the bottom of ulcers, especially characteristic of the colon.

It should be noted that both forms of the process can alternate in the same cases with areas of progressive gangrene, with typical unlimited tissue necrosis and masses of spirochetes breaking through the reactive shaft.

The third version of the process is the transition from typical gangrene to purulent inflammation of the usual form. Such gangrenous-purulent processes on the mucous membranes cannot be delimited from the transitional forms mentioned above, differing only in a more purulent character. This purulent character of the process is even better expressed in cases of fusospirochetosis infection of the cavities, for example, the middle ear, caverns in the lungs, etc. The purulent process in such cases has a specific smell and usually a dirty brownish color of purulent masses. Spirochete in these cases takes less part in the process, without penetrating into the surrounding tissue.

However, with a progressive form of the course, even with a pronounced purulent nature of the inflammation, spirochete is of predominant importance, penetrating far into normal tissue.

All gangrenous processes, despite their different localization and forms, should be combined into a special nosological group of diseases "fusospirochetosis," the main feature of which is the constant presence of the same bacterial forms, and the relationship between the anatomical features of the process and bacteriological findings is noteworthy, which indicates the undoubted importance of these bacteria in the etiology of gangrene. For the development of a progressive type of gangrene, spirochetes are of particular importance. The therapeutic effect of the action of salvarsan on the gangrenous process also supports this view. *B. fusiformis* most likely has the value of a symbiont needed for spirochetes, maybe it paves the way for the latter, producing an initial tissue disruption.

The predominance of *B. fusiformis* entails a more limited nature of the lesion, up to the complete disappearance of typical necrosis; on the contrary, spirochete and reactive lymphocytic leukemia seem to be mutually exclusive.

The role of *B. fusiformis* in the development of gangrenous processes can, apparently, sometimes be played by forms similar to commas (kommabacillen). However, there are no reasons to ascribe to threadlike forms great importance in the development of infectious gangrene with a mixed infection with pyogenic cocci, when the latter comes to the fore, the process takes on a purulent character. It is possible that a mixed infection with this kind of bacteria has an inhibitory effect on the development of gangrenous processes, causing a sharp inflammatory reaction from the tissues.

The most important of the predisposing moments is hunger in combination with vitamin deficiency.

In recent years, lung gangrene has also been detected extremely rarely, mainly on the material of military pathologists.

Macroscopically in typical cases of pulmonary gangrene, usually a single large focus is found, occupying a large portion of the lobe. In the case of attachment of gangrene to pneumonia, the gangrenous focus is located in the central part of the hepatized lobe, most often the lower. Changes are characterized, first of all, by the decay of tissue, acquiring a blackish, greenish, or brownish tint. The lesion produces a sharp nauseating smell. Subsequently, a cavity is formed at this place containing greenish—or brownish-black rag-like decaying masses.

Microscopic examination at the initial stages of the process reveals granular decomposition of the tissue, in the areas in which drops of fat, crystals of fatty acids, leucine, and tyrosine are detected. The argyrophilic framework gradually disappears, and even later elastic fibers are destroyed. These areas gradually turn into edematous tissue (Fig. 12.5). With less rapid progression of the process, one can see a shaft of neutrophils and macrophages. The lesion focus contains a huge number of microbes, the main place among which is occupied by spirochetes. They are determined both in necrotic tissue (especially in peripheral areas) and penetrate far

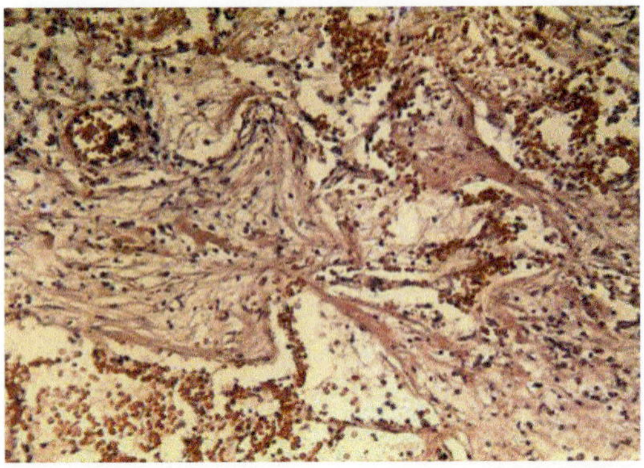

Fig. 12.5 Lung gangrene H.-E. ×100

into the surrounding edematous tissue. The spread of the process depends on the active introduction of spirochetes into tissues, which occurs especially easily in those that are poor in blood vessels.

Propagation of this species of spirochetes and their distribution throughout the tissues is possible only in the absence of a normal inflammatory, in particular leukocyte, reaction. With the intensification of the inflammatory process, the progression of gangrene stops, the pathogen disappears; the lesion is delimited by the cell shaft. With further progression of the disease, granulation tissue develops around foci of necrosis. Later, its maturation occurs, at this stage, the process becomes similar to fibrinous-cavernous pulmonary tuberculosis.

It is believed that the condition conducive to the development of lung gangrene is preliminary tissue necrosis, which, when the mycosis settles, undergoes putrefactive decay and passes into gangrene. This may be important for the reproduction of microbes at the beginning of the process, but is not mandatory and does not play a role in the further development of gangrene. The closure of the lumen of the bronchi during the organization of fibrinous exudate due to the deterioration of aeration can contribute to its occurrence and progression.

The instability of spirochetes in the body is also indicated by their death when they enter the bloodstream. In this regard, metastatic gangrenous lesions practically do not occur.

12.6 Other Pathogens Producing Pneumonia Especially in Immunosuppressed Host

There are data related to the possibility of other microorganisms to cause lung lesions: nocardia, rhodococcus, tropheryma whiplei, and others seem to be extremely rare and never diagnosed in our practice.

References

1. Wilson MG, Pandey S. Pseudomonas aeruginosa Stat Pearls. Treasure Island (FL): Stat pears Publishing; 2020. PMID 32491763.
2. FitzGerald ES, Luz NF, Jamieson AM. Competitive cell death interactions in pulmonary infection: host modulation versus pathogen manipulation. Front Immunol. 2020;11:814. https://doi.org/10.3389/fimmu.20.00814.
3. Krasnogorsky IN, Indikova MG, Zinserling VF, Boykov SG. Pathologic anatomy of pseudomonas infection in children. Arkh Patol. 1983;(10):9–14.
4. Leslie KO, Wick MR, editors. Practical pulmonary pathology. A diagnostic approach. 2nd ed. 2011. 828 p.
5. Zinserling AV, Zinserling VA. Modern infections: pathologic anatomy and issues of pathogenesis: a guide. SPb: Sotis; 2002. 346 p. (In Russian).
6. Kradin RL, editor. Diagnostic pathology of infectious diseases. Elsevier; 2018. 698p.
7. Zinserling VA, Boikov SG, Leenman EE, et al. Modern Klebsiellla pneumonia. Arkh Patol. 1991;(9):22–27. (In Russian).
8. Zinserling WD. Über die fuso-spirochätose Gangrän und einige verwandte Prozesse, vorzugsweiose bei Kindern. Jena. 1928.
9. Bazan OI. Pathology service in sieged Leningrad. Scientific analysis and reminiscence of specialist. 2nd ed. Moskwa, "Prakticheskaya meditsina"; 2020. 159 p. (In Russian).

13 Tuberculosis and Other Mycobacteriosis

13.1 General Considerations. The Role of Pathology in the Study of Tuberculosis

The first paleopathological findings associated with tuberculosis date back to 5000 BC. In the ancient world, up to seven synonyms of this disease were used. Already in Ancient Greece in the writings of Pericles, Homer, Aristotle, its manifestations were described, and its infectiousness was assumed. In the works of Paracelsus (1493–1541), lesions of internal organs were described, and Francis Silvius in 1650 first described tubercle in the lungs and other internal organs, in 1700 the term "miliary tuberculosis" was first used. The macroscopic changes described by many pathologists of the 17th–19th centuries in different organs were so diverse that the idea of tuberculosis as a single disease developed only in the works of Laennec and Schönlein in the middle of the 19th century. Subsequently, the outstanding pathologists Carl von Rokitansky and Rudolf Virchow made the greatest contribution to the study of structural changes in tuberculosis.

It is impossible to list all pathologists who were actively studying morphological changes and pathogenesis of tuberculosis. These were Buhl, Schüppel, Orth, Birch-Hirschfeld, Ghon, Ranke, Vorvald, Sweaney, Rich, Abrikosov, Strukov, Puzik, Shtefko, Ariel, Mandelstam, Raskina, Solovieva, Erokhin, Chistovich, and many others. Variants of structural changes in tuberculosis in different organs were described in detail, proposed pathogenetic concepts related primarily to allergic rearrangement of the body, several morphological classifications were specified later. There was a firm belief that the diagnosis of tuberculosis is based on the identification of "specific" changes by morphological methods. At the same time, significant progress in the methods of microbiological and molecular biological diagnostics of mycobacteriosis has led to their widespread adoption in everyday clinical practice, which significantly reduced the diagnostic role of morphological studies. In many modern fundamental manuals on phthisiology, even the section "morphological diagnostics" is missing; it is not even mentioned in many documents regulating the work of the TB service.

The tasks facing pathology in tuberculosis, in our opinion, can be divided into 4 groups, namely, (1) specification of approaches for the detection of mycobacteria in Tissues; (2) optimization of postmortem diagnosis of tuberculosis; (3) optimization of intravital differential diagnosis of tuberculosis and the development of methods for predicting its course; and (4) the study of the pathogenesis of tuberculosis in the light of modern ideas about the infectious process.

1. Clarification of approaches for the detection of mycobacteria in tissues

   Obviously, the morphological diagnosis of tuberculosis must necessarily include the

V. Zinserling, *Infectious Pathology of the Respiratory Tract*,
https://doi.org/10.1007/978-3-030-66325-4_13

detection of mycobacteria in the tissues. In the 1980s of the 19th century, Franz Ziehl (1857–1926) and Friedrich Neelsen (1854–1898) proposed the famous technique that allows the detection of acid-resistant mycobacteria both in smears and paraffin sections. In the case of detection of acid-resistant rods in relatively large quantities, everything is relatively simple. Despite its popularity, its numerous modifications are currently being used, none of which completely satisfy the researchers. Perhaps it is the reason, we were not able to find in the classical works on the pathology of tuberculosis a detailed histobacterioscopic evaluation of the pathogen.

However, when evaluating the results of this staining, one has to face several significant difficulties. So, in cases of indisputable tuberculosis, including those confirmed by PCR, acid-resistant bacilli may not be detected at all or only a very small amount with a repeated review of slices.

Despite the presence in the literature information about cocciform and not staining red according to Z-N forms of mycobacteria, this question is almost not considered by morphologists, and the negative results of staining of the slices are explained by the technological faults. The work of many researchers provides data on the negative results of detecting acid-resistant rods, even in cases of indisputable tuberculosis. In the literature, there are indications on the diagnostic value of single small cocciform Z-N-positive structures, and the reliability of the interpretation is based on the identification of single positive granules that are detected by immunohistochemical studies with a serum to antigens of mycobacterium tuberculosis complex. In addition, we should not forget that IHC is used mainly in research works and there are only a few publications with its use in diagnostic work [1]. In microbiological practice, luminescent microscopy with staining of smears with auramine–rhodamine has been used for quite a long time. There are only a few studies devoted to the analysis of the use of this method on paraffin sections. According to our data related to autopsy cases of fibro-cavernous TB when stained with auramine–rhodamine, the number of mycobacteria detected was significantly higher than by Z-N, and it was the largest during an IHC study [2, 3]. The localization of mycobacteria was exclusively extracellular. The proportion of typical rods when stained according to Z-N (88.13 ± 2.14), when stained with auramine–rhodamine (64.38 ± 4.24), when IHC (57.29 ± 2.78).

Substantial clinical and epidemiological clarification of the species and genotype of mycobacteria is also of importance. In world practice, for several decades, PCR research has been carried out, including formalin-fixed and paraffin-embedded tissues, to identify "atypical" mycobacteria: avium/intracellulare, kansasii, fortuitum, and others. Recently, several reports have appeared on the role of nontuberculous mycobacteria in the etiology of life-threatening lesions in HIV infection. Clinical and morphological manifestations of tuberculosis and nontuberculous mycobacteriosis in AIDS are very close. There are only indications that for the most common causative agent of nontuberculous mycobacteriosis (avium/intracellulare), the intracellular location of a large number of pathogens is more characteristic.

2. Optimization of Postmortem Diagnosis of Tuberculosis

Among both phthisiatricians and pathologists, the most common point of view is that the postmortem diagnosis of tuberculosis is relatively simple, which in typical observations, of course, is true. Unfortunately, a detailed analysis of mortality from tuberculosis, including the morphological characterization of the changes at autopsy, is not carried anywhere, and they say with satisfaction that clinical and pathological diagnoses in almost all cases coincide. However, it should be noted that in the vast majority of observations of tuberculosis, especially in combination with HIV infection, even with a formal coincidence of the pathological and clinical diagnosis, the latter is almost always specified and supplemented, often very significantly. In addition, current forms of tuberculosis cannot be adequately characterized using existing classifications. The reasons for this phenomenon are not entirely clear. The possibilities for the clinical diagnosis of tuberculous lesions of the liver, intestines, spleen, kidneys, thyroid gland, and adrenal glands are limited.

Cases of clinical hyperdiagnosis of tuberculosis are much less frequently analyzed. Without a doubt in some cases, the lifetime diagnosis of tuberculosis (especially with a question mark) in cases with HIV is not based on any objective data and it is assumed only due to their frequent combination. In addition, in single observations, we had to deal with such combinations of secondary infections that simulated both a radiological and a macroscopic picture of tuberculosis.

3. Optimization of lifetime differential diagnosis of tuberculosis and the development of methods for predicting its course. With HIV infection in the AIDS stage, it is often a matter of generalized forms of the disease with the widespread nature of the lesions, the diagnosis of which, especially by biopsy and surgical material, is extremely difficult due to the atypical microscopic picture, which is dominated by alterative changes without typical cellular and tissue reactions, in many cases, the diagnosis needs staining according to the Z-N method, which allows us to recommend it for wider use. However, it should be remembered that tuberculosis cannot be excluded even with its negative results, PCR remains the only reference method in such cases.
4. The study of the pathogenesis of tuberculosis in the light of modern views on the infectious process.

Classical ideas about the pathogenesis of tuberculosis are based on basic research mainly performed in the first half of the 20th century. Modern studies on the mechanisms of the development of this disease are based mainly on the study of the interaction of mycobacteria with cell cultures. Thus, one of the interested parties—host with different constitutional features, premorbid background, and immune status, completely disappears from the field of view, infinitely devaluating such studies. Many aspects of modern concepts of the pathogenesis of tuberculosis are controversial and require clarification.

Particular attention is paid to the "Beijing" strain (genotype B), which has been known since the 1990s as a W strain, identified in the USA, which has drug resistance and pronounced pathogenic properties. According to the results of a study conducted in the city of Irkutsk on the material of autopsies, this genotype was detected in 65% of cases, causing significant structural changes [4].

Another practically not discussed problem is that of mixed infections. In cases of tuberculosis combined with HIV infection this is quite obvious, in other clinical situations, the search for non-tuberculosis pathogens in patients with tuberculosis is practically not carried out. At the same time, our experience in the study of surgical, biopsy, and autopsy materials in many cases allows us to speak about the presence of lesions in the tissues associated with both DNA and RNA containing viruses, mycoplasmas, chlamydia, and fungi. The clinical significance of such coinfections is not always indisputable, but, of course, needs further comprehensive study. With HIV infection, observations are observed on our material with the simultaneous presence of many infections. Although it is obvious that all of them must somehow interact with each other, there is no evidence in this regard.

Speaking about the properties of the host, it should be remembered that along with the level of immunocompetent cells in the peripheral blood, local resistance and constitutional properties also belong to them. There are relatively few morphological studies aimed at local resistance of the respiratory tract, and with tuberculosis, such approaches were almost never used.

In our opinion, the results of molecular biological studies on the interaction of polymorphic loci of human genes with epidemic strains of *Mycobacterium tuberculosis*, which we obtained as part of the same study in Irkutsk, turned out to be important. Of particular interest was the DC-SIGN (Dendritic Cell-Special Intercellular adhesion molecule-3-Grabbing Non-integrin) gene of position—336A/G, better known as

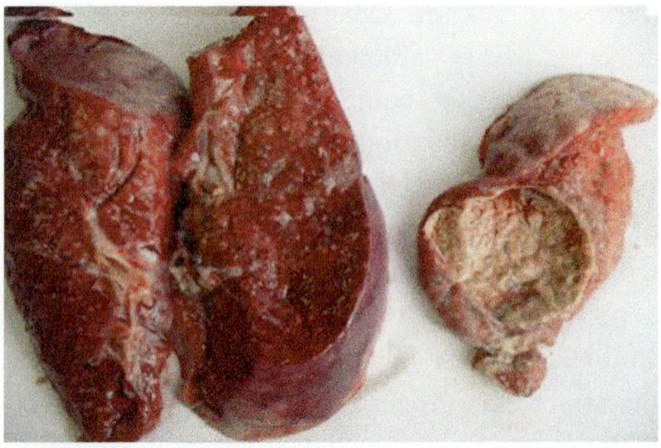

Fig. 13.1 Simultaneous miliary and cavernous changes in the same patient with HIV infection. Lung at the autopsy

CD209, which is responsible for the capture of infect [4]. It was found that in men with the G allele (genotypes AG and GG), the combination with the epidemic strain of genotype B (Beijing) was the most common. In the calculations, it turned out that the probability of developing a fatal outcome in this group, compared with the group of women of any genotype and men of genotype AA, was six times higher, while the odds ratio (OR) = (p = 0.0008, 1.9458–19.923 (95% CI)) [4].

Some facts that are inexplicable by existing concepts of TB pathogenesis also need to be studied (Fig. 13.1). First of all, the existence of isolated lesions of pia mater, vertebral bodies, and so on, in the absence of post-tuberculous changes in the area of a usual primary complex during postmortem examination.

Very promising are several works on the ability of mycobacteria to form biofilms, including in conjunction with other microorganisms [5]. Unfortunately, these studies, performed at the modern molecular biological level, lack comparisons with histobacterioscopy data.

13.2 Pathology of Lung Tuberculosis Without Immunodeficiency

The data presented in this chapter are partly based upon experiences of Russian phtisiopathology scientific school [6–8], partly own long-term experience of one of the authors (Yu. R. Zyuzya).

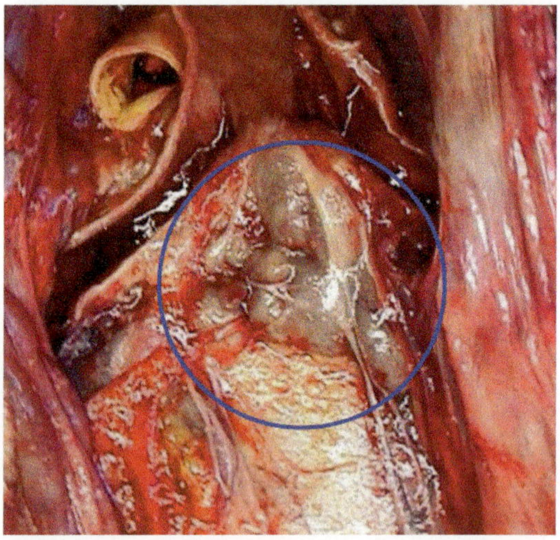

Fig. 13.2 Hyperplasia of intrathoracic bifurcation lymph nodes (circled). Unfixed macropreparation

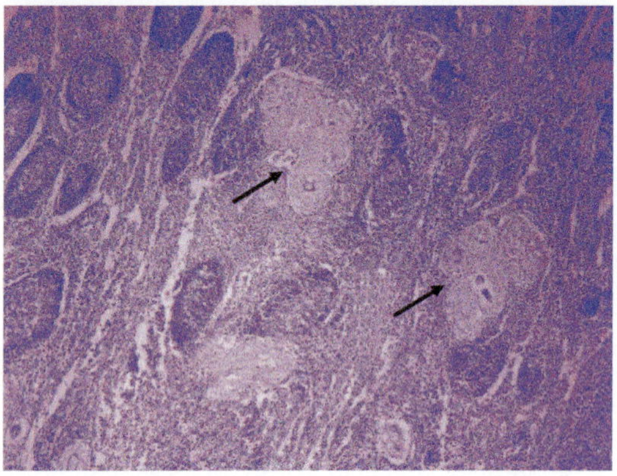

Fig. 13.3 Tuberculous granulomatous lymphadenitis (granulomas are indicated by arrows). H.-E. ×100

Tuberculosis of the intrathoracic lymph nodes: A form of primary tuberculosis, which is characterized by damage to various groups of lymph nodes, more often—tracheobronchial and bronchopulmonary groups. When primary infection by MBT occurs, the lymph nodes became hyperplastic (Fig. 13.2), tuberculous granulomas form in them (Fig. 13.3). The progression of tuberculosis leads to the replacement of the lymph node tissue by merging granulomas with areas of caseous necrosis and the formation of extensive necrotic foci with the formation of subtotal and total caseous lymphadenitis (Fig. 13.4).

Granulomatous inflammation can develop in the pleura, bronchi, and adjacent areas of the

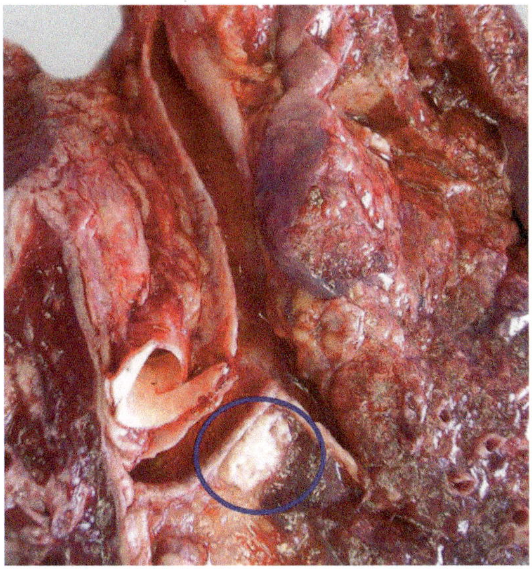

Fig. 13.4 Tuberculous total caseous lymphadenitis of intrathoracic bifurcation lymph nodes (circled). Non-fixed macro specimens

lung, the formation of bronchodilator fistulas takes place, esophageal–nodular fistulas are less common (Fig. 13.5). Suppuration and sequestration of necrotic masses in caseous lymphadenitis leads to the formation of lympho-glandular (lymphogenous) tuberculous caverns (Fig. 13.6). One of the most serious complications of caseous lymphadenitis of the intrathoracic lymph nodes is caseous mediastinitis, which develops when caseous masses are breaking into the mediastinal tissue. The enlarged lymph nodes, squeezing large bronchi, lead to the formation of segmental and lobar atelectasis of the lungs. In patients with immunosuppressive conditions, bronchogenic dissemination, lymphogenous, and hematogenous generalization of tuberculosis can be observed.

A manifestation of TB activity in the intrathoracic lymph nodes is also the development of the so-called paraspecific reaction. It is caused by the

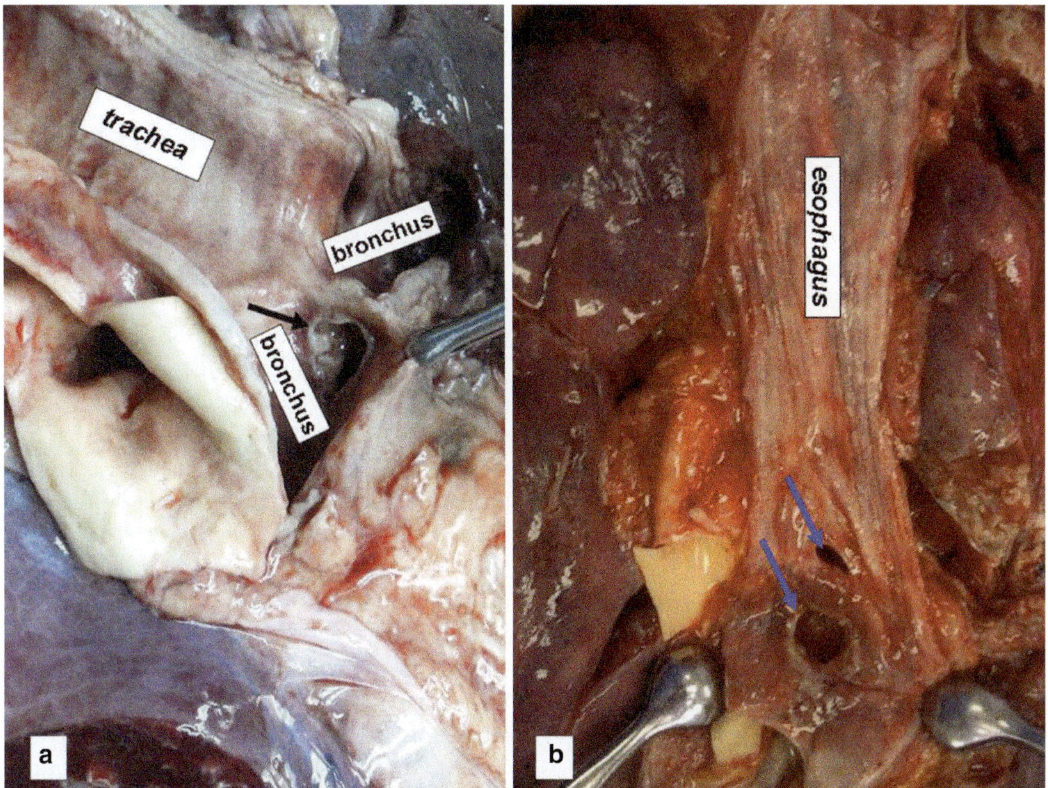

Fig. 13.5 Fistulas in tuberculosis caseous lymphadenitis of the intrathoracic lymph nodes: (**a**) Bronchonodular fistula; (**b**) esophageal–nodular fistulas. Non-fixed macropreparations (fistula mouths are indicated by arrows)

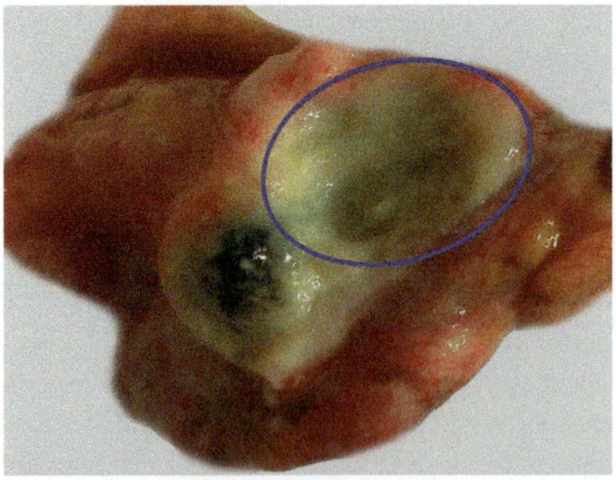

Fig. 13.6 Lymphogenic cavern of the intrathoracic lymph node (circled). Non-fixed macro specimens

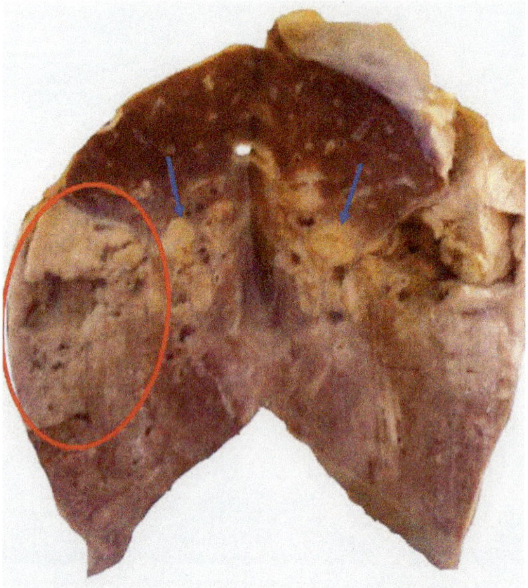

Fig. 13.7 Primary tuberculosis complex. The primary tuberculous affect of the lung is caseous segmentitis with a developing decay cavity (circled). Caseous bronchadenitis—total caseous lymphadenitis of regional (intrathoracic) lymph nodes (indicated by arrows). Fixed macropreparation

action of the MB antigen, but morphologically has the form of nonspecific inflammation, which develops in the pleura, perinodular fatty tissue, adjacent bronchi, blood vessels, and lung sites. The "paraspecific" reaction is histologically manifested by edema, plethora, lymphoid, and lymphoid–leukocyte infiltration, in the alveoli there is serous, macrophagous, fibrinous exudate.

Favorable outcomes of tuberculosis of the intrathoracic lymph nodes include fibrosis, hyalinosis, and calcification of necrotic masses.

Primary tuberculosis complex (Ranvier complex): The most severe form of primary tuberculosis, which develops when the host encounters an infection for the first time. Exudative–necrotic changes predominate, a tendency to hematogenous and lymphogenous generalization is noted, "paraspecific" reactions in the form of vasculitis, arthritis, polyserositis, and erythema nodosum are expressed. The respiratory organs are most often affected, although there are cases of primary tuberculosis complex of the intestine and skin.

Three components of the primary tuberculosis complex are distinguished namely, primary tuberculous affect (focus), tuberculous lymphangitis, and tuberculous lymphadenitis of the regional lymph nodes.

In 95% of cases, the primary tuberculosis complex develops in the lungs, with the aerogenic transmission of infection. The most typical localization of the process is the third segment (S3) of the right lung, with a subpleural location of the lesion. In addition, foci can be formed in SS 8, 9, and 10.

At the site of introduction of MBT into the lung tissue, when they multiply, a focus of inflammation develops, which spreads first to several alveoli, then to the adjacent respiratory bronchioles. Initially, inflammation has a serous or serous-fibrinous nature of the exudate, subsequently giving way to a "specific" phase with the development of caseous necrosis. When a large number of alveoli are involved in the process, primary pulmonary affect is formed in the form of acinous or lobular tuberculous (caseous) pneumonia (depending on the extent of the lesion—acinus, lobule) (Fig. 13.7).

The inflammatory process from the focus extends to the regional lymph nodes along the lymphatic paths in the interlobular septa, peribronchial, and perivascular. Along the lymphatic vessels, tuberculous lymphangitis is formed (Fig. 13.8).

Subsequently, regional bronchopulmonary lymph nodes with the development of subtotal

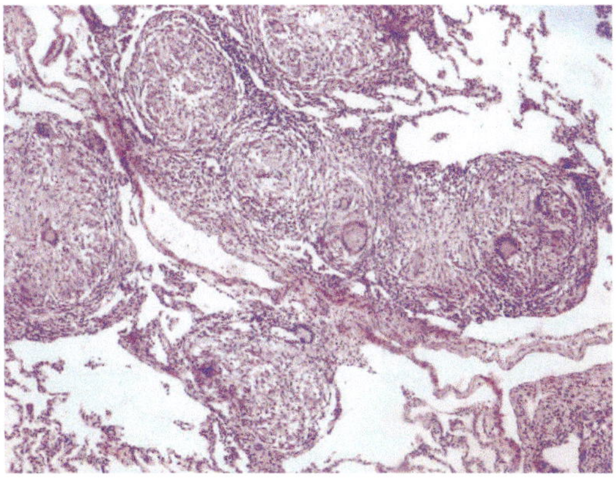

Fig. 13.8 Tuberculous lymphangitis. H.-E. ×100

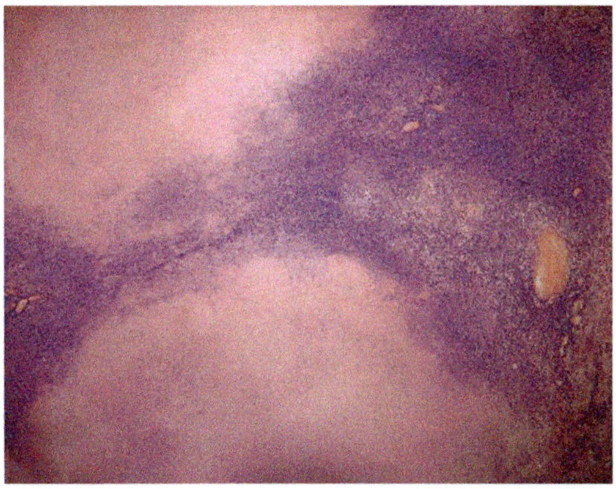

Fig. 13.9 Tuberculous caseous lymphadenitis. H.-E. ×100

and total tuberculous caseous lymphadenitis are involved in the infectious process (Fig. 13.9).

It is believed that with the aerogenic pathway of infection, MBT can penetrate through the intact mucous membrane of the bronchus into the peribronchial lymphatic plexuses and then into the intrathoracic lymph nodes. It is also considered a possible retrograde pathway with the spread of inflammation from the lymph node to the bronchial wall, followed by the penetration of MBT into the lung tissue and the formation of caseous necrosis.

The favorable outcomes include the healing of the process, and the adverse ones include progression and its chronic course.

During the healing of primary tuberculous affect, the perifocal exudate is resorbed with encapsulation, compaction, fibrosis, hyalinosis, and calcification of caseous masses (Fig. 13.10). The use of metaplasia in the organized focus of caseous necrosis can form bone tissue—ossification (Fig. 13.11). Organized primary tuberculous affect is called the focus of Gohn. The outcome of tuberculous lymphangitis is perivascular and peribronchial fibrosis. In the lymph nodes, the organization process is much slower, with an outcome in calcifications.

The progression of the primary tuberculosis complex develops in several ways, namely, hematogenous generalization (early, late), lympho-glandular (lymphogenous) generalization, growth of primary affect, and mixed forms.

For the progression, hematogenous generalization is the main characteristic. For early generalization, a large focal nature of dissemination is characteristic; it usually develops in the presence of an "active" primary affect. The foci of dissemination in various organs can be single and multiple. Screenings in various organs formed during generalization of the primary tuberculosis complex may subsequently play a role in the development of extrapulmonary tuberculosis. Early hematogenous screenings at the tops of the lungs are called foci of Simon. Unlike the foci of Gohn, they are usually symmetrical and multiple.

The late generalization of the primary tuberculosis complex is characterized by the presence of signs of organization in the focus of primary tuberculous affect and the miliary dissemination. Late hematogenous miliary generalization can occur with a small dimension of primary affect and its identification is very problematic.

During lymphogenous generalization, in addition to bronchopulmonary generalization, various groups of lymph nodes with the development of caseous lymphadenitis are involved in the tuberculosis process. With massive caseous bronchadenitis due to pronounced tuberculous changes in the vessels of the root zone of the lung and mediastinal tissue, massive bleeding may develop.

Another way of progressing the primary tuberculosis complex is increasing primary affect. Decay cavity, the so-called primary pulmonary cavity, can be formed there. In the chronic course of the primary tuberculosis com-

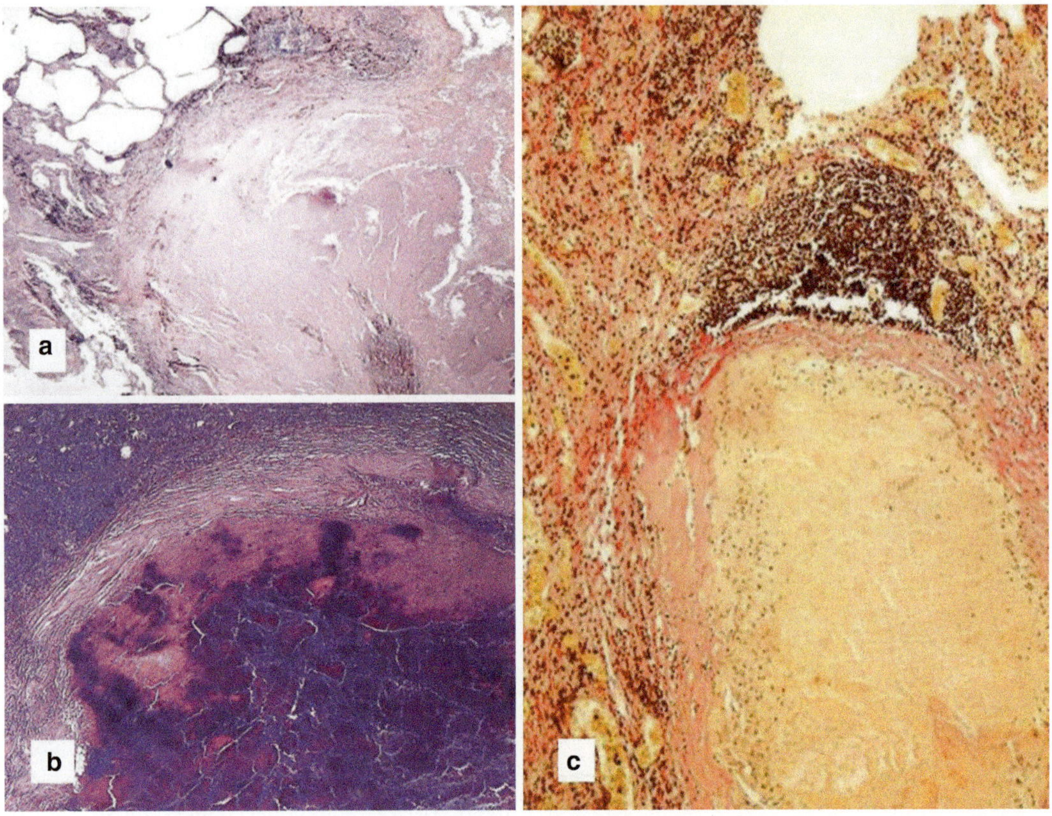

Fig. 13.10 The organization of the caseous tuberculous lesions. (**a**) Hyalinosis; (**b**) Calcification of necrotic masses; and (**c**) Encapsulation of the focus of caseous necrosis. (**a**, **b**) H.-E. and (**c**) van Gieson staining. ×100

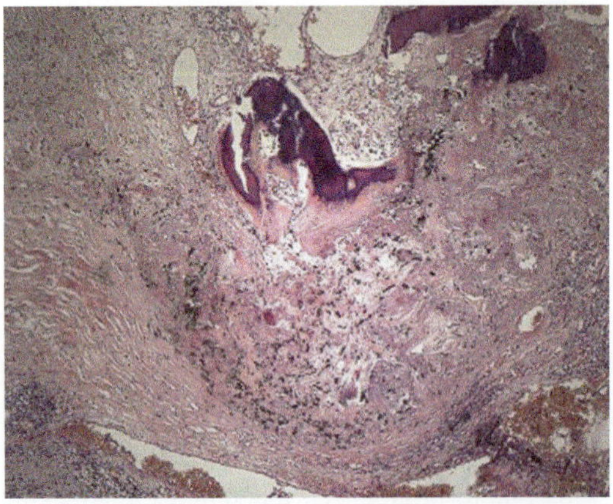

Fig. 13.11 Organization of the focus of tuberculosis inflammation. Ossification in a sclerosed necrosis site. H.-E. ×200

plex, a fibrous capsule forms around and the cavity acquires the structure of a chronic tuberculous cavity in the presence of caseous bronchadenitis.

Mixed forms of progression are usually noted with the presence of two or three of its variants (hematogenous, lymphogenous generalization, and growth of primary affect).

Adverse outcomes include the chronic course of the primary tuberculosis complex. With a healed primary affect, the tuberculous process in the lymph nodes comes to the fore. The course of tuberculous caseous lymphadenitis takes a slowly progressing course, with alternating exacerbations and remissions, the gradual involvement of new groups of lymph nodes.

The chronic course of the primary tuberculosis complex is accompanied by reactive "paraspecific" changes, which include polyserositis, vasculitis, nodular skin erythema, myocarditis, and rheumatism (rheumatoid) Ponce.

The disseminated form of pulmonary tuberculosis includes all varieties of the disease, which occurs with a predominance of dissemination phenomena over other manifestations of the tuberculosis process, combines processes of various genesis that developed as a result of the spread of MBT through the hematogenous, bronchogenic, and lymphogenous pathways.

The disseminated form of pulmonary tuberculosis can develop from the very beginning as an independent form and can also be a manifestation of the progression of any other form of tuberculosis (e.g., dissemination in the lungs in the presence of a chronic tuberculous cavity).

Dissemination in the lungs can be acute, subacute, and chronic. On the localization of foci of dissemination: one or two side process; according to the size of the foci: large focal (diameter of the foci >1 cm), small focal (diameter <1 cm). Separately, a miliary disseminated form of tuberculosis with a foci size of 1–2 mm is distinguished.

In the acute course of disseminated tuberculous in the lungs, multiple yellowish-white foci of caseous necrosis are determined, dissemination can be miliary, large focal, small focal, or of various sizes (from miliary to lobular) (Fig. 13.12). Among the foci of dissemination are distinguished acinous, confluent acinous, lobular, confluent lobular, nodose, and miliary. In large foci, sections of necrotic mass sequestration and decay can form with the formation of decay cavities (acute tuberculous caverns) (Fig. 13.13), there is a zone of exudative inflammation in the form of airless parts of the lung with a fine-grained surface.

Microscopically foci of caseous necrosis are revealed without signs of encapsulation, with leukocyte infiltration of caseous-necrotic masses (Fig. 13.14). Along the edge of necrosis, a mild productive reaction is detected in the form of a small number of epithelioid cells and giant multinucleated cells. The wall of the acute tuberculous cavity has a two-layer structure. The inner layer is purulent–necrotic, consists of caseous-necrotic masses with severe leukocyte infiltration. The outer layer is represented by tissue with pronounced exudative changes, scarce elements of granulomatous inflammation can occur. Signs of organization, for-

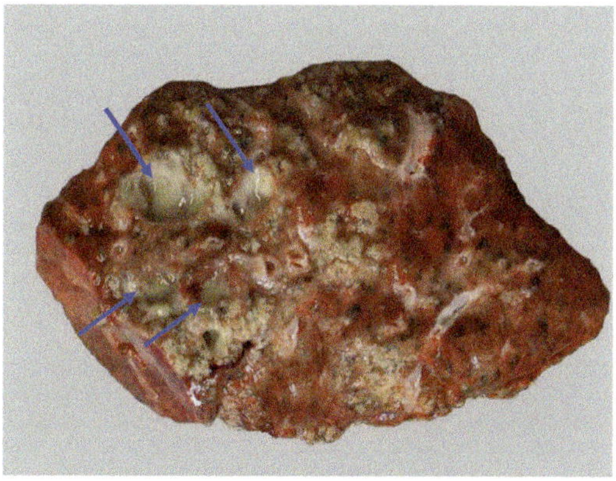

Fig. 13.13 Acute tuberculous cavities of the lung (indicated by arrows). Unfixed macropreparation

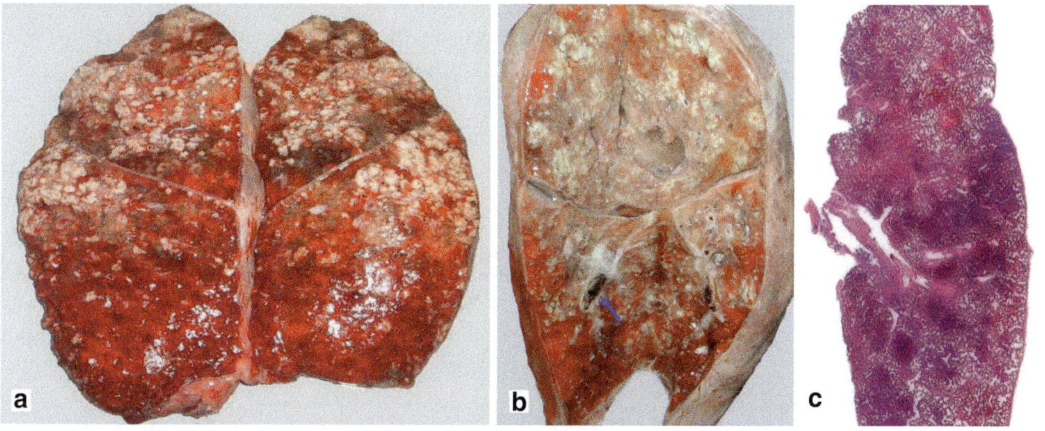

Fig. 13.12 Disseminated form of pulmonary tuberculosis. (**a**) Small-focal dissemination; (**b**, **c**) Large-focal dissemination. (**a**, **b**) Non-fixed macropreparations; (**c**) histotopogram according to Kristeller

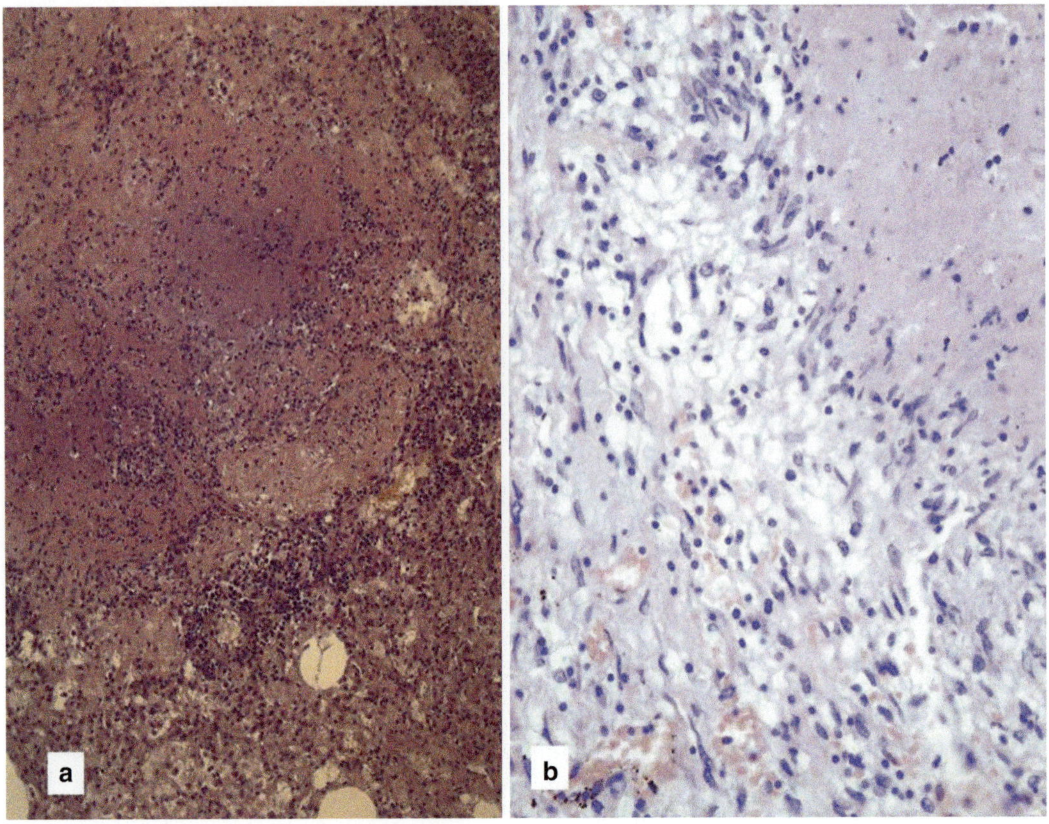

Fig. 13.14 Foci of caseous necrosis, progression of tuberculosis. H.-E. (**a**) ×100 and (**b**) ×400

mation of fibrous elements of the decay cavity wall are not determined (Fig. 13.15). Perifocal and pericavitary pronounced exudative or exudative granulomatous tissue reaction in the form of edema and plethora of vessels of the alveolar septum, serous, serous-fibrinous, and fibrinous-purulent exudate in the lumen. With fibrinous-purulent exudate in the area of perifocal inflammation, there is a need for a morphological differential diagnosis between tuberculosis with perifocal inflammation and a combination of tuberculosis with bacterial pneumonia. The simplest method is Z-N histobacterioscopy. The identification of acid-resistant bacteria in the exudate confirms the tuberculous etiology of the lesions (Fig. 13.16).

The area of perifocal inflammation can many times exceed the size of the focus of caseous necrosis, which increases the volume of lung tissue damage and exacerbates acute respiratory failure.

Acute progression of the tuberculosis process in some cases is complicated by DAD with the formation of parietal hyaline membranes in the lumen of the alveoli (Fig. 13.17).

The acute course of the disseminated form of the disease is characterized by the constant progression of the tuberculous process, due to the extensive damage to the lungs, many foci of destruction, a poorly expressed productive reaction, low activity of reparation, widespread damage to the vascular bed, manifested in the form of vasculitis and thrombovasculitis.

The direct cause of death in patients with massive pulmonary tuberculosis dissemination is the progression of tuberculosis, accompanied by severe intoxication with severe alterative changes in the parenchymal organs and respiratory failure, as well as bleeding from the acute decay cavities, vascular thrombosis with the development of pulmonary infarction.

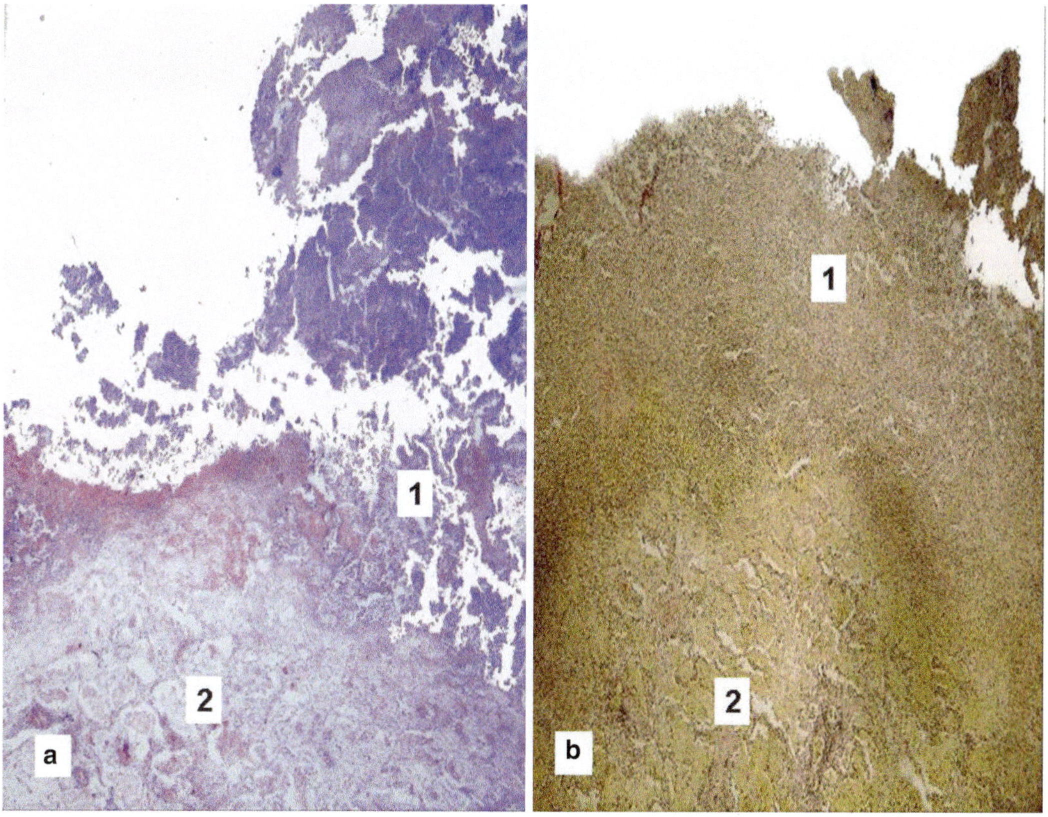

Fig. 13.15 Acute tuberculous cavern. Two-layer structure of the acute cavity wall: 1—purulent–necrotic inner layer; 2—lung tissue with exudative changes, the outer layer. (**a**) H.-E. and (**b**) van Gieson staining. ×100

The subacute course of disseminated pulmonary tuberculosis in the lungs is characterized by the gradual development of signs of disease progression. The phenomena of alteration and exudation are less pronounced, a productive (granulomatous) reaction is detected, and the phenomena of lymphangitis with the involvement of the deep and peripheral lymphatic network of the lung are noted. In addition to foci of tuberculous dissemination, thin-walled subacute and acute tuberculous caverns with a mild perifocal reaction can occur. These caverns are most often located in symmetrical sections of the lung and are called "stamped."

The chronic course of disseminated tuberculous process in the lungs is due to the predominance of hematogenous dissemination and the undulating course of the process. In the lungs, foci of different degrees of activity are determined, the productive nature of inflammation predominates (Figs. 13.18 and 13.19). At the same time, apical–caudal distribution of the process is noted, which is confirmed by more pronounced signs of fibrosis in the foci of the overlying sections, while in the underlying sections, the foci are more recent, without organization phenomena. The predominant lesion of the cortico-pleural and dorsal parts of the upper lobes, due to the manifestations of hemo- and lymphostasis expressed in this zone is characteristic. The process has a bilateral symmetrical character with the involvement of blood and lymph vessels, the development of emphysema, interstitial, peribronchial and perivascular mesh, and focal pneumosclerosis with deformation of the lung tissue. In the lungs, caverns can be found in the form of sharp and subacute decay cavities, including symmetrical (so-called "stamped," "spectacled") caverns (Fig. 13.20).

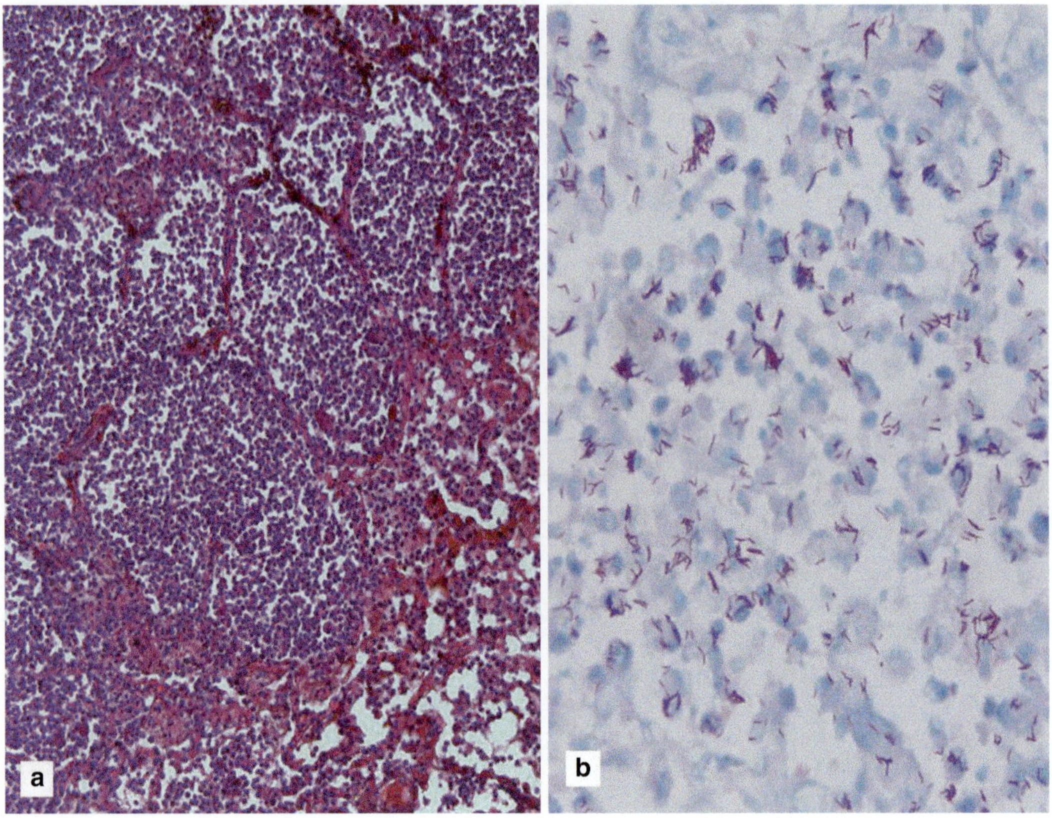

Fig. 13.16 Perifocal exudative reaction. (**a**) In the lumen of the alveoli adjacent to the focus of caseous necrosis, serous-fibrinous and fibrinous-purulent exudate; (**b**) an abundance of acid-resistant bacteria in the perifocal exudate. (**a**) H.-E. ×200 and (**b**) Z-N staining. ×1000

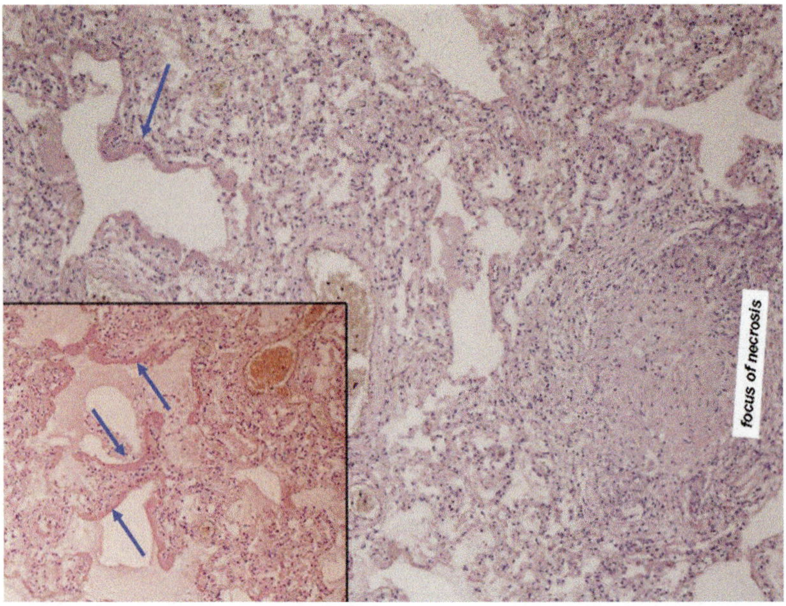

Fig. 13.17 Diffuse alveolar lung injury, acute phase with the formation of hyaline membranes (indicated by arrows) in the progressive tuberculosis process. H.-E. ×200

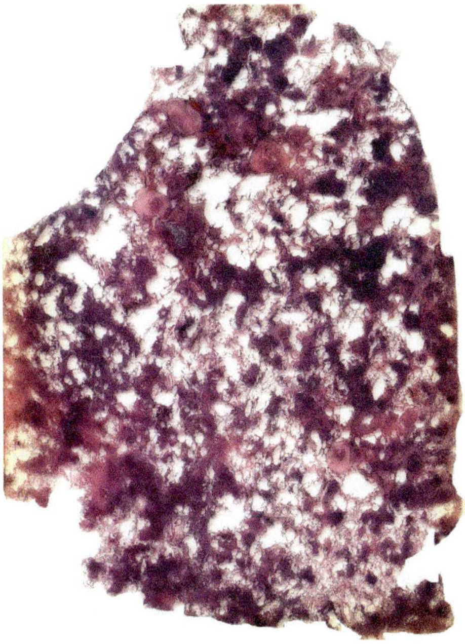

Fig. 13.18 Disseminated pulmonary tuberculosis, chronic course. Multiple acinous and nodous foci of caseous necrosis of various ages. Histotopographic section according to Kristeller

The chronic course of disseminated pulmonary tuberculosis is characterized by the development of pulmonary hypertension and the formation of a "pulmonary heart." The causes of death in a chronic course are usually decompensation of the chronic pulmonary heart, progres-

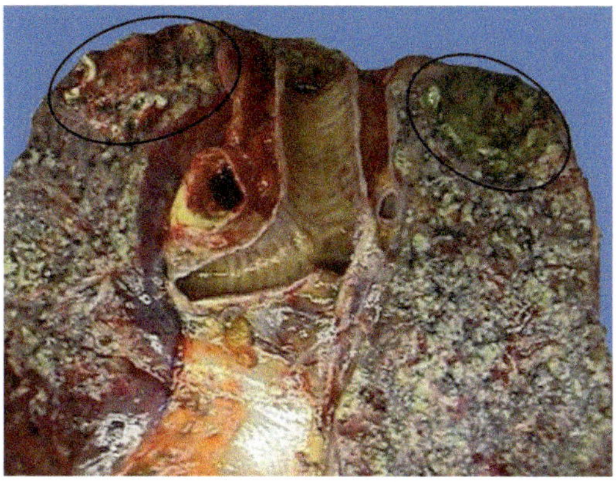

Fig. 13.20 Disseminated tuberculosis, chronic course. Symmetrical "spectacled" caverns in the tops of the lungs. Fixed macropreparation

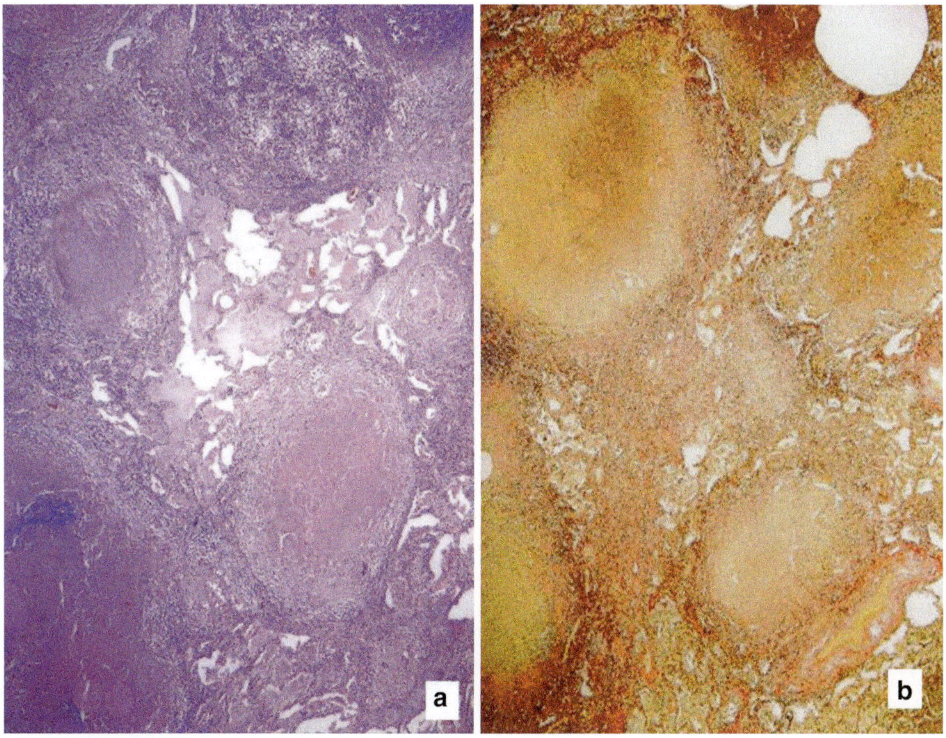

Fig. 13.19 Undulating course of the tuberculosis process. Foci of tuberculosis dissemination of various ages in the lung. (**a**) H.-E. and (**b**) van Gieson staining. ×100

sion of a specific process, pulmonary hemorrhage, generalization of the process, and amyloidosis of internal organs.

Acute and subacute forms of disseminated pulmonary tuberculosis can turn into chronic, subacute caverns can transform into chronic ones, and the development of severe cirrhotic changes in the lungs is also noted.

An acute course with the formation of multiple small foci (tubercles) with a diameter of 1–2 mm is usually characteristic of a *miliary disseminated tuberculosis*. Against the background of weakened immunity, the acute course of the miliary process with massive hematogenous dissemination often leads to a generalization with damage not only to the lungs but also to many organs. Acute miliary dissemination develops with a decrease in antituberculosis immunity and massive bacteremia with increased vascular permeability, which contributes to the penetration of MBT into the interalveolar septa.

Miliary dissemination is usually characterized by bilateral, almost simultaneous, development in the lungs along the capillaries of multiple monomorphic millet rashes, from the appearance of which the name of this form originated ("millium"—millet, lat.). Rashes in the lungs with a miliary character of dissemination have the appearance of tubercles, denser to the touch, grayish-white or yellowish-white, rounded in shape, with a diameter of 1–2 mm (Fig. 13.21). The exudative and necrotic reaction quickly changes into a productive one, and therefore fusion of foci does not occur.

Microscopically, the foci of miliary dissemination are granulomas from epithelioid cells, macrophages, lymphocytes, neutrophilic leukocytes, and single multinuclear giant Langhans

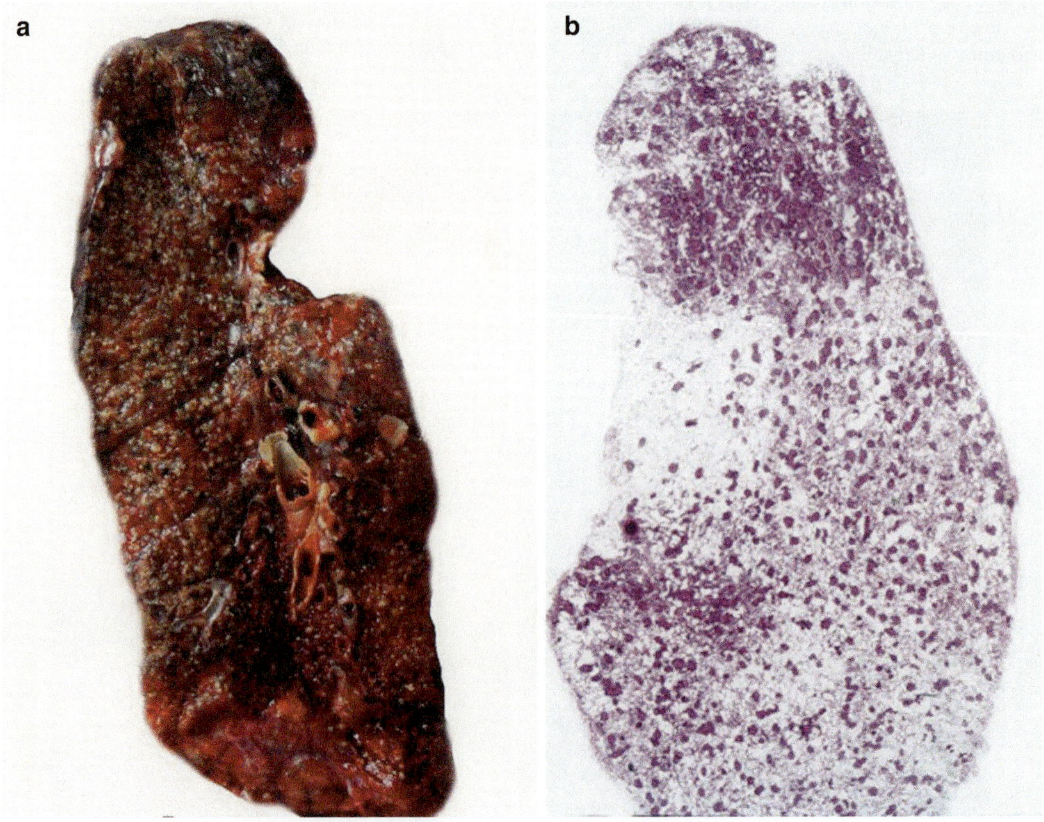

Fig. 13.21 Miliary tuberculosis of the lungs. (**a**) Non-fixed macropreparation and (**b**) histotopogram according to Kristeller

cells (productive tubercles). Caseous necrosis is quite often noted in the center of granulomas, with an active course, almost the entire miliary foci are replaced by necrotic masses (necrotic tubercles) (Fig. 13.22). Foci of miliary dissemination are located perivascular or in the wall of the vessels. Usually, all foci of a monomorphic microscopic structure. In some cases, part of them is fibrosed, and in other foci, there are no signs of organization, which indicates a wave-like nature of the process.

With a favorable course, compaction and scarring of the foci of inflammation occur with the formation of small scars or calcifications, diffuse net pneumosclerosis. With proper antituberculosis therapy, complete resorption of miliary foci may occur. With a progressive course, miliary tuberculous dissemination in the lungs can transform into a large focal lesion or go into a generalized form of lesion.

Focal pulmonary tuberculosis is a form of tuberculosis combining various pathogenesis, morphological, and clinical–radiological manifestations of the lesion, in which the diameter of each pathological formation is not more than 12 mm, i.e., does not exceed the transverse size of the pulmonary lobule, localized in individual isolated pulmonary lobules of one to two segments. Focal tuberculosis can develop as an independent form or in the outcome of hematogenously disseminated, infiltrative pulmonary tuberculosis.

Macroscopically in the lung, one or more grayish or yellowish-white rounded lesions, encapsulated or without capsule, up to 1 cm in diameter, localized more often in one to two segments of the lungs and located within one or two segments, is determined (Fig. 13.23).

A focus of caseous necrosis surrounded by a layer of specific granulation tissue or a fibrous capsule is detected microscopically. Fresh foci,

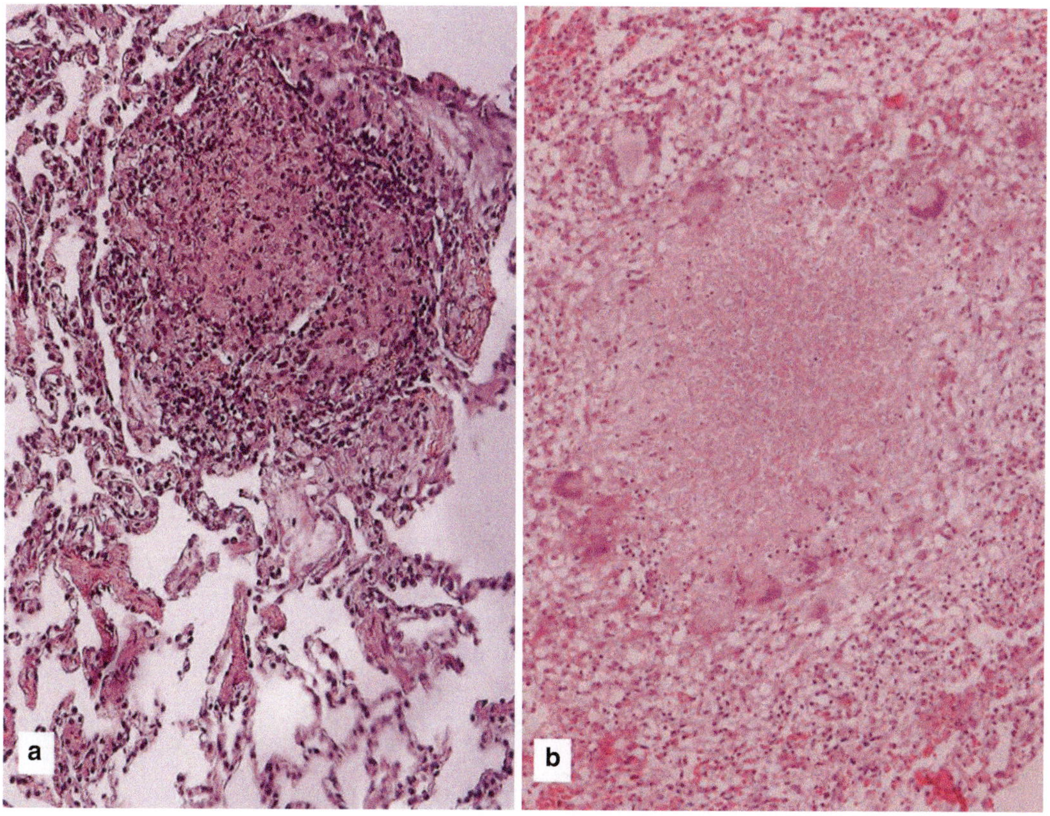

Fig. 13.22 Miliary tuberculosis of the lungs. (**a**) tubercle of a productive nature and (**b**) tubercle of a necrotic nature. H.-E. ×200

which are caseous intralobular endo- and panbronchitis with developing around intralobular caseous pneumonia and perifocal exudative reaction, are called Abrikosov foci (Fig. 13.24). When tuberculous inflammation subsides, the leukocyte infiltration of caseous-necrotic masses decreases and disappears, calcium salts are deposited in them, perifocal exudate is absorbed and fibrous capsule forms, fibrosis of the lesion (Aschoff–Puhl foci) (Fig. 13.25).

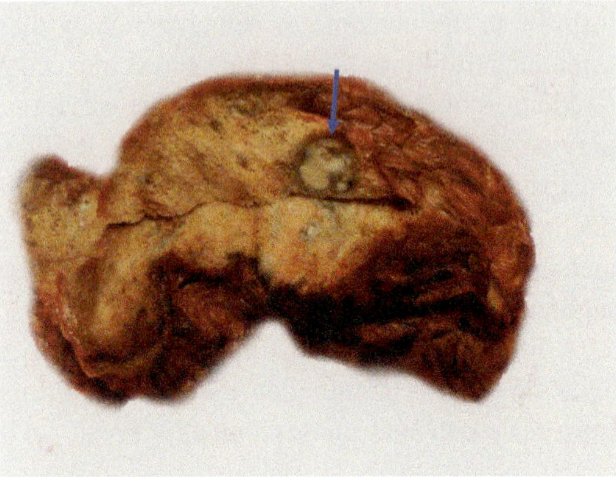

Fig. 13.23 Focal tuberculosis of the lung. Fixed micropreparation

With the progression of the process, caseous-necrotic masses are infiltrated with polynuclear leukocytes, followed by sequestration and purulent fusion of caseosis, with the spread of leukocyte infiltration to the fibrous capsule and adjacent lung tissue. A zone of exudative inflammation is formed perifocal with the involvement of the adjacent bronchi in the process with the development of specific inflammation in them and subsequent bronchogenic dissemination (Fig. 13.26). The molten caseous masses are removed through the draining bronchus with the transformation of the focus into the decay cavity. Thus, focal tuberculosis can be transformed into cavernous and fibro-cavernous pulmonary tuberculosis, as well as into tuberculoma, infiltrative tuberculosis, and, with massive dissemination, into disseminated pulmonary tuberculosis.

Pulmonary tuberculoma is a form of tuberculosis in which an encapsulated caseous-necrotic

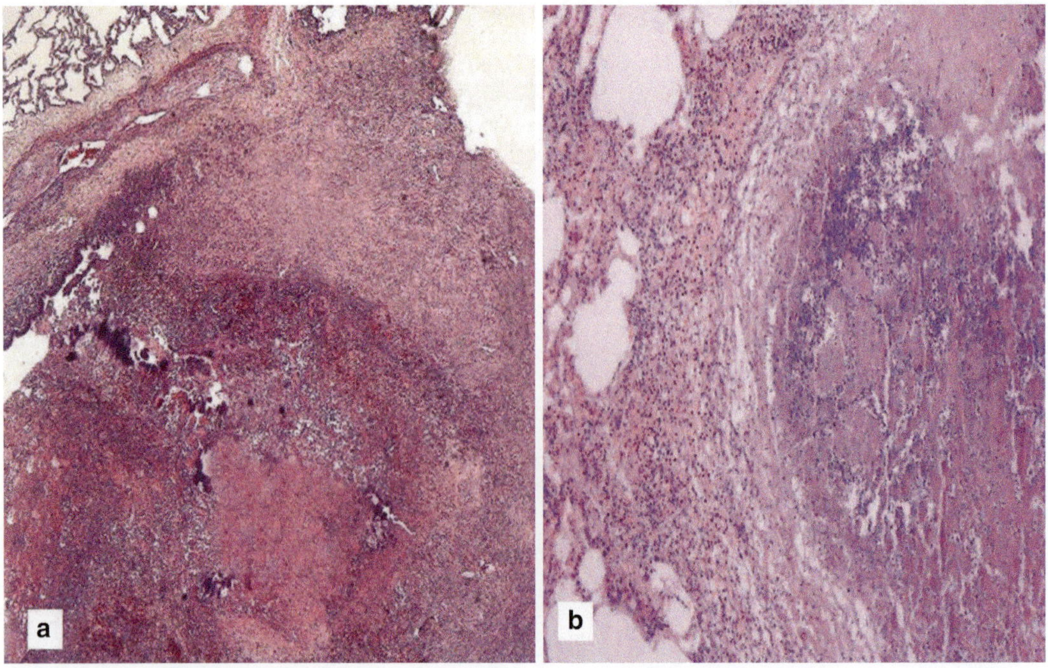

Fig. 13.24 Focal tuberculosis of the lung (Abrikosov's focus). (**a**) In the lumen of the draining bronchus (upper part of the microphoto)—caseous-necrotic masses; (**b**) leukocyte infiltration of caseous-necrotic masses in the focus, perifocal exudative reaction. H.-E. ×100

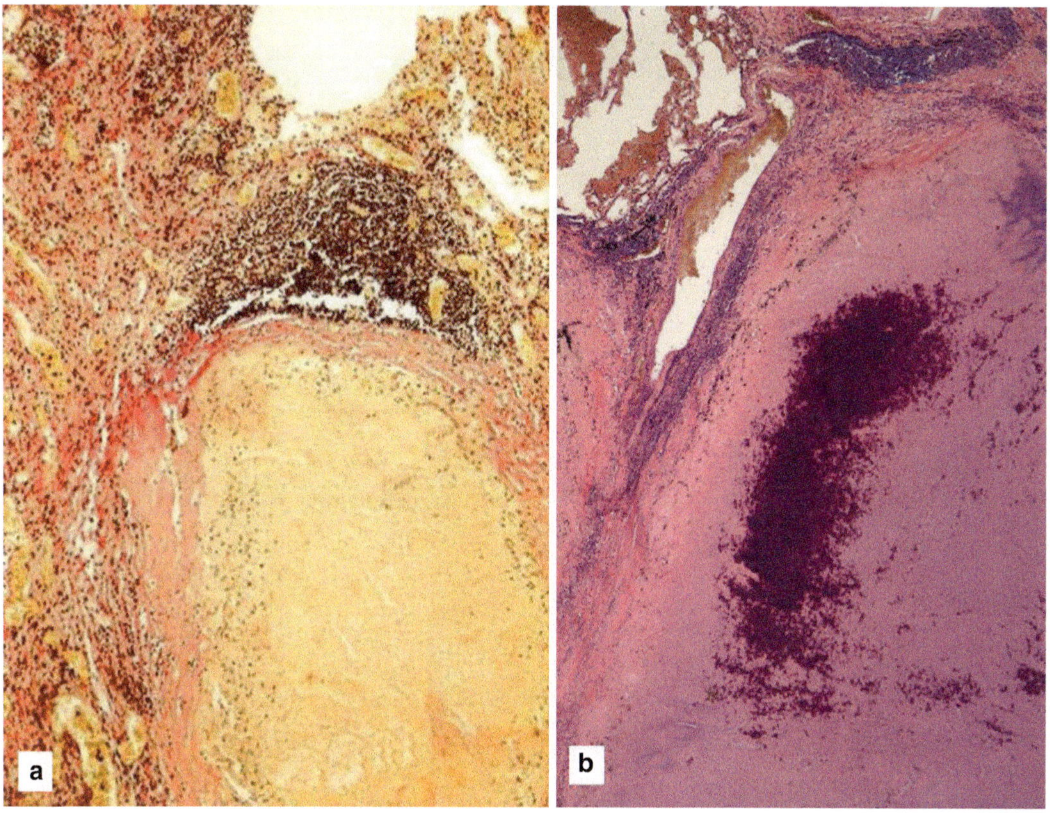

Fig. 13.25 Focal tuberculosis of the lung (Aschoff–Puhl focus). (**a**) Encapsulation of the focus of caseous necrosis; (**b**) Calcification of caseous-necrotic masses. (**a**) van Gieson staining; (**b**) H.-E. ×100

mass is formed in the lung with a diameter of more than 12 mm (exceeds the transverse dimension of the pulmonary lobule), delimited from the adjacent lung tissue by a two-layer capsule.

By the number of foci, tuberculomas are divided into solitary (single) and multiple. According to the morphological structure, homogeneous, layered, conglomerate, infiltrative-pneumonic, and the type of filled caverns (pseudotuberculomas) are distinguished. In size, small (up to 2 cm in diameter), medium (up to 4 cm) and large (more than 4 cm) tuberculomas are distinguished (Fig. 13.27).

Homogeneous tuberculoma is a grayish-white homogeneous focus of rounded caseous necrosis, clearly distinguished from the surrounding pulmonary parenchyma by a thin fibrous capsule. Subcapsularly, on the border with caseous necrosis, there is a predominantly narrow layer of specific granulation tissue with the presence of epithelioid cells, macrophages, giant cells Langhans, and foreign body types, sometimes forming small single and fused granulomas. Macroscopically, the focus has a homogeneous appearance, but remains of the elastic fibers of the alveolar septa are revealed (Fig. 13.28).

Layered tuberculoma is characterized by a concentric arrangement of caseous masses, alternating with annular or arched strands of collagen fibers, indicating previous exacerbations of the tuberculous process, accompanied by an increase in tuberculosis in size, and remission with the formation of a new fibrous capsule. On a section, the structure of layered tuberculoma somewhat resembles a cross-sectional drawing of a tree with "annual rings." The lamination of the structure is well determined microscopically with histological stains on the connective tissue (e.g., according to van Gieson) (Figs. 13.29 and 13.30).

Conglomerate tuberculoma has an irregular shape since it consists of several closely located

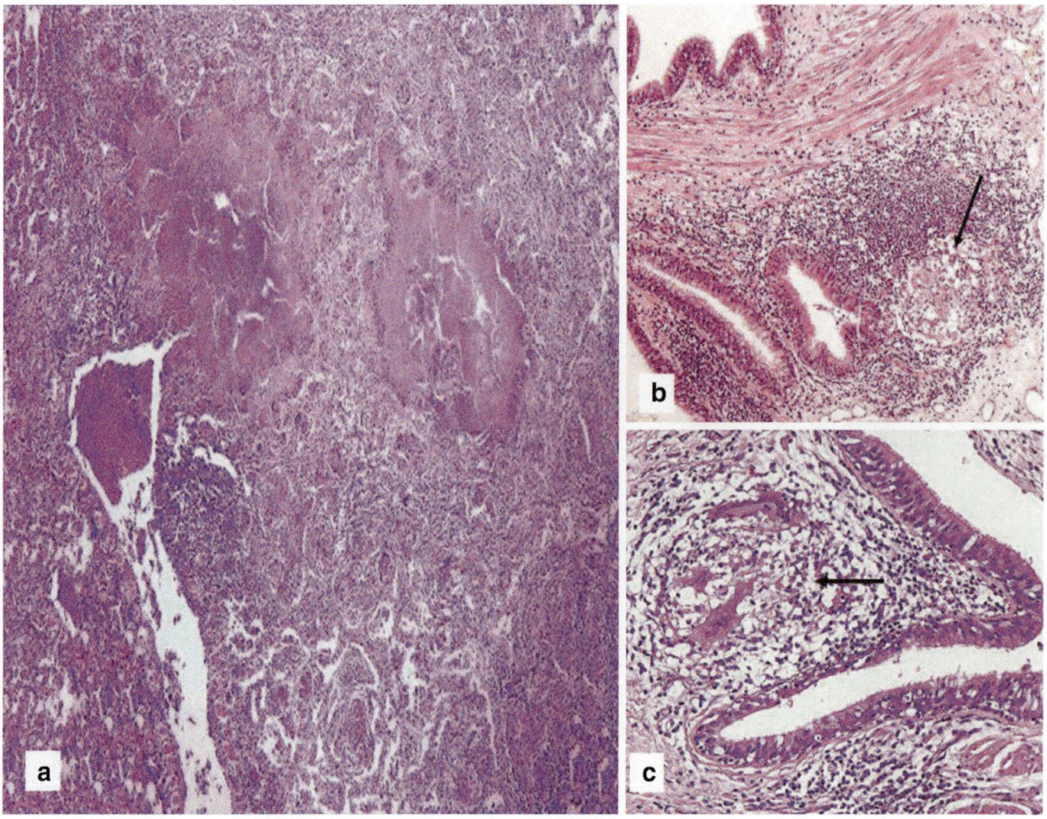

Fig. 13.26 Tuberculosis of a bronchus. (**a**) Draining bronchus and (**b**, **c**) tuberculosis lesion of the draining bronchus (granulomas are indicated by an arrow). H.E. (**a**) ×100; (**b**, **c**) ×200

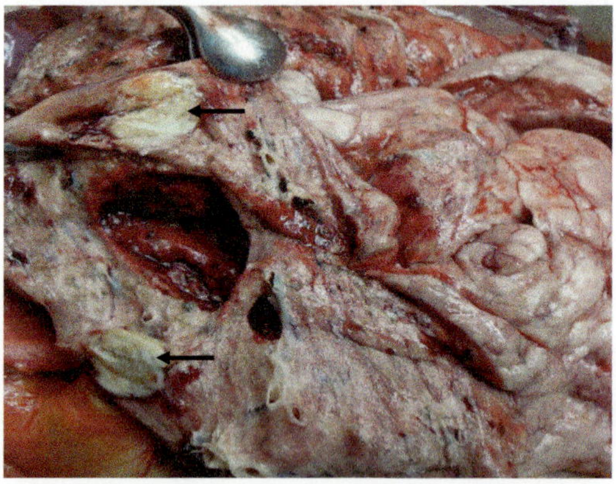

Fig. 13.27 Tuberculoma of the lung (indicated by arrows) cut. Unfixed macropreparation

foci of caseous necrosis, united by a common fibrous capsule (Figs. 13.31 and 13.32).

Infiltrative-pneumonic tuberculoma is the outcome of infiltrative pulmonary tuberculosis with its partial resorption and delimitation. This type of pulmonary tuberculosis is a rounded circular focus of tuberculous pneumonia, consisting of foci of granulomatous inflammation, areas of exudative–productive reaction in the presence of exudative alveolar reaction with exudative alveolar reaction and granulomas in the interalveolar septa, small foci of caseous necrosis, and connective tissue fibers between them (Fig. 13.33).

Tuberculoma as a filled cavity (pseudotuberculoma)—It is formed from a chronic tuberculous cavity during obliteration of the lumen of the draining bronchus. Obliteration develops in the outcome of chronic inflammation (post-tuberculous stenosis of the bronchus), the lumen of the bronchus can be obstructed by compacted or calcified caseous-necrotic masses, bronchiolitis. The lumen of the cavity is gradually filled with caseous masses, which are compacted and dehydrated, and takes the form of a round encap-

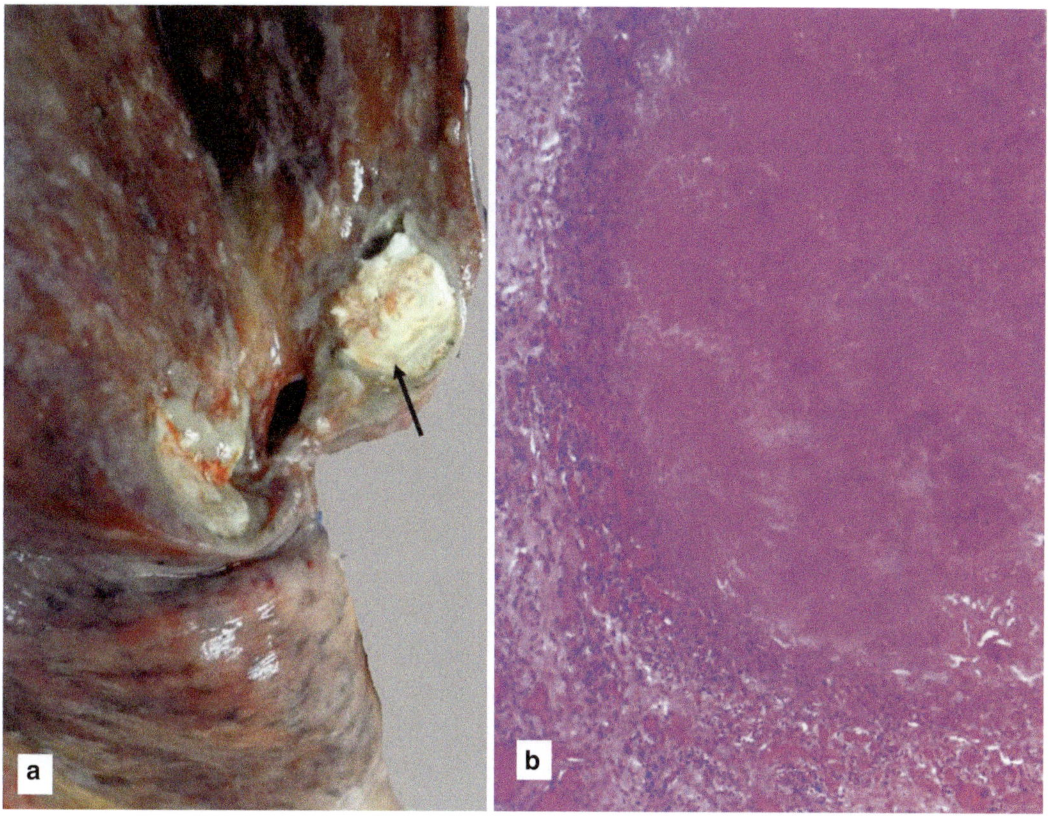

Fig. 13.28 Solitary homogeneous pulmonary tuberculoma. (**a**) Non-fixed macro specimens and (**b**) the edge of tuberculoma of the lung stained H.-E. ×100

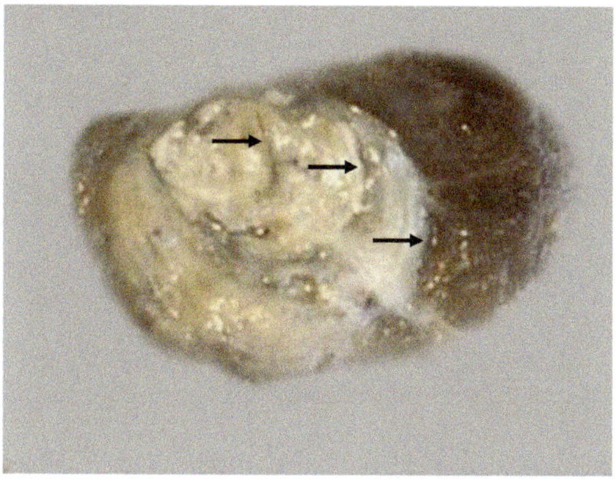

Fig. 13.29 Layered pulmonary tuberculoma. Fixed macropreparation. Layers are indicated by arrows

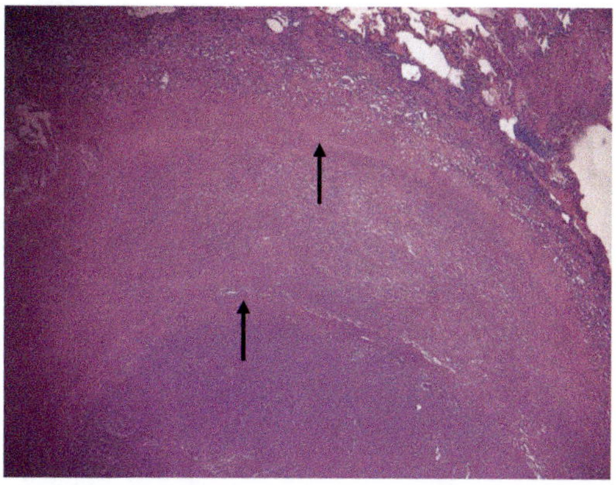

Fig. 13.30 Layered pulmonary tuberculoma. Layers are indicated by arrows. Stained H.-E. ×100

sulated caseous focus. Unlike focal tuberculosis and other types of tuberculosis, in this case, the foci capsule is dense, wide, represented by coarse-fibrous connective tissue with hyalinosis, with radiant fibrous strands in the adjacent lung tissue, that is, it has the structure of a capsule of a chronic tuberculous cavity. When stained with picrofuchsin and fuchseline or when impregnated

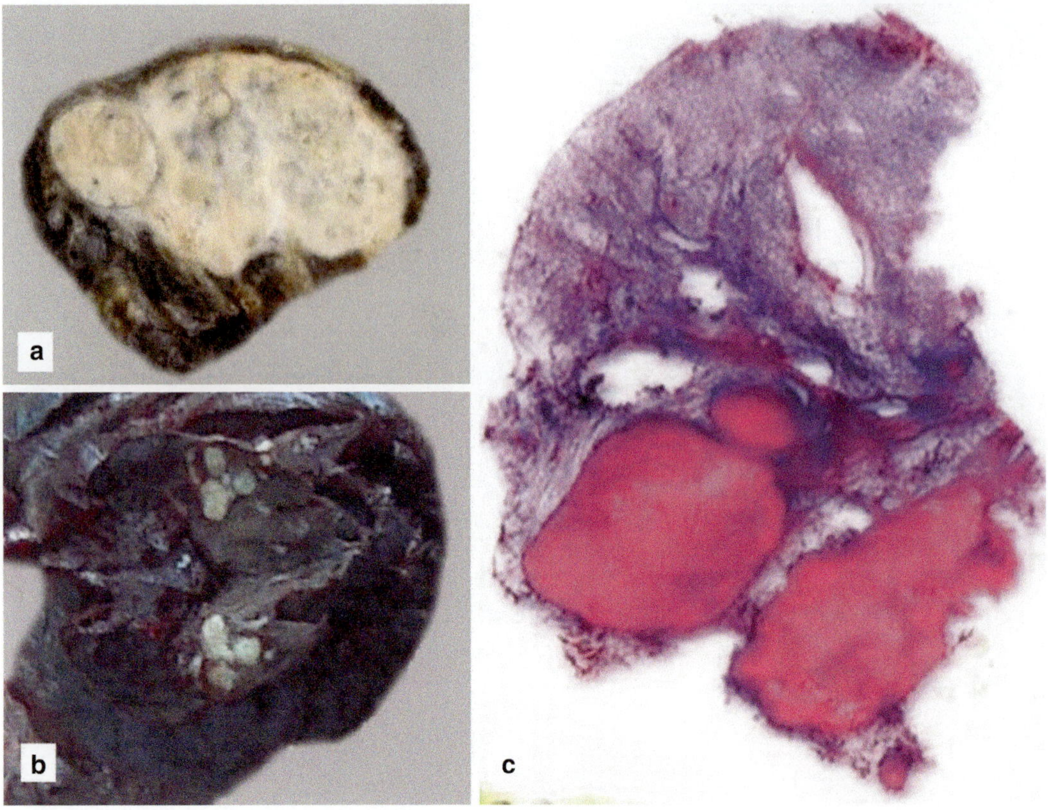

Fig. 13.31 Conglomerate's a tuberculoma of the lung. (**a**) Fixed macropreparation; (**b**) non-fixed macropreparation; and (**c**) histotopogram (slice according to Kristeller)

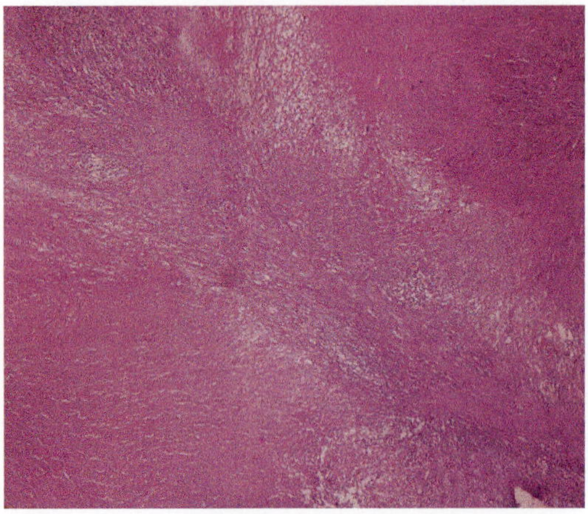

Fig. 13.32 Conglomerate's a tuberculoma of the lung. Closely located foci of caseous necrosis. Stained H.-E. ×100

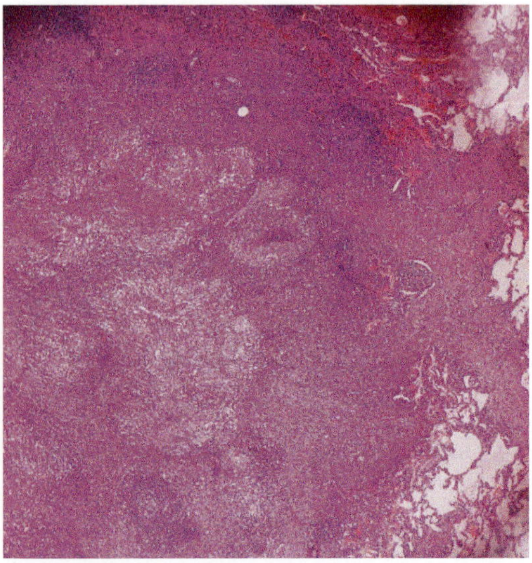

Fig. 13.33 Emerging infiltrative-pneumonic tuberculoma of the lung. Stained H.-E.. ×100

with silver in caseous masses, the contours of the alveolar stroma of the lung are not detected; caseosis in such foci is rarely calcified.

Around tuberculoma there can be secondary foci, most often bronchogenic and lymphogenic, the size and condition of which depend on the phase of the process. With progression around tuberculoma, a perifocal exudative reaction appears, a specific perifocal inflammation that spreads to the adjacent lung tissue with an increase of its size. Caseous necrosis melts, more often at the border with the capsule in the lower medial zone and is excreted through the draining bronchi (Fig. 13.34). Tuberculous inflammation can spread to the walls of the draining bronchi, leading to the development of bronchogenic dissemination and the appearance of secondary acinous, acinous–lobular, lobular, confluent lobular caseous foci.

One of the ways to heal tuberculoma can be the release of caseous masses through the draining bronchus, as a result of which the tuberculoma is cleaned and scarred. With the development of healing processes, perifocal inflammation resolves, the leukocyte infiltration of the capsule and necrotic masses decreases and gradually disappears. Collagen fibers from the side of the capsule grow into caseous masses. In addition to fibrosis in caseous-necrotic masses,

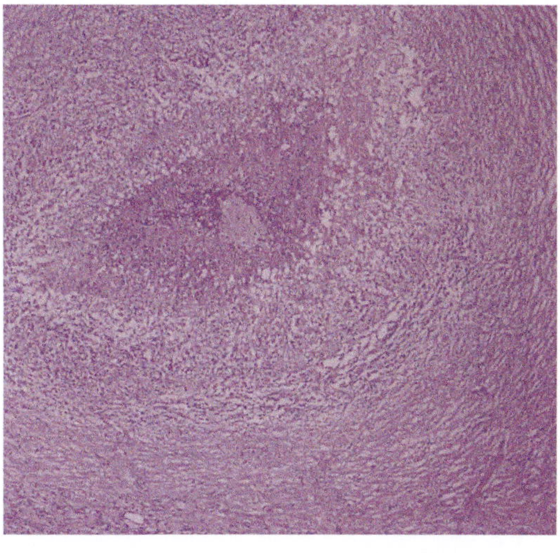

Fig. 13.34 Pulmonary tuberculosis, progression. Leukocyte infiltration of caseous-necrotic masses. Stained H.E. ×100. See also Fig. 13.24b

focal calcification can be observed (Fig. 13.35), deposition of cholesterol crystals. Reparative processes in medium and large tuberculomas are usually quite weak. Tuberculomas in the future can be a source of disseminated pulmonary tuberculosis, caseous pneumonia, and cavernous pulmonary tuberculosis.

The allocation in the domestic Russian classification of such forms of tuberculosis as "small" forms of tuberculosis is due to the patient monitoring regimen, antituberculosis chemotherapy, and indications for surgical treatment.

Infiltrative pulmonary tuberculosis develops in the presence of specific hypersensitivity of the lung tissue and is characterized by the predominance of exudative tissue reaction in the focus of inflammation. Infiltrative pulmonary tuberculosis develops as an independent form but maybe a result of progression of focal tuberculosis with the rapid development of perifocal inflammation around both fresh and old foci. This form of tuberculosis is characterized by rapid progression of the process with widespread lung damage.

Infiltrative pulmonary tuberculosis is single- and bilateral; broncholobular (two to three lung segments), segmental, polysegmental, lobar, distinguished by the volume of pulmonary parenchyma lesion. The development of infiltrative changes along the interlobar fissure is called periscissuritis.

Macroscopic examination of the area of the lung is densified, without clear boundaries, yellowish-gray in color, granular in appearance,

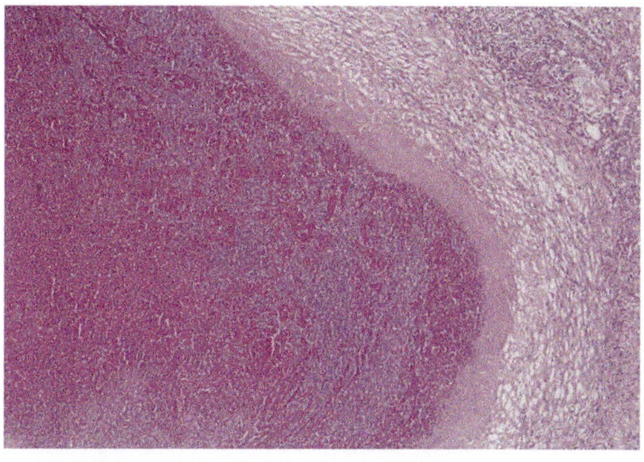

Fig. 13.35 Pulmonary tuberculosis, organization. Calcification of necrotic masses. Stained H.-E. ×100

with interspersed foci of yellowish–whitish necrosis of irregular shape (Fig. 13.36). Microscopically, the areas of exudative changes with filling the lumen of the alveoli with serous fluid, fibrin, desquamated alveolar epithelium, with an admixture of macrophages, epithelioid cells, lymphocytes, and leukocytes are determined. In addition, fusing epithelioid-giant cell granulomas are detected. With TB progressing, foci of caseous necrosis appear in the center of specific infiltration sites. With infiltrative pulmonary tuberculosis, a predominance of exudative reaction and granulomatous inflammation over alterative (necrotic) changes is noted (Fig. 13.37). With the active course of tuberculosis, sequestration of necrotic masses with subsequent decay (infiltrate with decay) and the formation of destruction cavities of various sizes are noted. With further progression, infiltrative pulmonary tuberculosis can transform into caseous pneumonia, cavernous, and fibro-cavernous pulmonary tuberculosis.

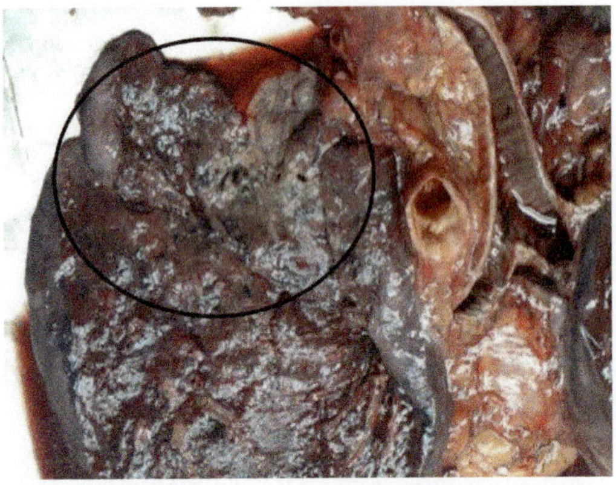

Fig. 13.36 Infiltrative pulmonary tuberculosis. Unfixed macropreparation

During the healing of infiltrative tuberculosis, perifocal inflammation resolves, delimitation and densification of caseous foci occur, their encapsulation, fibrosis with the formation of a star or

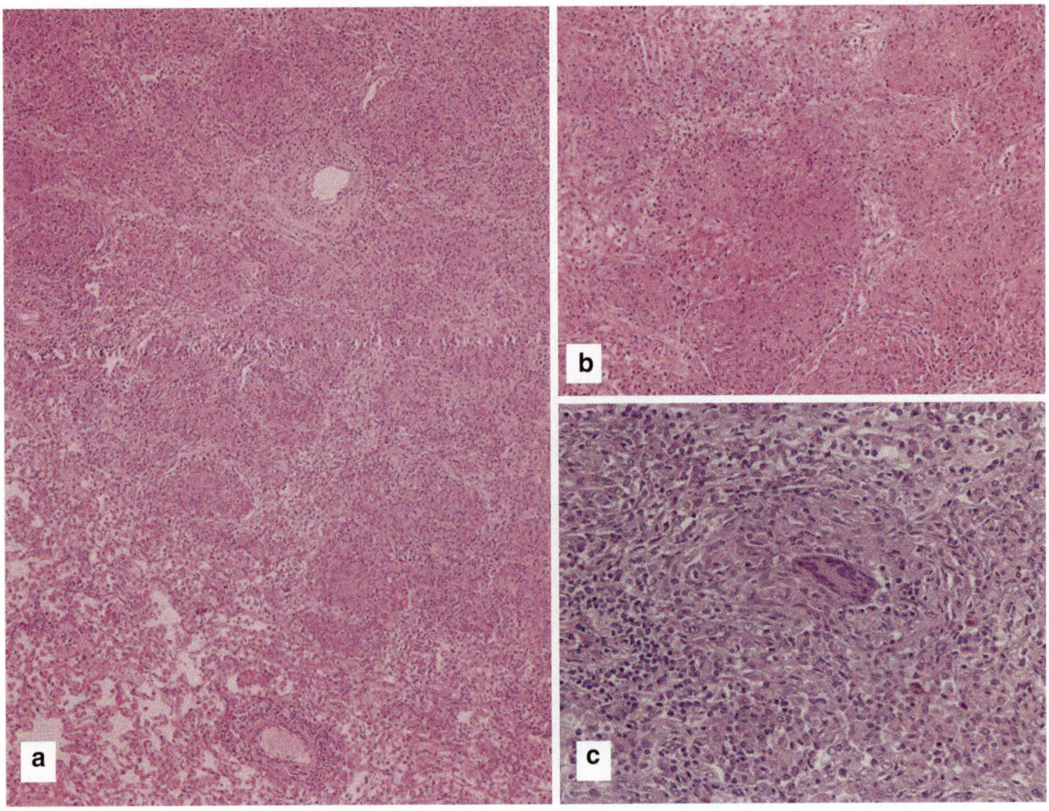

Fig. 13.37 Infiltrative pulmonary tuberculosis. Stained H.-E. (**a**, **b**) ×100 and (**c**) ×200

linear scar, and petrification (calcification). When organizing, the outcome of this form of the disease is focal pulmonary tuberculosis, tuberculomas, or residual tuberculous changes in the lungs (often in 1–2 SS of the right lung).

The most severe form of pulmonary tuberculosis is *caseous pneumonia*. The inflammatory and destructive process in the lungs is characterized by a high spread rate, severe clinical symptoms of respiratory failure, and severe intoxication. The predominance of exudative–necrotic tissue reactions with extensive caseous transformation of lung tissue, acutely progressive course, and the early development of destruction sites with the formation of pneumoniogenic caverns are noted.

Macroscopically in the pulmonary parenchyma, grayish-yellow necrotic foci are determined with the formation of caseous segmentitis, lobitis, bilobitis, damage to the entire organ, or both lungs. Against this background, large and small areas of melting of necrotic masses with the formation of acute decay cavities are visible (Figs. 13.38 and 13.39). Perifocal pulmonary parenchyma is airless, with signs of infiltration.

Microscopically, tuberculous inflammation is observed in the form of extensive areas of caseous necrosis with significant leukocyte infiltration, a weak productive granulomatous cell reaction at the periphery, and pronounced perifocal exudative changes (Fig. 13.40). The course of the process is accompanied by the melting and sequestration of caseous masses, the formation of acute pneumoniogenic caverns. Vasculitis and thrombovasculitis in the affected area are detected, pronounced signs of increased permeability of the vascular walls, which is the reason for the exudative tissue reaction. Thrombovasculitis can result in the development of foci of ischemic pulmonary infarction in areas of caseous pneumonia, which increases the volume of pulmonary parenchyma lesion and aggravates respiratory failure (Fig. 13.41). Bronchi of all generations are also actively involved in the pathological process with the development of total caseous panbronchitis, foci of bronchogenic dissemination, and bronchogenic caverns. Decay cavities with caseous pneumonia in some cases are subsequently transformed into chronic caverns, pronounced cirrhotic changes can form in the lung.

Two variants of caseous pneumonia are distinguished: primary caseous pneumonia as an independent form of tuberculosis, and secondary caseous pneumonia as the main morphological manifestation of the progression of other forms of pulmonary tuberculosis. So, with the progression of tuberculosis with the presence of chronic caverns, with the predominance of large focal bronchogenic dissemination, multiple acinous and lobular foci screenings can merge with each other, forming caseous segmentitis, lobitis, or bilobitis.

Cavernous changes in tuberculosis are characterized by the presence of decay cavities in the

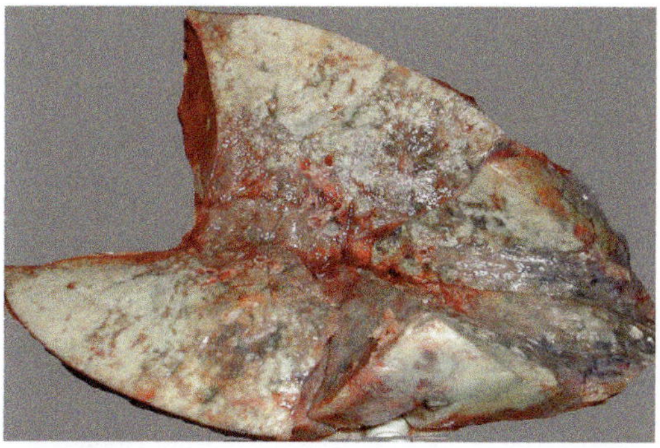

Fig. 13.38 Caseous pneumonia. Non-fixed macro specimens

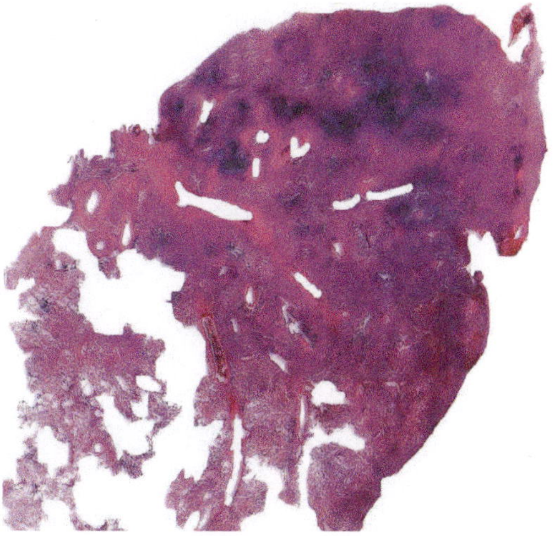

Fig. 13.39 Caseous pneumonia. Histotopogram (slice according to Kristeller)

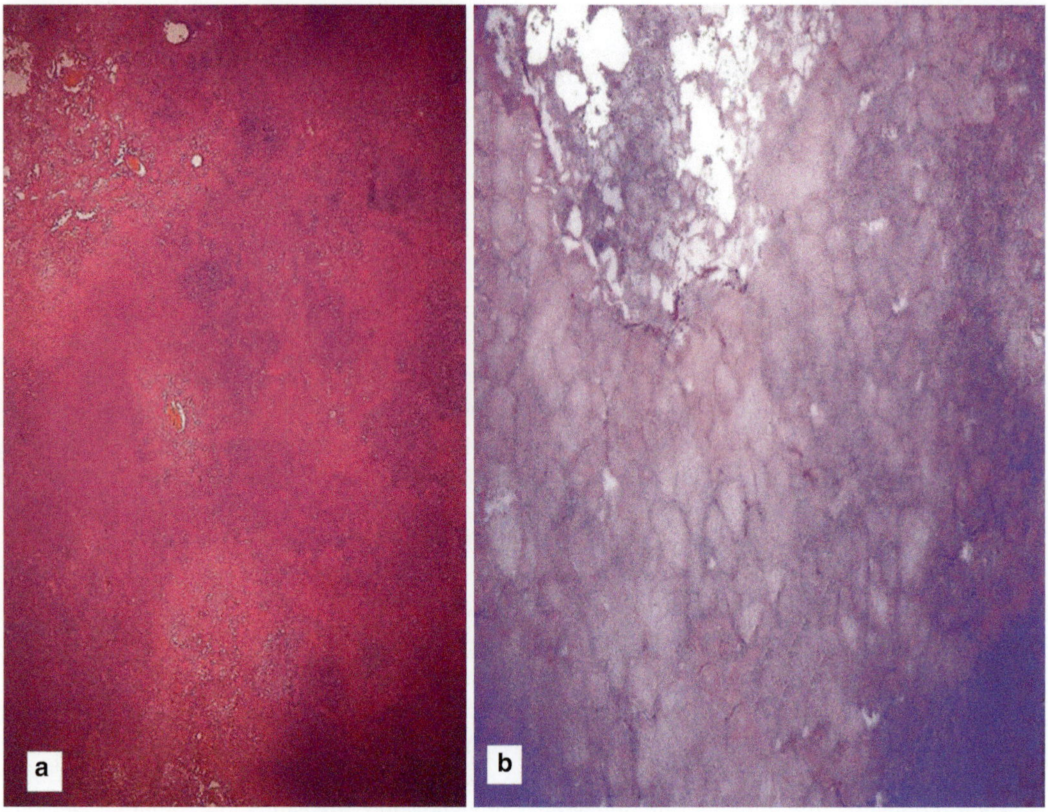

Fig. 13.40 Caseous pneumonia. Stained H.-E. ×100

Fig. 13.41 Caseous pneumonia. Reactive thrombovascular emerging ischemic infarction of the lung. Stained H.-E. ×100

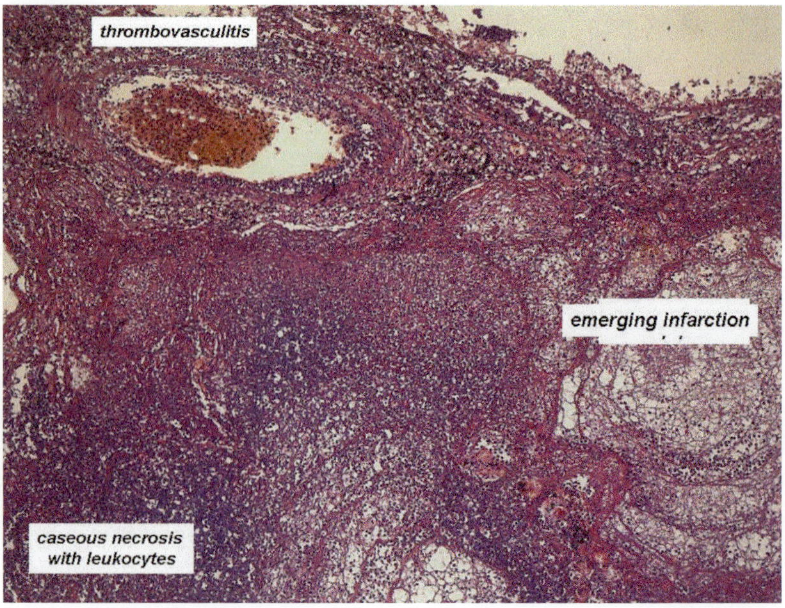

lung. An isolated tuberculous cavity without marked fibrotic changes in the surrounding tissue may be observed. In case of long-term destructive tuberculosis, the process is characterized by the formation in the lungs of one or several chronic caverns with a wide fibrous capsule, against the background of widespread pulmonary fibrosis and screening foci of various genesis and prescription (according to the Russian classification of tuberculosis, this form is called *"fibro-cavernous pulmonary tuberculosis,"* lethality it takes first place among all forms of tuberculosis).

The process can be either one-sided or two-sided; mono- and polycavernous (up to the complete destruction of the lung). In addition to the chronic cavity or caverns, subacute and acute tuberculous decay cavities can be simultaneously determined. Caverns are localized in any parts of the lungs, but more often in SS 1, 2, and 6. Small caverns (up to 2 cm in diameter), medium (up to 4 cm), large (up to 6 cm), and gigantic (more than 6 cm in diameter) are distinguished by size.

Caverns are divided into pneumoniogenic and bronchogenic. Under the action of leukocyte proteolytic enzymes, caseous-necrotic masses melt and are partially resorbed by macrophages. Due to the rejection of caseosis through the draining bronchi, a decay cavity is formed—a *pneumoniogenic tuberculous cavity*. In the formation of a *bronchogenic cavity*, the process begins with damage to the bronchus, the development of caseous panbronchitis, followed by the destruction of adjacent lung tissue with the formation of a decay cavity. Another way of developing a bronchogenic tuberculous cavity is to spread the tuberculous process to preexisting bronchiectasis, bronchogenic cyst.

Macroscopically affected segments or lungs are dense, pleura with fibrous adhesions, thickened, hyalinized, often cartilaginous density, especially in areas adjacent to the chronic cavity. The visceral and parietal pleural sheets are fused together; lumped cavities of tuberculous empyema and pleuro-bronchial fistulas may form. On a cut in the lungs, coarse, grayish fibrous-type layers of fibrous tissue, single or multiple cavities of an irregular rounded or slit-like shape are determined. Caverns can form a system of communicating cavities. The inner surface of the caverns is uneven, with yellowish-white crumbly cheesy appearance or pus-like overlays. Disk-shaped whitish-gray formations up to 2–4 mm in size on the inner surface of the wall of the decay cavity, the so-called Koch lenses, are clusters of colonies of mycobacterium tuberculosis. The walls of the chronic tuberculous cavity are dense, sometimes cartilaginous, whitish, stiff, do not fall off when pressed. Multiple foci of dissemination of various sizes and prescription, infiltrates, including with decay (Figs. 13.42 and 13.43).

Microscopically, the wall of the chronic tuberculous cavity consists of three layers (in contrast to the two-layer acute tuberculous cavity). The inner layer is caseous-necrotic, represented by necrotic masses, often with leukocyte infiltration. The middle layer is a layer of specific granulation tissue with the presence of epithelioid cells, macrophages, giant multinucleate cells such as Langhans, or foreign bodies, with the formation of granulomas. The outer layer is a wide fibrous capsule of coarse-fibrous connective tissue with hyalinosis (Fig. 13.44). From the fibrous layer radially deep into the lungs depart fibrous cords that deform the adjacent lung tissue.

The width of the caseous-necrotic and granulation layers of the chronic cavity varies and depends on the phase of the process—progression or healing. With progression, the caseous layer with massive leukocyte infiltration prevailing, spreading to the layer of specific granulations, fibrous capsule, and adjacent lung tissue (Fig. 13.45). With purulent expansion of the fibrous capsule, an increase in the size of the cavity occurs. Another reason for the increase in the size of the decay cavity is the difficulty of air movement from the cavity due to obstruction of the lumen of the draining bronchus with tuberculous granulations.

During remission, the walls of the cavity may collapse, while the cavity becomes slit-shaped and the result may be the formation of a linear or rough stellate scar. However, complete healing in a chronic tuberculous cavity with cavity closure

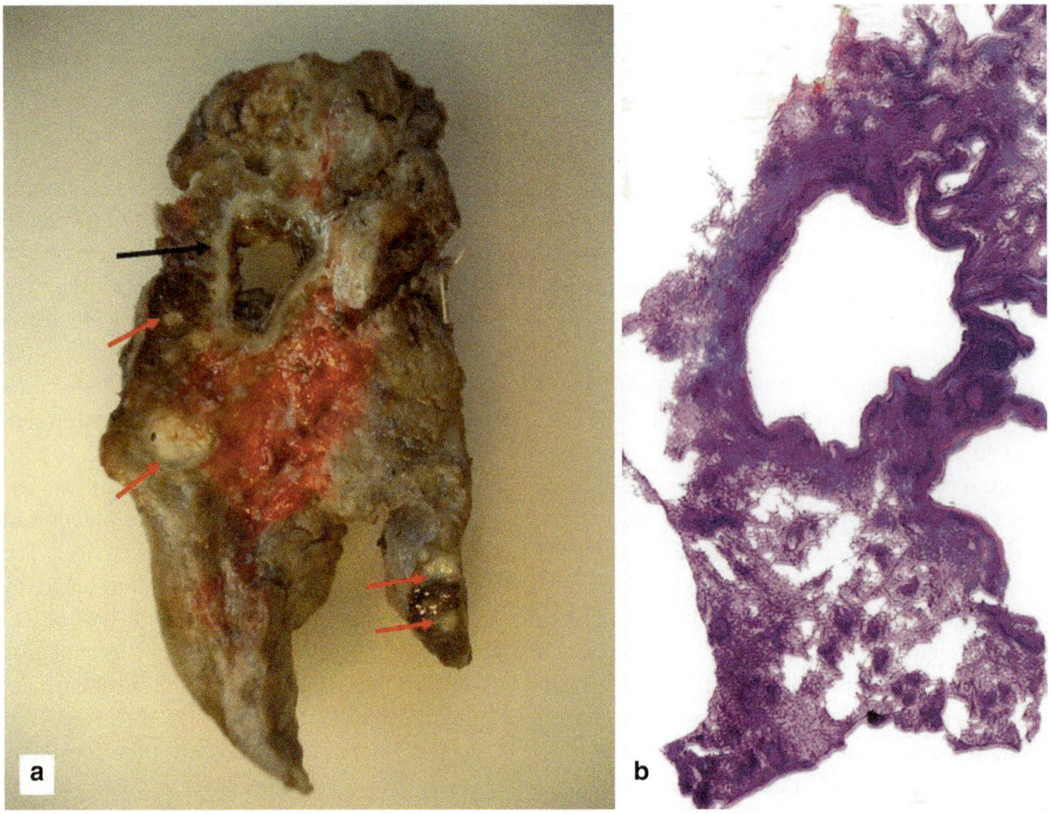

Fig. 13.42 Fibrous-cavernous pulmonary tuberculosis. (**a**) Fixed macropreparation (chronic cavern is indicated by a black arrow, foci of dissemination are indicated by red arrows) and (**b**) histotopogram (slice according to Kristeller)

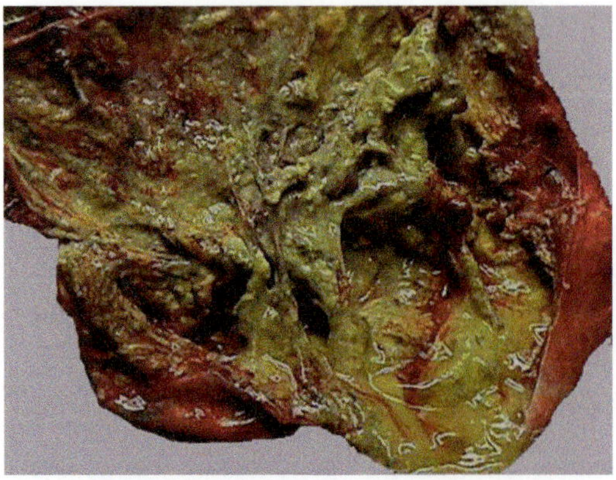

Fig. 13.43 Fibrous-cavernous pulmonary tuberculosis. A collapsed lung. Unfixed macropreparation

is rare. The cavity also heals by growing granulation tissue into the lumen. In some cases, an encapsulated focus is formed at the site of the cavity. This occurs with obstruction or stenosis of the draining bronchial cavity with a gradual filling of the decay cavity with caseous-necrotic masses. The outcome of the cavity is also a residual cystic cavity (Fig. 13.46). During epithelization from the draining bronchus of the inner surface of the wall of the cleaned cavity, a lung cyst is formed (Fig. 13.47).

Granulomatous and caseous *endo-, meso-, and panbronchitis* develop in the bronchi of various generations. Signs of the formation of bronchogenic foci are the identification of bronchial wall elements (fragments of the destroyed hyaline cartilage of the bronchial wall, bundles of smooth muscle fibers, scraps of bronchial epithelium) in caseous masses or small fragments of the bronchial wall along the edge of the forming screening site.

The immediate cause of death in the described form of tuberculosis is the progression of the tuberculosis process, massive pulmonary hemorrhage, decompensation of the chronic pulmonary

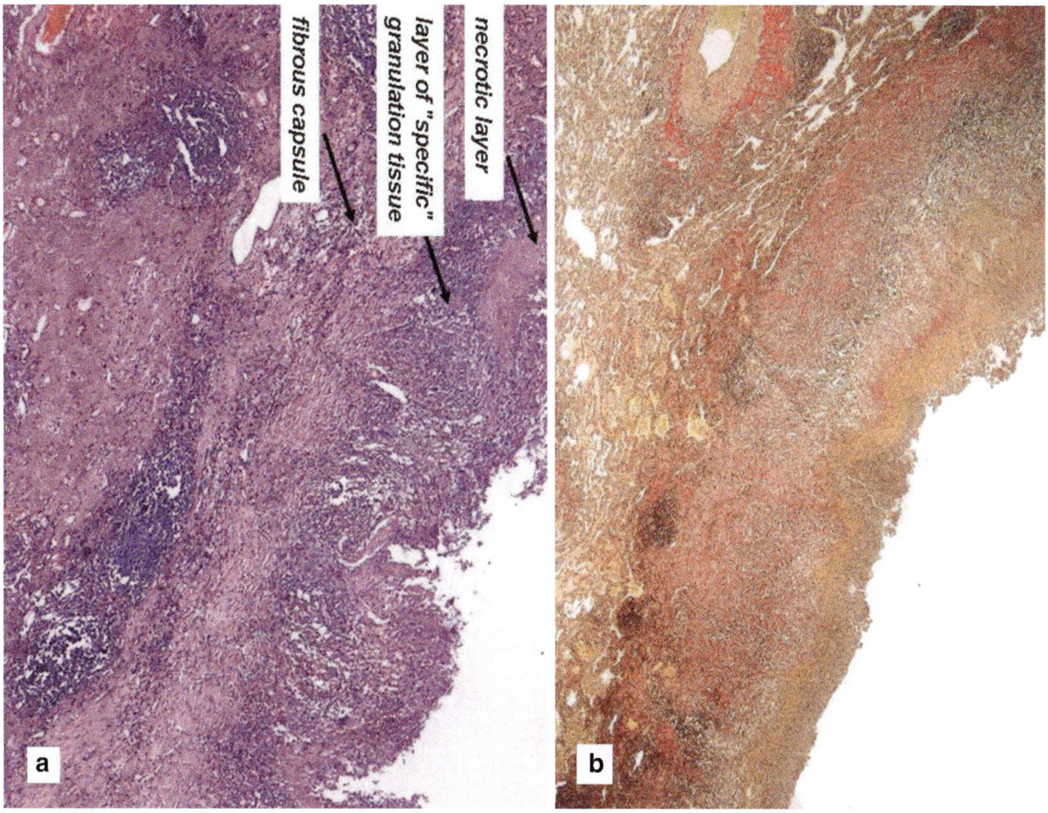

Fig. 13.44 Fibrous-cavernous pulmonary tuberculosis. The wall of a chronic tuberculosis cavern. The inner caseous-necrotic layer, the middle layer—"specific" granulation tissue, the outer layer—a fibrous capsule. (**a**) H.-E. and (**b**) van Gieson staining. ×100

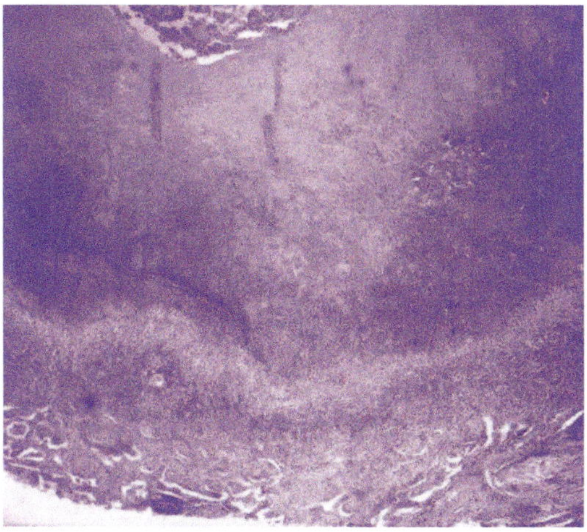

Fig. 13.45 Fibrous-cavernous pulmonary tuberculosis. The wall of a chronic tuberculosis cavity, the progression of tuberculosis. A wide inner caseous-necrotic layer that is many times larger than the width of the "specific" granulation tissue layer (the granulation tissue layer is in the form of a light eosinophilic strip under the necrotic layer). Stained H.-E.. ×100

heart, and uremia in the complication of chronic destructive tuberculosis with amyloidosis of the kidneys.

With pulmonary hemorrhage, the lungs are compacted, variegated due to the alternation of grayish–pinkish sections of the pulmonary parenchyma and reddish foci. In the lumen of the trachea, bronchi and caverns are located blood bundles that obstruct their lumen (Fig. 13.48). The source of bleeding is an arosive blood vessel in the wall of the cavity (both chronic and acute), which can be detected by a thorough examination of the decay cavity. Unchanged blood found in the lumen of the esophagus, stomach, proximal small intestine is reflexively swallowed by patients with massive pulmonary hemorrhage and is not a manifestation of gastrointestinal bleeding, since there are no ulcerative defects in these sections of the gastrointestinal tract. Microscopically in the lumen of the alveoli and

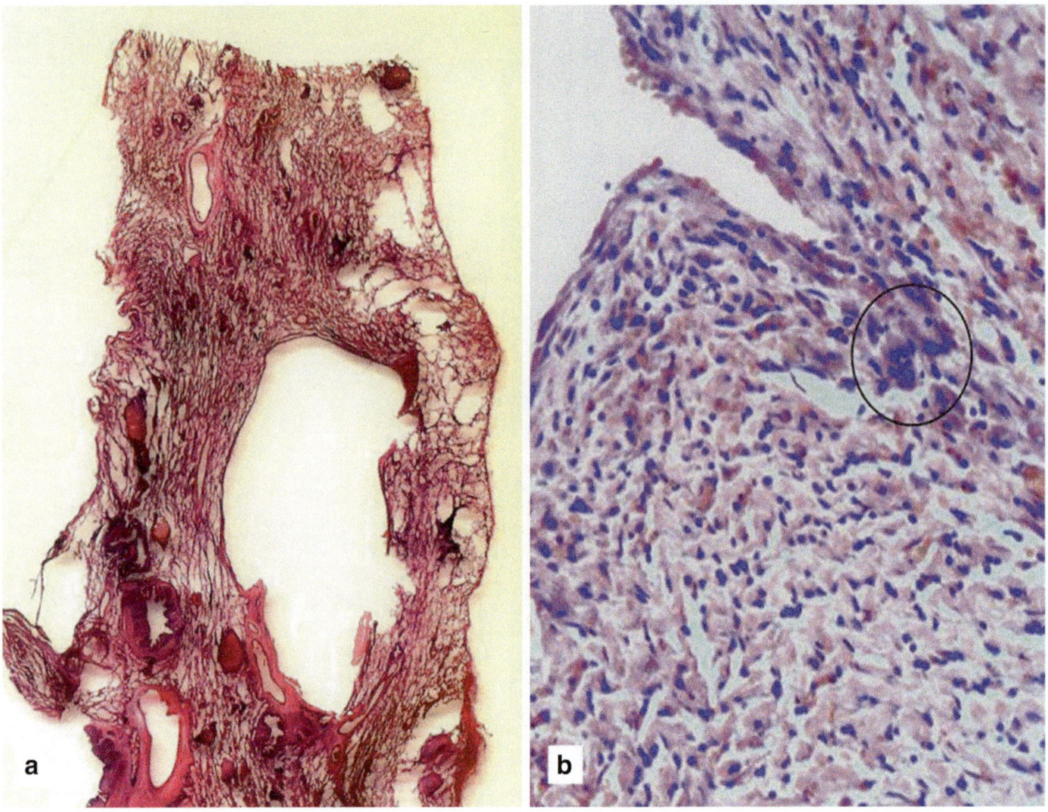

Fig. 13.46 Cystic cavity—the outcome of fibrotic cavernous pulmonary tuberculosis. (**a**) A thin-walled cavity without epithelial lining; (**b**) the walls of the post-tuberculosis cyst cavity, without epithelial lining, single giant multinucleated cells are surrounded by a round frame. (**a**) Slice according to Kristeller (**b**) H.-E. ×400

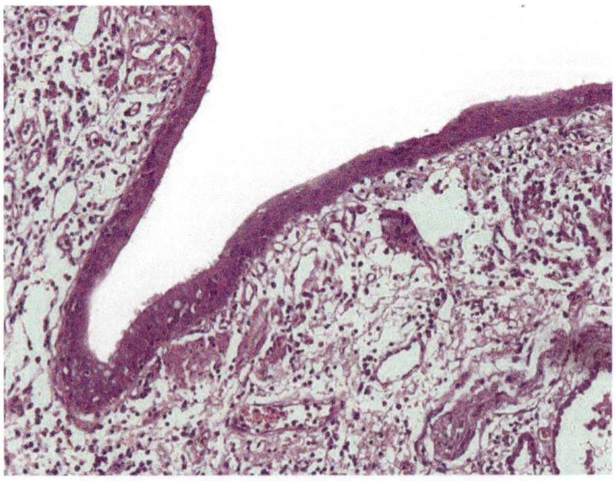

Fig. 13.47 Lung cyst—the outcome of fibro-cavernous pulmonary tuberculosis. The internal epithelial lining of the mosaic type is an alternation of multilayered flat non-keratinizing and respiratory epithelium. Stained H.-E. ×400

bronchi of all generations, non-hemolyzed red blood cells are detected; fresh blood bundles are located on the inner surface of the decay cavities (Fig. 13.49). After suffering a pulmonary hemorrhage, the patient can subsequently die from aspiration pneumonia, microscopically having the form of fibrinous–purulent bronchopneumonia with a hemorrhagic component in the exudate.

With a prolonged course of the chronic destructive form of tuberculosis, fibrotic and cirrhotic changes in the lungs increase (Fig. 13.50). Cirrhotic changes develop due to inferior involution of tuberculous inflammation and are characterized by severe deforming fibrosis in the lung with restructuring of the pulmonary parenchyma, a significant predominance of fibrotic changes over specific ones ("*cirrhotic tuberculosis*") (Fig. 13.51).

Among the massive fibrotic growths that propagate peribronchial, perivascular along the interlobular and intersegmental septa, signs of tuberculosis are determined in the form of purified caverns without signs of progression, cystic

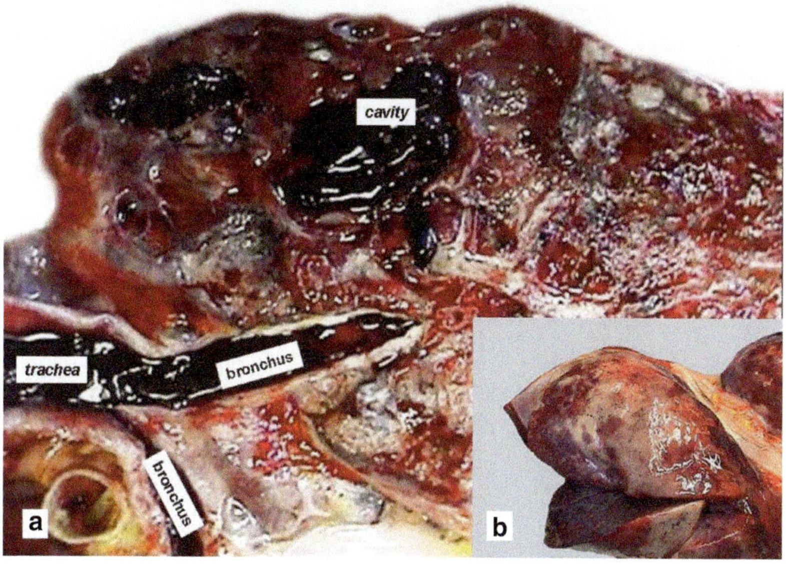

Fig. 13.48 Massive pulmonary hemorrhage. (**a**) Obturation of the trachea and bronchi with blood clotting, blood coagulation in the cavity of the tuberculous cavern and (**b**) acute emphysema of the lung, variegation of the lung tissue with dark red areas of hemaspiration. Non-fixed macropreparations

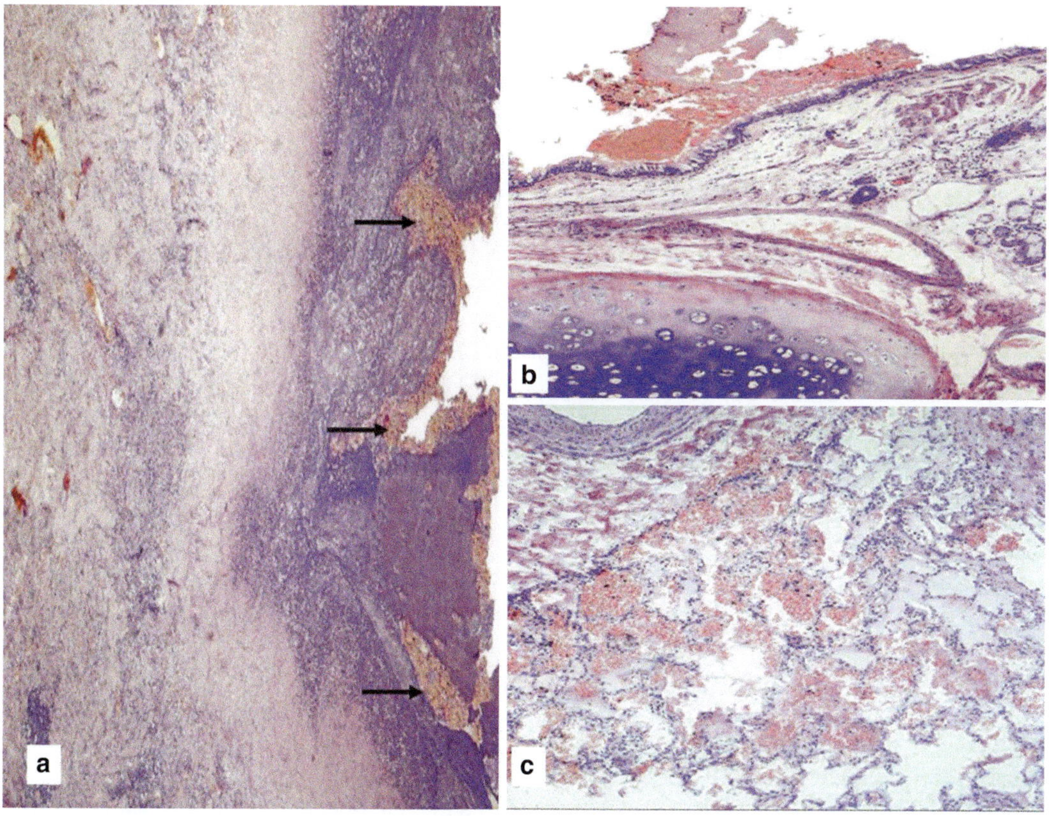

Fig. 13.49 Pulmonary hemorrhage. (**a**) The wall of a chronic tuberculosis cavern (progression of tuberculosis) with parietal blood clots (indicated by arrows); (**b**) parietal blood clot in the bronchus; (**c**) Hemaspiration—non-hemolysed red blood cells in the lumen of the alveoli. Stained H.-E. (**a**, **c**) ×100 and (**b**) ×200

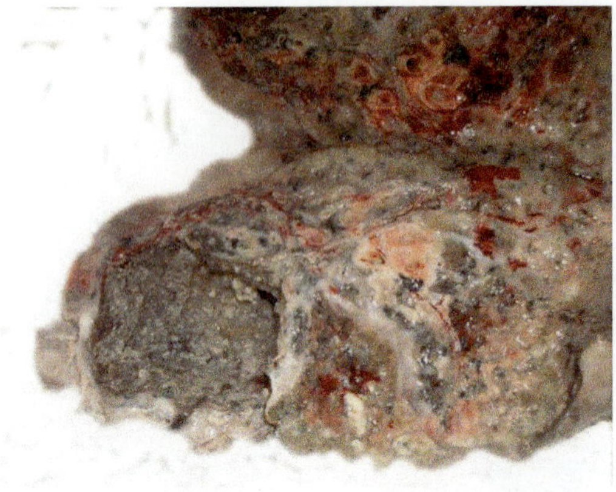

Fig. 13.50 Fibrous-cavernous tuberculosis on the background pronounced cirrhotic changes. Fixed macro specimen

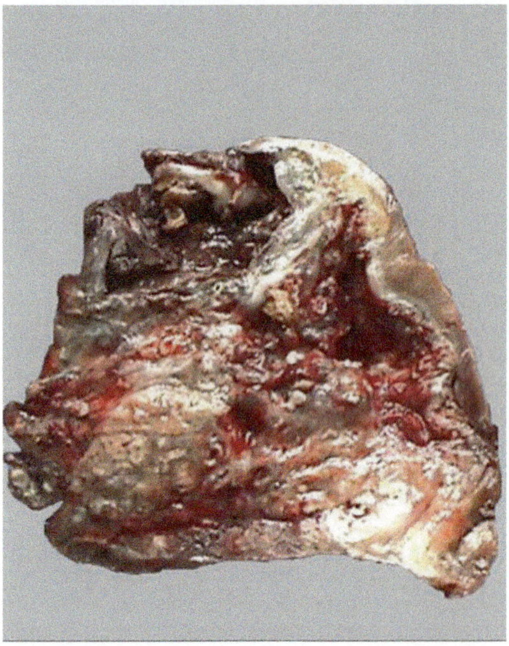

Fig. 13.51 Cirrhotic tuberculosis of the lung. The lung is significantly reduced in size, pronounced pleuropneumosclerosis, restructuring and deformity of the lung, cystic cavities, foci of tuberculosis dissemination. Fixed macropreparation

cavities and cysts, organized caseous lesions, bronchiectasis, emphysema bullous. Small vessels of the lung are obliterated, arteriovenous anastomoses, and angioectasis are formed, which can become a source of pulmonary bleeding.

The most common immediate cause of death in tuberculosis with severe cirrhotic changes is the decompensation of chronic pulmonary heart disease.

Tuberculous pleurisy—acute, subacute, or chronic and recurrent tuberculous inflammation of the pleura. Pleural tuberculosis can develop in any period of the tuberculosis process. It can occur as an independent form of tuberculosis of the respiratory organs and can act as a complication of other forms of pulmonary tuberculosis. Ways of development of tuberculous pleurisy can be different—lymphogenous, hematogenous, and contact.

Localization of tuberculous pleurisy can be one- and two-sided, in terms of prevalence—limited (only in the projection of tuberculous inflammation in the lung) and common with damage to both pleura sheets. It can be combined with damage to the serous membranes of the pericardium and abdominal cavity, which indicates the development of tuberculous polyserositis. By the nature of the exudate, pleurisy can be serous, serous fibrinous, serous hemorrhagic, and caseous.In allergic pleurisy, which develops with a hyperergic reaction of the pleura to a tuberculosis antigen, which is usually found in primary tuberculosis and proceeds with hypersensitivity of tissues (including serous membranes), exudate is serous or serous fibrinous, with an admixture of lymphocytes, leukocytes, and eosinophils. In this case, signs of specific inflammation are absent or minimal. In the pleura, edema, hyperemia, lymphostasis, focal lymphoid reaction can be present. The phenomena of exudation can be pronounced and lead to lung collapse.

Perifocal pleurisy refers to cases of contact lesion of the pleura when the source of inflammation in the pleura is a subpleurally located area of tuberculous inflammation. The process in the pleura is initially local, in the projection of the site of tuberculous lesion of the lung, with the subsequent development of serous or fibrinous exudate.

With the lymphogenous and hematogenous pathways of the infection, multiple millet-like, dense, grayish-white tuberous eruptions form in the pleura. Exudation is detected in the pleural cavity, which, in the case of the reverse development of the tuberculous process, resolves. The pleura leaves are fibrosed, thicken, solder together with partial or complete obliteration of the lumen of the pleural cavity.

With the contact path of the development of tuberculosis of the pleura, two options are distinguished. In the first case, pleurisy develops with subpleural localization of the site of tuberculous inflammation with the spread of the process from the lung tissue to the adjacent pleura. In the second variant, the infected material enters the pleural cavity from the lung affected by tuberculosis, for example, when the contents of the subpleural tuberculous cavity break through into the pleural cavity or when the subpleurally located caseous-necrotic focus disintegrates.

Acute tuberculous empyema of the pleural cavity develops, with the presence of pus-like exudate with caseous contents in it (Fig. 13.52). The exudate consists of molten caseous masses, fibrin, among which are lymphocytes, macrophages, leukocytes, and giant multinucleated cells. There are caseous overlays on the surface of the pleura, infiltrates from lymphocytes, histiocytes, neutrophilic leukocytes are formed in the pleura, there may be scattered epithelioid cells, and granulomas are formed in a small amount. This type of pleurisy is treated as tuberculous empyema of the pleura.

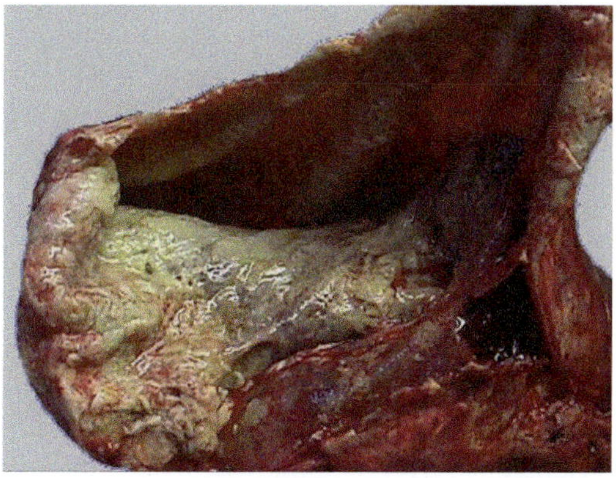

Fig. 13.52 Tuberculous empyema of the pleural cavity. Non-fixed macro specimen

With long-term communication between the cavity of the tuberculous cavity and the pleural cavity, the process becomes chronic—*chronic tuberculous empyema* of the pleural cavity with bronchopleural fistula. The pleura leave sharply thicken due to the development of fibrosis and hyalinosis. On the surface, there are caseous overlays with the underlying layer of specific granulation tissue. In the thickness of fibrosis, small sections of caseous necrosis and granulomas can be found (Fig. 13.53).

Chronic tuberculous empyema of the pleural cavity leads to the development of pleuropneumosclerosis, chest deformity, the development of bronchopleural and pleuro-thoracic fistulas, "armored" lung. Patients die from chronic pulmonary heart failure, severe intoxication and exhaustion, and amyloidosis.

Tuberculosis of the trachea and bronchi macroscopically manifests itself in the form of edema and wall infiltration with narrowing of the lumen (infiltrative form), the formation of tuberculous ulcerative defects (infiltrative-ulcerative form), and tubercular miliary rashes on the mucous membrane.

Histologically, with the infiltrative form of trachea and bronchial tuberculosis, the following symptoms are characteristic: squamous metaplasia of the respiratory epithelium, dense diffuse lymphoid or lymphoid–leukocyte infiltrate in the own plate of the mucous membrane, replacement of the own plate with specific granulation tissue with the presence of epithelioid giant cell reaction and caseous necrosis (Fig. 13.54). There are granulomatous and caseous tuberculous bronchitis (Fig. 13.55), and, depending on the location in the bronchial wall, endo-, meso-, peri-, and panbronchitis. In the case of infiltrative-ulcerative tuberculosis of the trachea and bronchi, erosive-ulcerative changes with signs of tuberculous inflammation in the area of defects are detected.

Tuberculosis of the trachea and bronchi can also develop with the formation of *broncho (tracheo)—nodular fistulas*, which is noted with caseous bronchadenitis.

Complications of tuberculosis of the trachea and bronchi are bleeding from tuberculous ulcers,

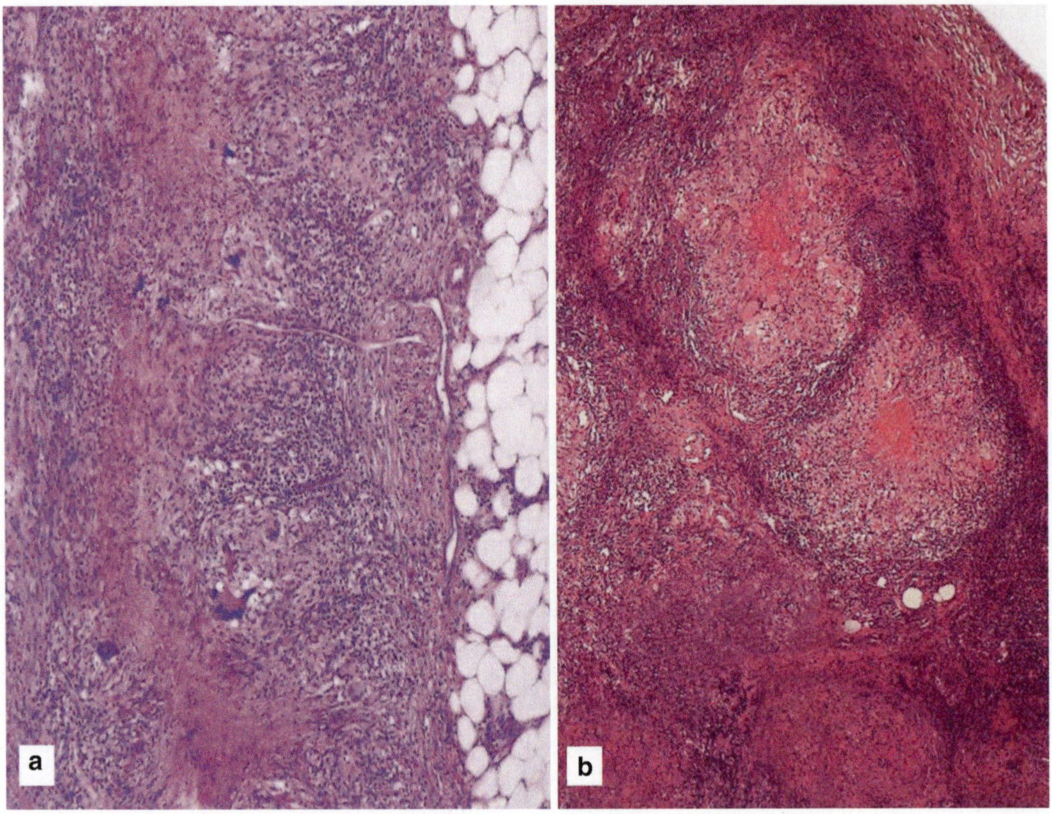

Fig. 13.53 Tuberculosis of the pleura. Multiple merging granulomas with necrosis in the center. Stained H.-E. (**a**) ×100 and (**b**) ×200

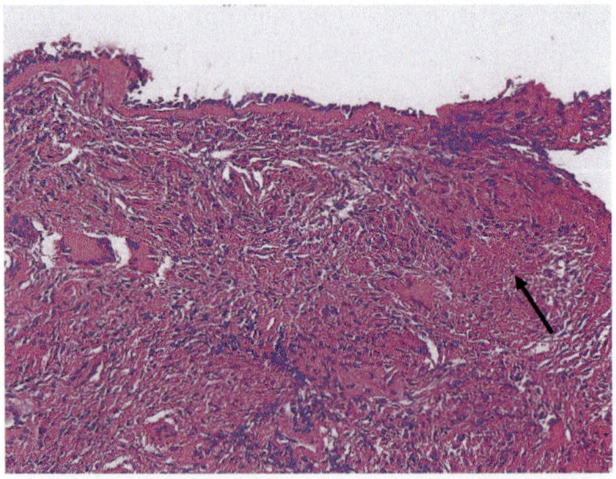

Fig. 13.54 Infiltrative tuberculosis of the bronchus. There are indistinct merging granulomas in the center of the mucosal lamina, including those with micronecrosis in the center (indicated by an arrow). Stained H.-E.. ×200

stenosis of the trachea and bronchi. If all layers of the wall of the airways are affected, the tuberculosis process can spread to adjacent tissues.

Konyotuberculosis, silicotuberculosis—pneumoconiosis (the most severe form of dust pathology—silicosis) associated with tuberculosis, usually developing endogenously due to the interaction of silicon dioxide and MBT. Tuberculosis in silicosis is secondary and is usually caused by the reactivation of previously healed tuberculous lesions in the lungs and intrathoracic lymph nodes.

The morphological picture is a combination of specific tuberculous changes and silicotic granulomas. The basis of the lesion is fibro-hyalinized silicotic nodules and silicotuberculous necrotic foci of various degrees of maturity, including hyalinized. The foci and caverns of silicotic origin are colored black due to the deposition of dust pigments (Fig. 13.56).

Silicotic nodules are localized in the lumen of the alveoli, alveolar passages, in place of the lymphatic vessels and are polycentrically or

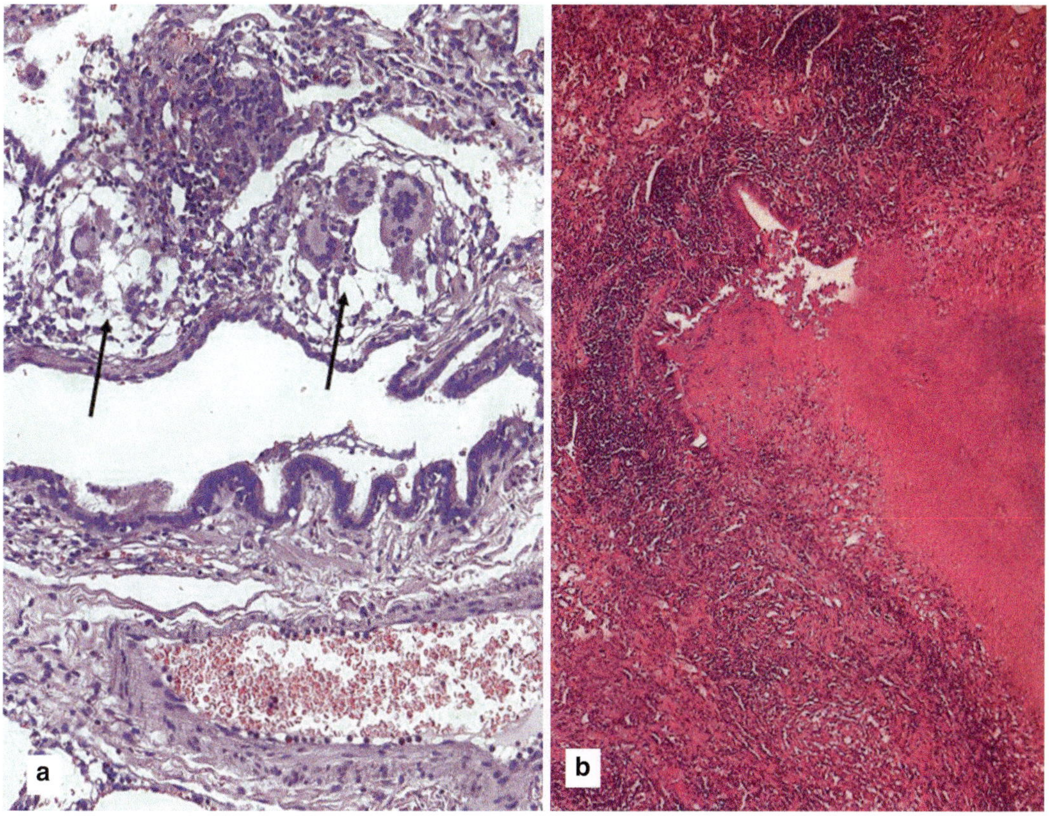

Fig. 13.55 Tuberculosis of the bronchus. (**a**) Granulomatous tuberculosis bronchitis (granulomas are indicated by arrows) and (**b**) Caseous bronchitis. Stained H.-E.. (**a**) ×200 and (**b**) ×100

vortex-shaped collagen fibers, with the presence of coniophages, in the cytoplasm of which dust particles are found extracellularly (Fig. 13.57). The decay of nodes leads to the formation of silicotic caverns. The nodular and diffuse sclerotic forms of lesions are distinguished, as well as the tumor-like form of silicosis—a variant of the nodular when the silicotic nodules merge into large conglomerates.

In addition to the described changes, tuberculous caseous-necrotic foci with bronchogenic dissemination and the formation of caverns are simultaneously detected (Fig. 13.58). In silicotuberculosis foci, destructive changes can be combined with calcification.

The following clinical and anatomical forms of silicotuberculosis are distinguished: isolated silicotuberculous lymphadenitis; disseminated silicotuberculosis; caseous pneumonia; focal silicotuberculosis; conglomerate silicotuberculosis; destructive (cavernous) silicotuberculosis.

Summarizing the data on the morphology of tuberculosis we find it necessary to evaluate changes allowing to judge about the activity of the process.

Microscopic signs of tuberculosis progression:

- leukocyte infiltration in foci of caseous necrosis
- absence of signs of the organization of secondary foci (lack of capsule, fibrosis)
- perifocal exudative, exudative–productive, or granulomatous reaction
- mild granulomatous (including epithelioid cell) reaction along the periphery of the foci of caseous necrosis
- foci of bronchogenic, lymphogenous, and hematogenous dissemination away from the main lesion
- parietal subcapsular purulent fusion of caseous necrosis in the secondary site

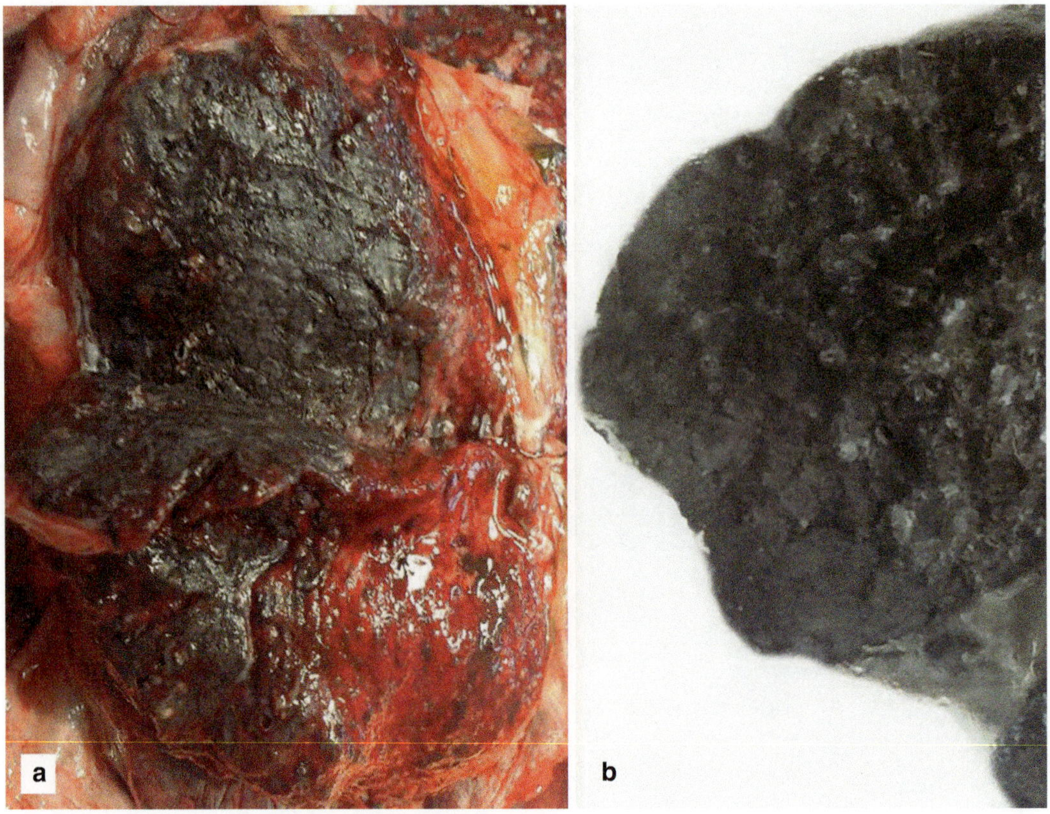

Fig. 13.56 Lung silicosis. (**a**) Non-fixed macropreparation and (**b**) fixed macropreparation

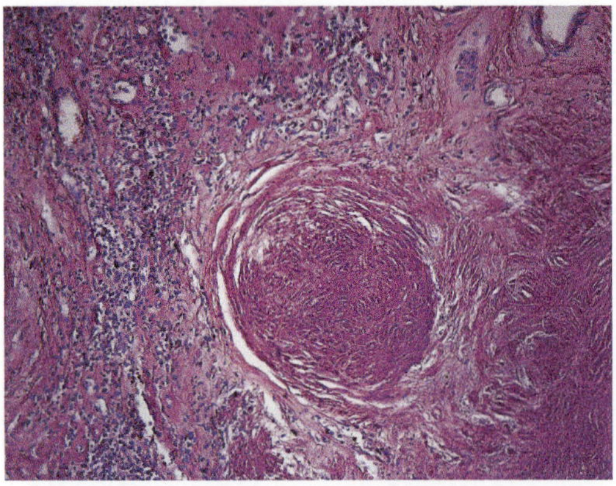

Fig. 13.57 Silicosis nodule in the lung. Stained H.-E.. ×100

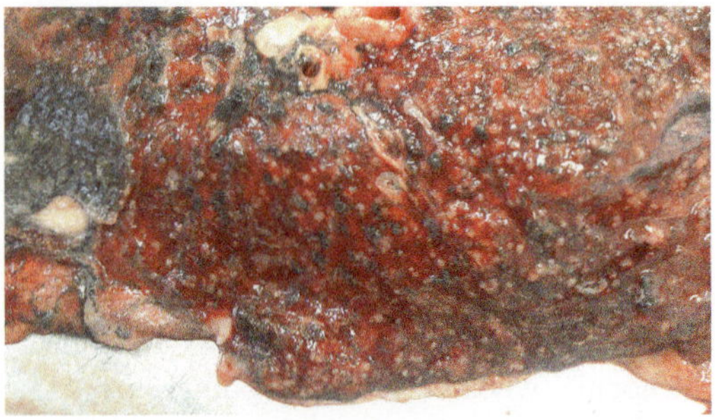

Fig. 13.58 Silicotuberculosis. Non-fixed macro specimens

- spread of specific inflammation in the capsule of the focus of caseous necrosis and outside the capsule of the focus of caseous necrosis (in adjacent areas)
- tuberculous inflammation of the draining bronchus
- the presence of acute tuberculosis caverns
- for a chronic tuberculous cavity—a wide inner layer of caseous necrosis, exceeding the width of a layer of specific granulation tissue; leukocyte infiltration of caseous masses; the spread of leukocyte infiltration to the layer of specific granulation tissue, fibrous capsule, adjacent lung tissue; purulent fusion of the outer fibrous capsule; pericavitary exudative, exudative–productive, granulomatous reaction.

Microscopic signs of stabilization in tuberculosis:

- encapsulation of the focus of caseous necrosis
- fibrosis of the focus of caseous necrosis
- hyalinosis of the focus of caseous necrosis
- calcification (petrification) of the focus of caseous necrosis
- ossification of the focus of caseous necrosis
- lack of leukocyte infiltration of necrotic masses
- lack of perifocal exudative or granulomatous reaction
- the absence of signs of tuberculous inflammation in the draining bronchi (there may be productive inflammation in the form of lymphoid infiltrate)
- for a chronic tuberculous cavity—cleansing the cavity of the cavity from caseous-necrotic masses, reducing the width of the caseous-necrotic layer (the caseous necrosis layer is equal to or less than the specific granulation tissue layer in width), the absence of leukocyte infiltration of necrotic masses, the absence of leukocyte infiltration of fibrotic capsule, fibrous capsule caverns, absence of pericavitary exudative or exudative granulomatous reaction

13.3 Peculiarities of Tuberculosis in Combination with HIV in AIDS Stage

The data presented in this chapter are partly based upon the experience of Russian phtisiopathology scientific school [9–25], partly own long-term experience of one of the authors (Yu. R. Zyuzya).

At stages 1 and 2 of HIV infection (according to CDC classification) the macro- and microscopic picture is identical to tuberculosis without HIV infection. The structure of mortality from tuberculosis in the early stages of HIV infection is comparable to that in people without HIV infection.

When HIV-associated tuberculosis develops at stage 3 of HIV infection, autopsy studies revealed a significant predominance of the generalized form (up to 90% of deaths), with lung damage in all cases. With generalized tuberculosis in 98% of cases, disseminated lung damage was observed with a predominance of small focal and miliary dissemination, which was observed in 75.5% of the dead. Dissemination, except for the lungs, develops in almost all internal organs (kidneys, liver, spleen, brain, testes, epididymis, adrenal glands, thyroid, pancreas, prostate gland, ovaries, uterus, heart, bones, joints, skin, etc.). All groups of lymph nodes are also involved in the pathological process.

Macroscopic examination in all segments of the lungs reveals multiple whitish-yellow lesions with a diameter of 1–2 mm with miliary dissemination to 1 cm (small focal dissemination) (Fig. 13.59). Severe congestion and pulmonary edema can impede the visualization of miliary foci. Large focal dissemination in the form of whitish-yellow confluent acinous, acinic–lobular, lobular, confluent lobular foci (whose diameter exceeded 1 cm), is much less common.

Foci of tuberculous dissemination have no signs of organization: there is no capsule on the periphery of necrotic foci, calcified, fibrosed, or hyalinized foci, and areas of pneumosclerosis are not detected. In some cases of recurrent tuberculosis or death after prolonged antituberculosis therapy in the study of the lungs, one can find a slight cicatricial deformation of the tops of the lungs, thin grayish strands of connective tissue, a faintly forming capsule around individual foci of dissemination.

In 40% of the cases of HIV-associated disseminated pulmonary tuberculosis, the formation

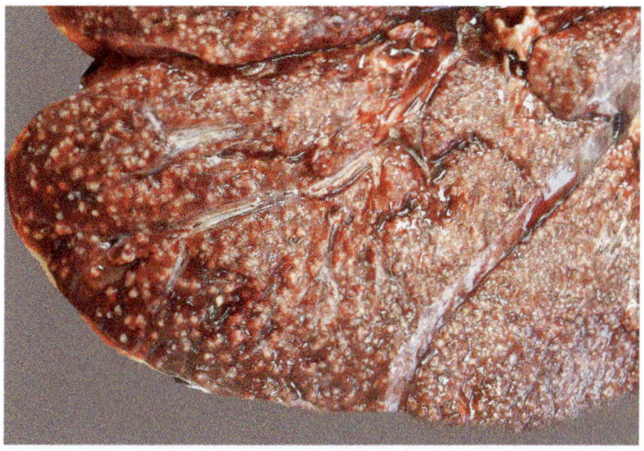

Fig. 13.59 Miliary dissemination in the lungs in HIV-associated tuberculosis. Unfixed macropreparation

of decay cavities (acute tuberculous caverns) was detected, and the development of acute caverns was also observed in small foci of caseous necrosis, the size of which did not exceed 1 cm. The walls of acute tuberculous caverns are thin, soft, elastic, easily fall off when the lung is compressed. The inner surface is covered with yellowish–whitish caseous-necrotic masses of a cheesy appearance, in the lumen of the cavity is a yellowish pus-like content with sequestered caseous masses (Fig. 13.60).

In isolated cases, pulmonary tuberculosis was characterized by the formation of extensive confluent caseous and necrotic foci, occupying a segment, lobe, or entire lung, with bronchogenic foci screenings and multiple acute caverns (the so-called caseous pneumonia).

It is also rare, in separate observations, in the late stages of HIV infection that chronic tuberculous caverns are found, localized mainly in the upper lobes—in one, two, and three segments. A "polycavernous" lesion with the presence of two or more caverns is possible, while in addition to chronic caverns, acute and subacute caverns of various sizes are formed. Chronic tuberculous caverns with dense rigid walls, which do not collapse upon palpation. They have a dense grayish fibrous fibrous outer capsule; the internal contents of the cavity are whitish masses of a cheesy appearance, located both parietally and in the cavity of the cavity. The acute progression of this form of tuberculosis during HIV infection is characterized not only by the development of extensive large-focal bronchogenic dissemination, caseous segmentitis, or lobitis with multiple acute cavities but also by the appearance of miliary pulmonary dissemination, which is one of the signs of hematogenous spread of tuberculosis.

Lymph nodes of all groups (peripheral, intrathoracic, mesenteric, retroperitoneal, etc.) are enlarged, with a whitish opaque capsule, dense, soldered into conglomerates (Fig. 13.61). In the section, the lymph node tissue is replaced by whitish–grayish, crumbly curdled necrotic masses with their sequestration, purulent fusion, and the formation of decay cavities—lympho-glandular caverns (Fig. 13.62). The inflammatory process extends to the adjacent soft tissues, which leads to the development of tuberculous periadenitis, external and internal tuberculous fistulas. Due to the rapid progression of the tuberculous process and the predominance of the exudative phase of inflammation, the external fistula can be purulent without whitish curd caseous-necrotic inclusions, which makes it similar to the fistulous form of bacterial purulent lymphadenitis caused by pyogenic microflora. Caseous lymphadenitis of the intrathoracic lymph nodes is accompanied by the formation of broncho-nodular and esophageal-nodular fistulas (Fig. 13.63).

Microscopic examination in most cases noted the predominance of the alternative (necrotic) and exudative (vascular) phases of inflammation with almost complete inhibition of the productive (granulomatous) component. This determines the absence of signs of delimitation and organization of foci of inflammation, as well as the development of a pronounced perifocal exudative tissue reaction.

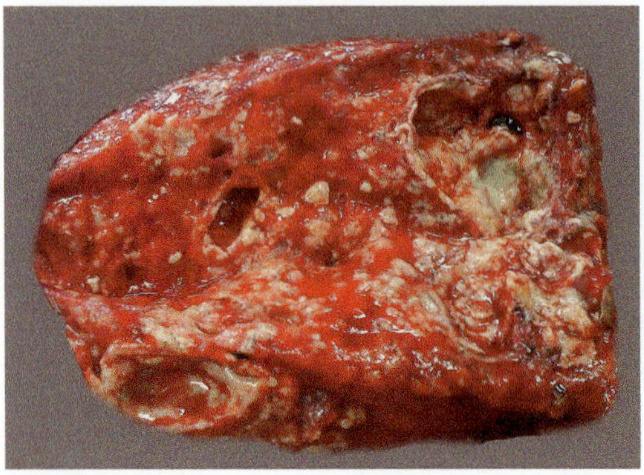

Fig. 13.60 Dissemination in the lungs with the formation of acute cavities in HIV-associated tuberculosis. Unfixed macropreparation.

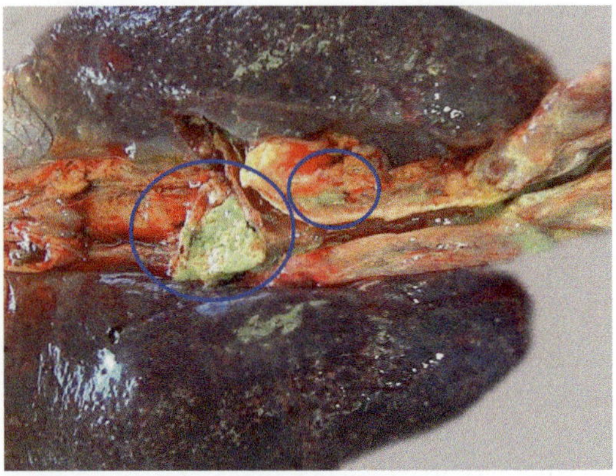

Fig. 13.61 Miliary dissemination in the lungs and caseous lymphadenitis of the intrathoracic lymph nodes (the lymph nodes are circled) in HIV-associated tuberculosis. Non-fixed macro specimens

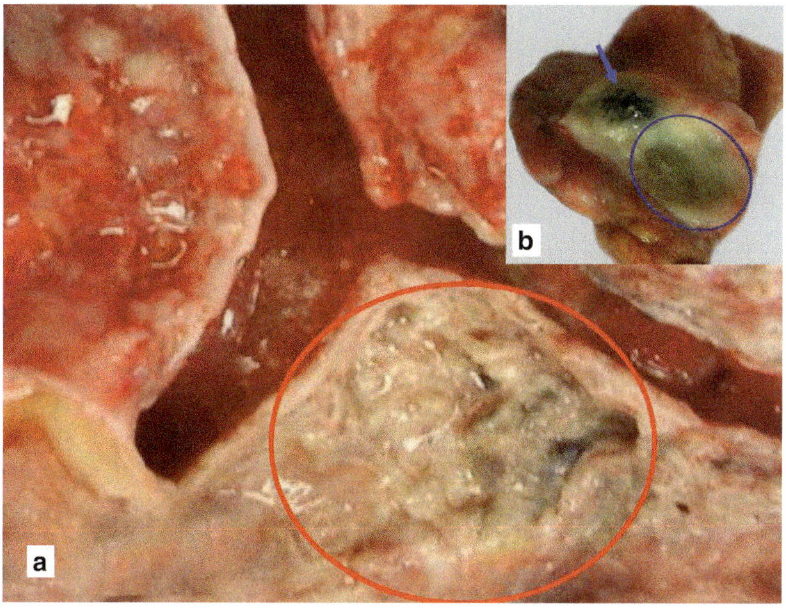

Fig. 13.62 (**a**) Total caseous lymphadenitis of the bifurcation lymph node (marked with a red round frame) with sections of necrotic mass sequestration; (**b**) lymphogenic (lymphoelesic) cavern of the intrathoracic lymph node (outlined with a blue round frame), the arrow indicates the adjacent lymph node with anthracosis and whitish foci of caseous necrosis. Unfixed macropreparations

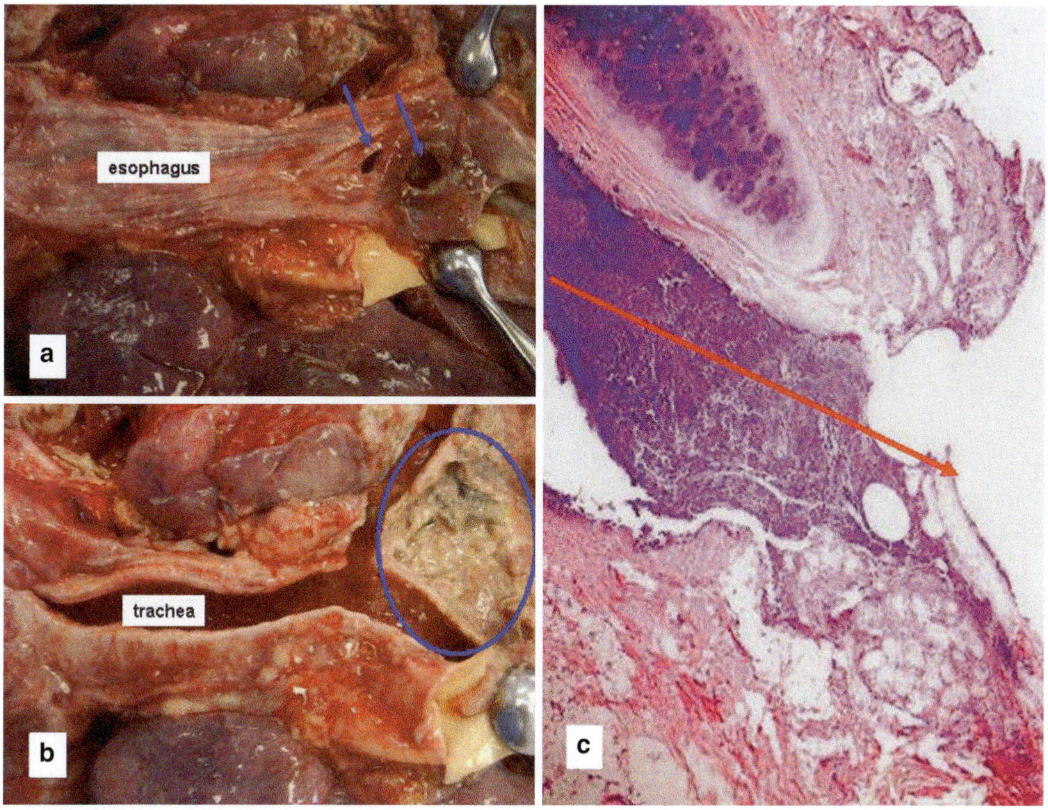

Fig. 13.63 Tuberculous fistulas. (**a**) Esophageal–nodular fistulas (indicated by arrows); (**b**) esophagus separated, visible bifurcation lymph node with total caseous lymphadenitis and sequestration of necrotic masses (circled by a round frame); (**c**) bronchodular fistula (red arrow indicates the direction of the fistula in the wall of the cartilaginous bronchus), in the lumen of the fistula caseous-purulent masses. (**a**, **b**) Unfixed macropreparations and (**c**) H.-E.. ×100

The foci of tuberculous inflammation are represented by necrotic masses with abundant neutrophilic leukocyte infiltration, with purulent spreading of necrotic masses. The foci in HIV-associated tuberculosis have the appearance of purulent-necrotic, identical to septic pyemic foci (Fig. 13.64). Signs of granulomatous inflammation are either completely absent or there is a very meager productive reaction in the form of single epithelioid or multinucleated giant cells; the perifocal lymphoid reaction is sharply inhibited.

There are no signs of a wave-like course of the process characteristic of tuberculosis. The purulent necrotic foci of tuberculous inflammation have a monomorphic structure corresponding to the same prescription of the process and indicating the swiftness of its progression and generalization (Figs. 13.65 and 13.66).

The "erasure" of granulomatous inflammation, the formation of purulent necrotic foci in the lungs that are atypical for tuberculosis can lead to an incorrect assessment of the pathological process and can be mistakenly regarded as bacterial pneumonia with abscess formation, as manifesta-

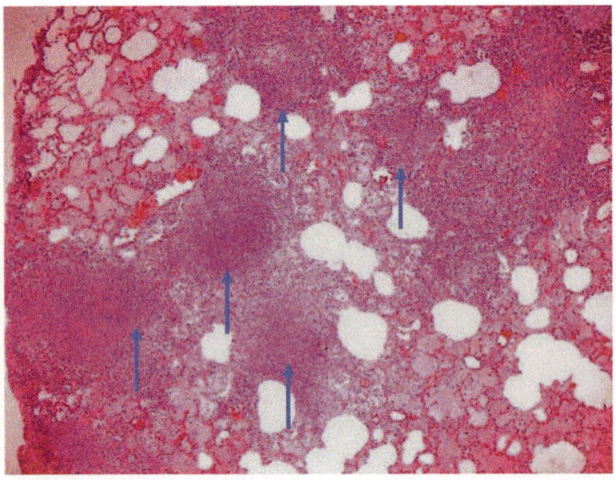

Fig. 13.65 HIV-associated tuberculosis. Monomorphic miliary and subsidiaries tuberculous foci in the lung (indicated by arrows) in acute progression of tuberculosis. H.-E. ×100 (for comparison, see Fig. 13.19)

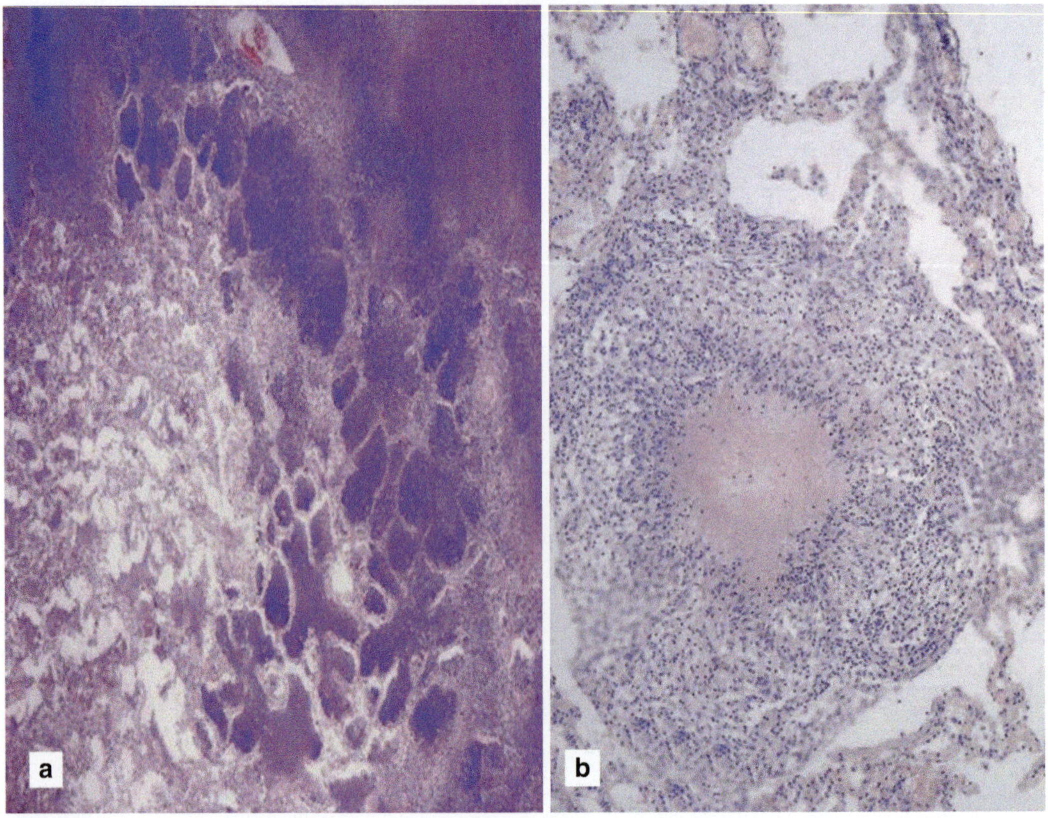

Fig. 13.64 (**a**) HIV-associated tuberculosis. Perivascular purulent-necrotic focus of tuberculosis inflammation in the lung in the absence of granulomatous reaction; (**b**) For comparison, tuberculosis without HIV infection. A typical tubercular lesion in the lung. H.-E. ×100

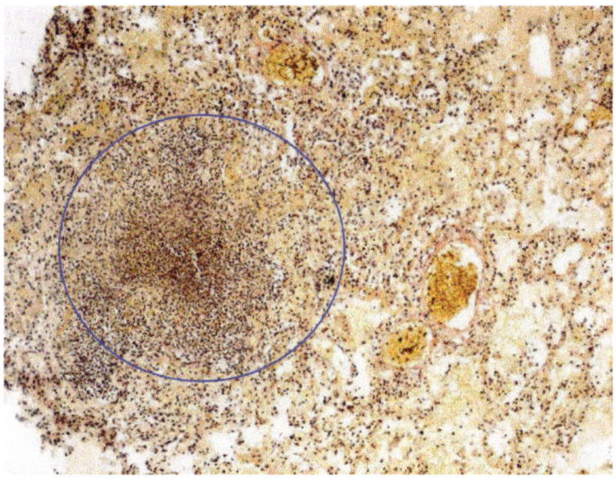

Fig. 13.66 HIV-associated tuberculosis. Miliary tuberculous purulent-necrotic lesion in the lung, without signs of the organization (circled by a round frame). Stained by van Gieson. ×200

tions of a septic process, purulent abscessed lymphadenitis, etc. (Fig. 13.67).

In addition to small focal and miliary dissemination, foci of inflammation are revealed histologically, the size of which was less than miliary (the so-called submiliary dissemination, which is almost indistinguishable by macroscopic examination of organs). Given the severity of exudative changes with the development of pulmonary edema, sharp venous congestion, the microscopic detection of miliary and "submiliary" foci can be extremely difficult (Fig. 13.68).

The localization of foci of tuberculous inflammation is predominantly perivascular (Fig. 13.69), which is one of the signs of hematogenous generalization of the process. There are also signs of

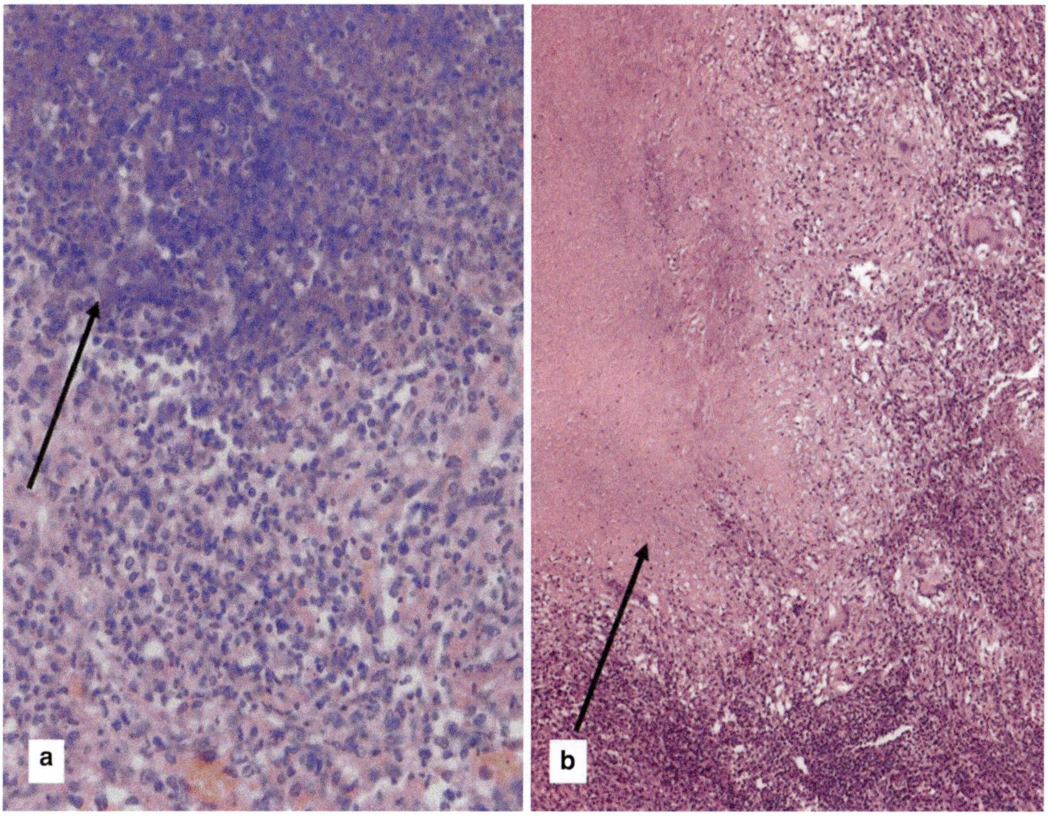

Fig. 13.67 (**a**) HIV-associated tuberculosis lymphadenitis, a purulent-necrotic focus without granulomatous reaction on the periphery and without signs of the organization (the microscopic picture is identical to purulent abscessing lymphadenitis caused by a purulent microflora); (**b**) for comparison—tuberculosis lymphadenitis without HIV infection, a focus of caseous necrosis with a granulomatous reaction on the periphery. Necrotic foci are indicated by arrows. H.-E. ×200

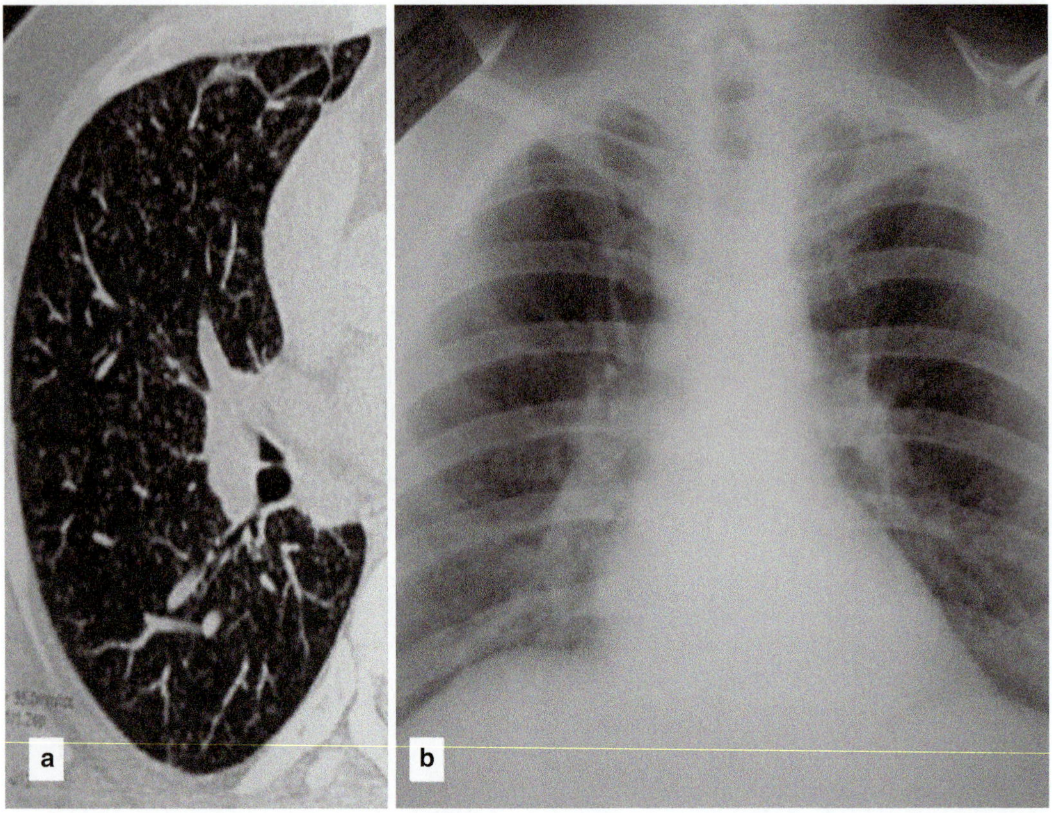

Fig. 13.68 HIV-associated tuberculosis. (**a**) Computed tomography of the chest organs with pronounced miliary and submiliary dissemination in the lungs and (**b**) overview radiography of the lungs in the same patient, signs of increased vascular pattern, dissemination is not determined

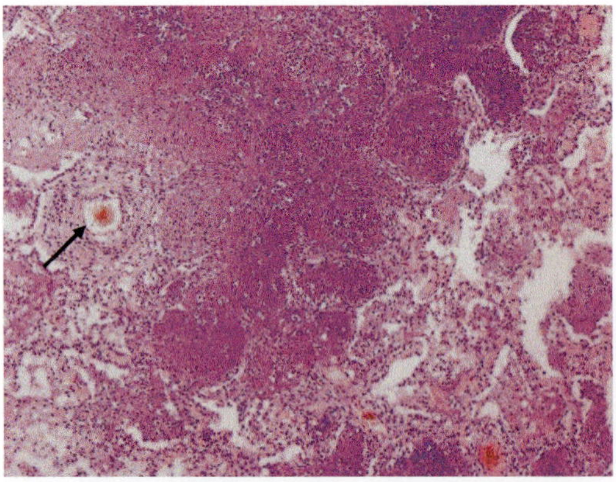

Fig. 13.69 HIV-associated tuberculosis. Perivascular localization of the focus of tuberculosis inflammation (the vessel is indicated by an arrow). H.-E. ×100

lymphogenous dissemination. Bronchogenic dissemination, which is usually detected with large foci of tuberculous inflammation, is less commonly noted.

In a microscopic examination, in addition to alterative (necrotic) reactions, there is a pronounced exudative component of inflammation, which indicates the involvement of the pathological process of blood vessels. This is confirmed by the presence of various types of vasculitis: endo-, panvasculitis, thrombovasculitis. The most common development is panvasculitis with severe polymorphic cell infiltration of all layers of the vascular wall with a predominance of neutrophilic white blood cells and purulent destructive endovasculitis. Acid-resistant bacteria were detected in the Z-N stain in the necrotic masses and cytoplasm of neutrophilic leukocytes of the vascular wall and thrombotic masses, as well as in perivascular leukocytes, which confirms the infectious (tuberculous) nature of vasculitis and may indicate hematogenous generalization of the process (Figs. 13.70, 13.71, and 13.72).

In addition to tuberculous vasculitis, inflammatory changes in vessels of a reactive nature

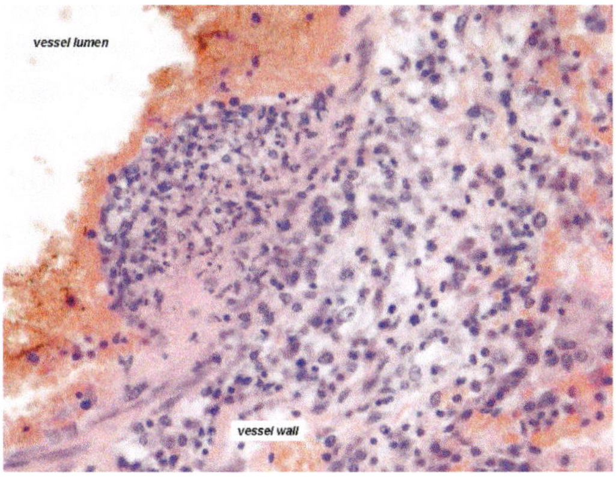

Fig. 13.70 HIV-associated tuberculosis vasculitis (diffuse polymorphic cell infiltration of the vascular wall, absence of signs of granulomatous inflammation, forming parietal thrombus). H.-E. ×200

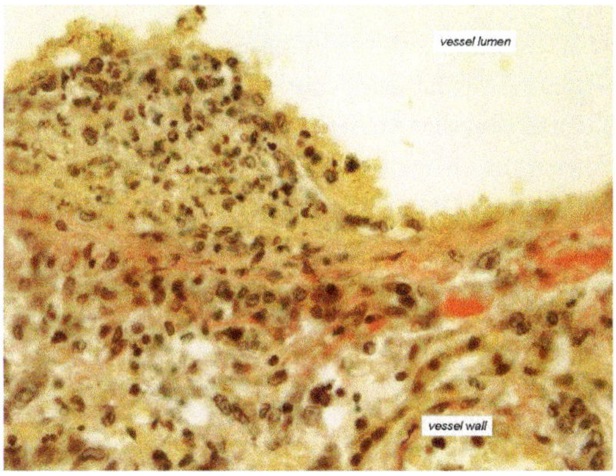

Fig. 13.71 HIV-associated tuberculosis vasculitis (same fragment), no signs of organization. Stained by van Gieson. ×200

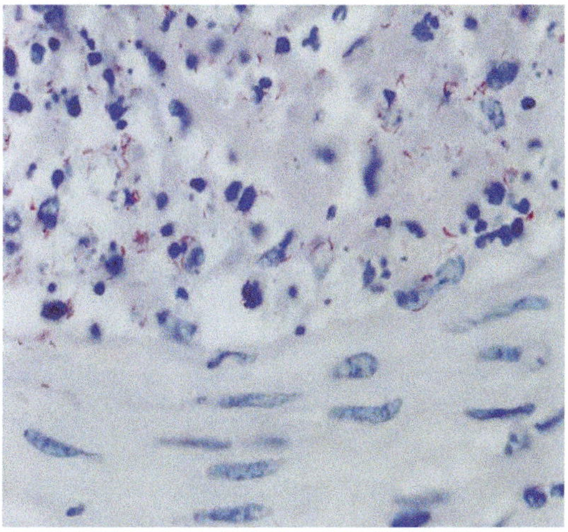

Fig. 13.72 HIV-associated tuberculosis vasculitis (same fragment), abundance of acid-resistant bacteria in the vascular wall infiltrate. Stained by Z-N. ×1000

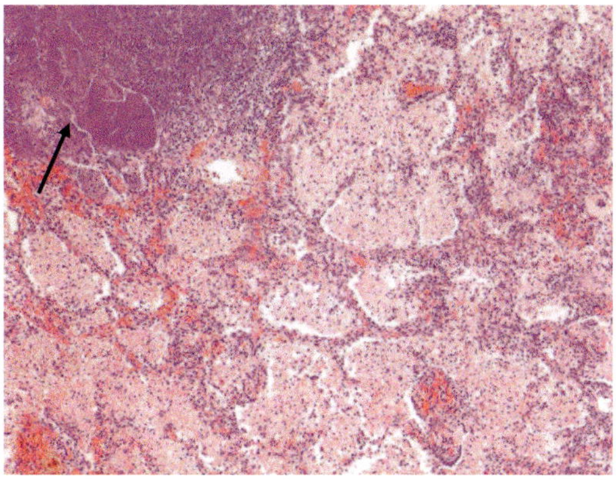

Fig. 13.73 Pronounced perifocal exudative reaction around the focus of caseous necrosis (the focus is indicated by an arrow). H.-E. ×100

have been identified, usually developing outside the foci of tuberculous inflammation. In the vascular wall, swelling, edema, plasma soaking, infiltration by mononuclear cells with an admixture of neutrophilic leukocytes are observed. When staining according to Z-N and IHC studies with tuberculosis antibodies, acid-resistant bacteria and mycobacteria are not detected.

The defeat of the vascular bed, caused by tuberculosis and reactive vasculitis, leads to the development of extensive circulatory disorders. Involvement in the pathological process of the vascular bed with the development of vasculitis of various origins, the addition of vascular disorders caused by DIC, local circulatory disorders (during surgery), strengthens severe exudative tissue reactions and is an unfavorable factor.

Around the foci of tuberculous inflammation, a pronounced extensive exudative reaction is formed, moreover, significantly exceeding the size of the focus. The nature of the exudate can be the most diverse—serous, fibrinous, serous–fibrinous, serous–hemorrhagic, fibrinous–purulent. In the lungs, the perifocal reaction, with the presence in the alveoli around the focus of tuberculous inflammation of fibrin and leukocytes, must be differentiated from fibrinous–purulent bacterial pneumonia, which can be combined with tuberculosis (Fig. 13.73).

A histobacterioscopic examination with staining of slices according to Z-N allows you to identify bacteria of the acid and alcohol resistant family, which include MBT. In HIV-associated tuberculosis, acid-resistant bacteria were local-

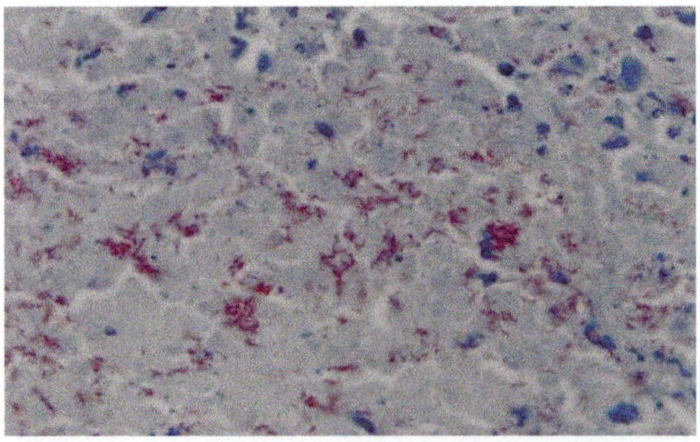

Fig. 13.74 HIV-associated tuberculosis. A large number of acid-resistant bacteria (colored red) in necrotic masses, in the cytoplasm of neutrophilic leukocytes, around destroyed white blood cells. Stained by Z-N. ×1000

ized in purulent–necrotic masses, in the cytoplasm of neutrophilic leukocytes, including destroyed ones (Fig. 13.74). The effectiveness of histobacterioscopy using Z-N stain in the study of tuberculosis associated with HIV reaches 80% and allows the use of this method as a screening method. It should be noted that most acid-resistant bacteria are in the form of sticks. Cocciform and atypical forms (better detected by luminescence microscopy when stained with auramine–rhodamine and IHC reactions) are relatively few in comparison with chronically current destructive forms of tuberculosis without HIV infection. In contrast to the above, in cases of tuberculosis without HIV infection, acid-resistant bacteria are localized in the cytoplasm of macrophages, as well as in the cytoplasm of neutrophilic leukocytes and are freely located in caseous-necrotic masses. The effectiveness of staining according to Z-N in individuals with a preserved immune status is quite low and reaches 40%.

An IHC study using monoclonal tuberculosis antibodies confirms the belonging of acid-resistant bacteria to the genus Mycobacterium identified by Z-N histobacterioscopy (Fig. 13.75).

Species identification of mycobacteria in the native material is carried out using bacteriological culture and polymerase chain reaction (PCR) with the detection of Myc. tuberculosis DNA. Isolation of MBT DNA can be carried out in the material from paraffin blocks.

In 7–62% of cases (according to various authors) with HIV-associated tuberculosis diffuse alveolar lung damage develops, and this condition is often not diagnosed clinically.

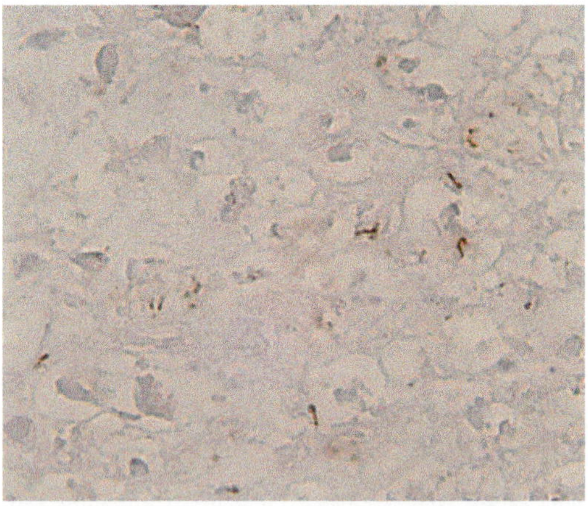

Fig. 13.75 Mycobacteria in the focus of tuberculosis inflammation (stained brown). IHC reaction with *M. tuberculosis* mouse monoclonal antibody. ×1000

Usually morphologically observed changes characteristic of the acute, early (exudative) phase of diffuse alveolar damage to the lungs, with the formation of hyaline membranes. Common distelectases, edema and plasma impregnation, moderate infiltration by neutrophilic leukocytes and mononuclear cells of the alveolar septa, stasis of red blood cells and capillary microthrombosis, hemorrhage in the alveolar septum, erythrocytes in alveoli, endothelial swelling, and necrosis of the individual. In the lumen of the alveoli, serous fluid, fibrin filaments, macrophages, lymphoid cells, plasmocytes, neutrophilic leukocytes, desquamated alveolar epithelium are formed. Hyaline membranes are formed in the lumen of the air alveoli in the form of parietal homogeneous eosinophilic masses (Fig. 13.76).

Changes in the pleura are often exudative: plethora, edema, polymorphic cell, or marked leukocyte infiltration with the formation of purulent–necrotic foci or the development of inflammation in the form of diffuse fibrinous-purulent pleurisy, with the detection of acid-resistant bacteria with Z-N histobacterioscopy. Small fuzzy granulomas may form.

Subtotal or total caseous lymphadenitis with purulent fusion of necrotic masses and the formation of extensive purulent-necrotic foci predominates in the intrathoracic lymph nodes. With sequestration of necrotic masses, acute tuberculous lympho-glandular caverns are formed. A productive reaction is absent or is extremely scarce in the

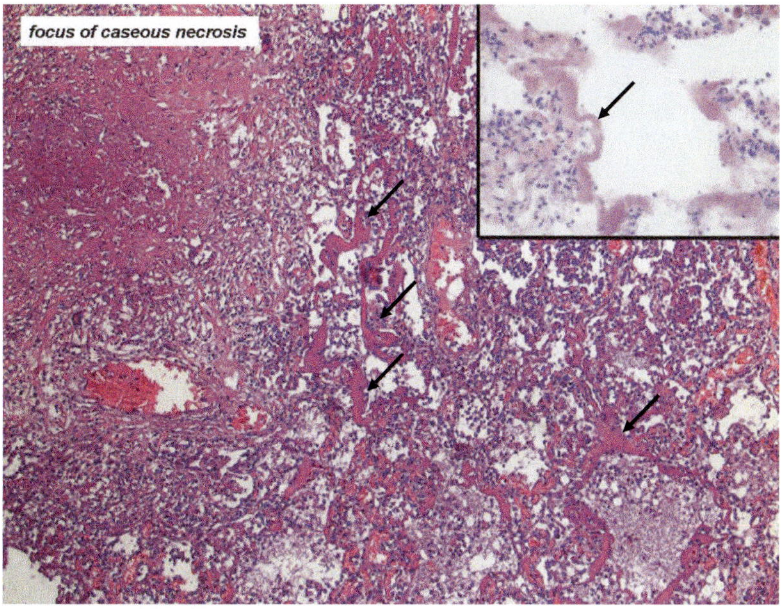

Fig. 13.76 Diffuse alveolar lung injury in HIV-associated tuberculosis. Acute phase of DAPL with the formation of hyaline membranes (indicated by arrows) in perifocal areas. H.-E.. ×200; inset ×400

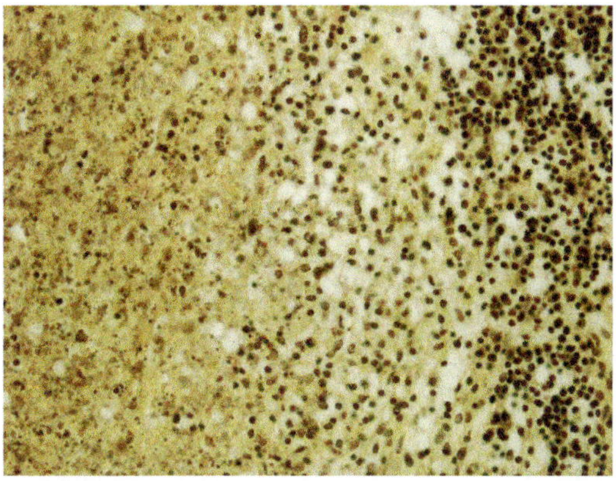

Fig. 13.77 HIV-associated tuberculous lymphadenitis. Caseous purulent-necrotic focus without signs of organization. Stained by van Gieson. ×200 (see Fig. 13.67a)

form of single epithelioid cells randomly located on the edge of the foci of inflammation. There are no signs of delimitation of the focuses of inflammation and capsule formation (Fig. 13.77). Tuberculous periadenitis with internal and external fistulas is characteristic. The microscopic picture of tuberculous lymphadenitis in HIV-associated tuberculosis is often very similar to purulent abscessed lymphadenitis caused by pyogenic flora, and Z-N histobacterioscopy is necessary for differential diagnosis of these processes.

In the small preserved areas of the lymph node, a marked reduction in follicular structures was observed up to lymphoid depletion.

A cytological examination in most cases determines the cytological picture of severe purulent inflammation in the form of a significant number of neutrophilic leukocytes, most of which were in a state of severe dystrophy, with the decay and death of cells, extensive sections of caseous necrosis with an abundance of neutrophilic leukocytes. Signs of granulomatous inflammation, lymphoid elements, and macrophages were not found. When staining cytological preparations according to Z-N, acid-resistant bacteria are detected, mainly in the leukocyte cytoplasm, as well as around destroyed leukocytes and in necrotic masses (Fig. 13.78).

Thus, for HIV-associated tuberculosis, which develops in conditions of a deep immunodeficiency state, an acute progressive course of generalized tuberculosis is characteristic, with hematogenous and lymphogenous generalization, involving all organs and systems of the host, and lung damage in all cases. Alterative–exudative tissue reactions develop with the complete loss of the productive component of inflammation, which prevents the delimitation of foci of tuberculous inflammation and contributes to the active course of the process.

When HIV enters the host, it provides a cytopathic effect on CD4+ cells with their subsequent death, thus eliminating the fundamental link—T--helpers, which play a key role in the formation of

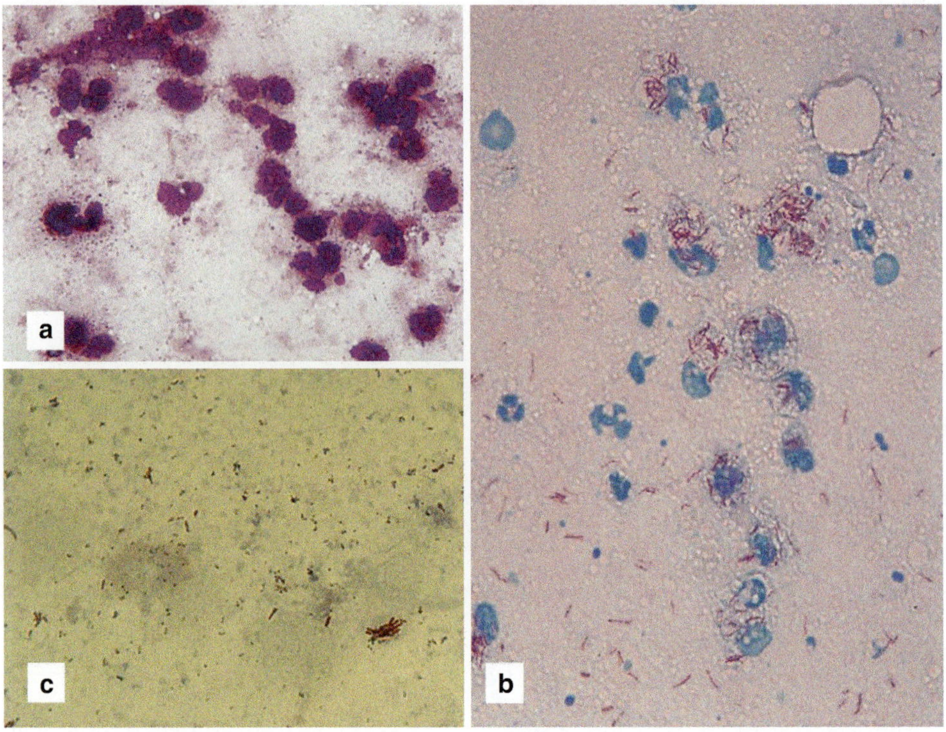

Fig. 13.78 HIV-associated tuberculosis. (**a**) Abundance of neutrophilic white blood cells; (**b**) acid-resistant bacteria in the cytoplasm of white blood cells, outside of destroyed white blood cells, in necrotic masses; (**c**) mycobacteria. Cytological preparations. (**a**) Romanovsky–Giemza coloration; (**b**) Z-N staining; (**c**) immunocytochemical study with *M. tuberculosis* mouse monoclonal antibody. ×1000

a cellular immune response. At the same time, there is a violation of their functional activity, early activation of apoptosis, a decrease in the duration of activity of other immune cells, the appearance of autoantibodies to lymphocyte membranes, a decrease in the number, and complete elimination of CD4+ T-lymphocytes.

Under conditions of extremely severe immune deficiency due to the cytopathic effect on CD4+ lymphocytes and macrophages, the ability of the host to form a cellular immune response to the effects of any infection, including mycobacterium tuberculosis, is lost. The absence or extremely small number of T-lymphocytes leads to the inability to adequately present the antigen by macrophages.

The cytopathic effect of HIV on cells of the macrophage link leads not only to their death, but also to disrupt differentiation and the maturation of both phagocytic and secretory macrophages. "Immature" phagocytic macrophages are not provided with a developed phagolysosomal apparatus. This leads to incomplete phagocytosis of mycobacterium tuberculosis. In addition to macrophages, incomplete phagocytosis of mycobacteria is carried out by neutrophilic leukocytes. Death due to the production of TNF-α neutrophilic leukocytes containing MBT in the cytoplasm is accompanied by damage to the host's own tissues. In addition, with intensive multiplication of MBT with ineffective phagocytosis, a toxin has a necrotizing effect on adjacent tissues, which also leads to the development of necrosis. The absence of a factor of suppression of leukocyte migration with a sharp decrease in the number of T-lymphocytes provokes the involvement of neutrophils in the inflammation focus, which enhances the destructive process due to the activation of an oxygen explosion that occurs when the object of phagocytosis is absorbed.

An extremely scarce or completely absent epithelioid cell reaction in the foci of inflammation in HIV-associated tuberculosis indicates a decrease in the number and violation of the structure and function of secretory macrophages. The absence of epithelioid cells that regulate cell interactions in the granuloma, activates and controls the process of fibrillogenesis, leads to a sharp decrease and complete inhibition of the synthesis of collagen fibers by fibroblasts, the lack of delimitation of the focus of tuberculous inflammation, and the progression of the infectious process.

Differential morphological diagnosis of HIV-associated tuberculosis and opportunistic infections is extremely difficult, due to many factors. Secondary infectious diseases at stage 3 of HIV infection acquire a generalized character with lymphogenous and hematogenous dissemination, with lung damage in the vast majority of cases, have an acutely progressive course with a worn morphological picture, polymorphism of tissue reactions. The purulent–necrotic foci, the perifocal exudative tissue reaction in many cases have identical macro- and microscopic characteristics, which determines the difficulties of the pathological differential diagnosis of HIV-associated infections and tuberculosis (Fig. 13.79).

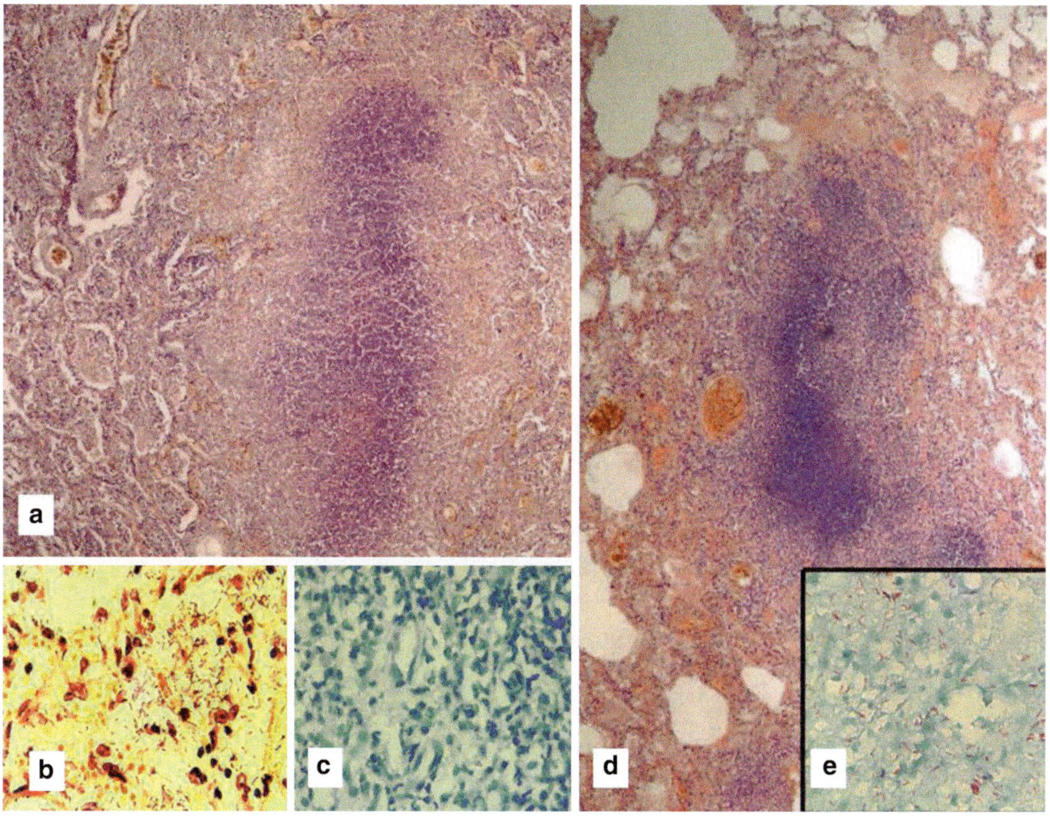

Fig. 13.79 (**a**–**e**) Differential diagnosis of bacterial pneumonia and tuberculosis in HIV infection; (**f**–**j**) differential diagnosis of pneumocystic pneumonia and tuberculosis in HIV infection. (**a**) Bacterial pneumonia; (**b**) Gram-positive microflora in the inflammation; and (**c**) the absence of acid-fast bacteria in the inflammation; (**d**) inflammation in the lung in HIV-associated tuberculosis, is almost identical to the site of inflammation during bacterial pneumonia; and (**e**) acid-fast bacteria in the foci of tuberculous inflammation. (**f**) The source of destruction of the alveolar walls and PCP with the presence of a small calcification, which gives the similarity with the microscopic picture in tuberculous inflammation; (**g**) in the area of destruction around the calcification positive IHC reaction with antibody to pneumocystis; (**h**) miliary focus when pneumocystosis similar to miliary necrotic foci in tuberculosis; (**i**) a positive PAS reaction in miliary focus of pneumocystosis; (**j**) a positive IHC reaction with antibodies to pneumocystis in miliary focus of pneumocystosis. (**a**, **d**, **f**, **h**) Hematoxylin and eosin staining; (**b**) Brown–Hopps staining; (**c**, **e**) Z-N staining; (**g**, **j**) IHC reaction with monoclonal mouse anti-pneumocystis Jiroveci. (**a**, **d**, **f**) ×100; (**h**) ×40; (**g**) ×200; (**i**, **j**) ×400; (**b**, **c**, **e**) ×1000

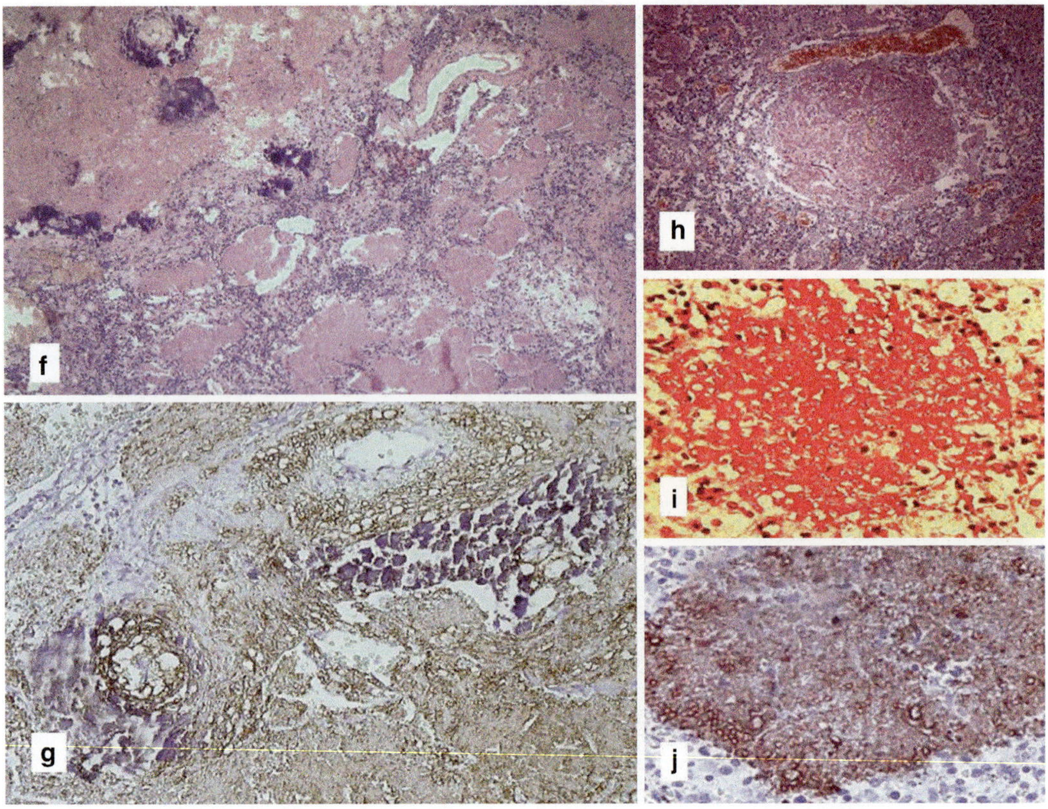

Fig. 13.79 (continued)

Destructive inflammatory processes in the lungs with the formation of decay cavities have been established with HIV infection in more than 50% of cases. This requires a morphological differential diagnosis of disseminated pulmonary tuberculosis with the formation of caverns and other infections in which decay cavities are formed. In addition, in the lungs, the formation of decay cavities was observed in secondary (opportunistic) diseases, which occur without negative destructive processes with negative HIV status—pneumocystic pneumonia, nontuberculous mycobacteriosis of MAC, cryptococcosis (Fig. 13.80).

Lesions of the lungs and other organs caused by various pathogens—bacteria, viruses, fungi, protozoa, are similar in macro and microscopic picture to tuberculosis. This dictates the need for a microscopic differential diagnosis of a thorough analysis of the nature of necrotic foci, the type and prevalence of damage to the vascular bed, perifocal changes, and other morphological features.

For pathological differential diagnosis of opportunistic infections, the most important is the identification of an infectious agent (pathogen), which requires a comprehensive morphological study using a wide range of material research methods (bacteriological, cytological, histobacterioscopic, immunohistochemical, and molecular diagnostic methods) (see Chaps. 8, 14, and 15).

Combined infectious opportunistic lung lesions in the late stages of HIV infection often develop not only in different organs but also in one organ, in particular, in the lungs. This reveals a wide range of diseases caused by bacteria, viruses, fungi, protozoa, and their various combinations (see also Chap. 16).

For example, in the lungs, such combined infectious lesions as tuberculosis and cytomegalovirus infection, pneumocystis pneumonia and cytomegalovirus infection, tuberculosis and bacterial pneumonia are most common. In addition, combinations of bacterial and pneumocystis pneumonia, bacterial pneumonia and cytomegalovirus infection, tuberculosis and pneumocystis pneumonia were identified; tuberculosis and nontuberculous mycobacteriosis, cytomegalovirus infection and mycotic lesions; nontuberculous mycobacteriosis and bacterial pneumonia, and many others. There are cases due to not only two, but also three, four, and even more infections. With combined lung lesions, tuberculosis appeared in half of the cases (Figs. 13.81, 13.82, and 13.83).

Pathological changes with a combined lesion are localized in one or both lungs, can alternate in different segments of one lung, and can also be detected in one microscopic field of view.

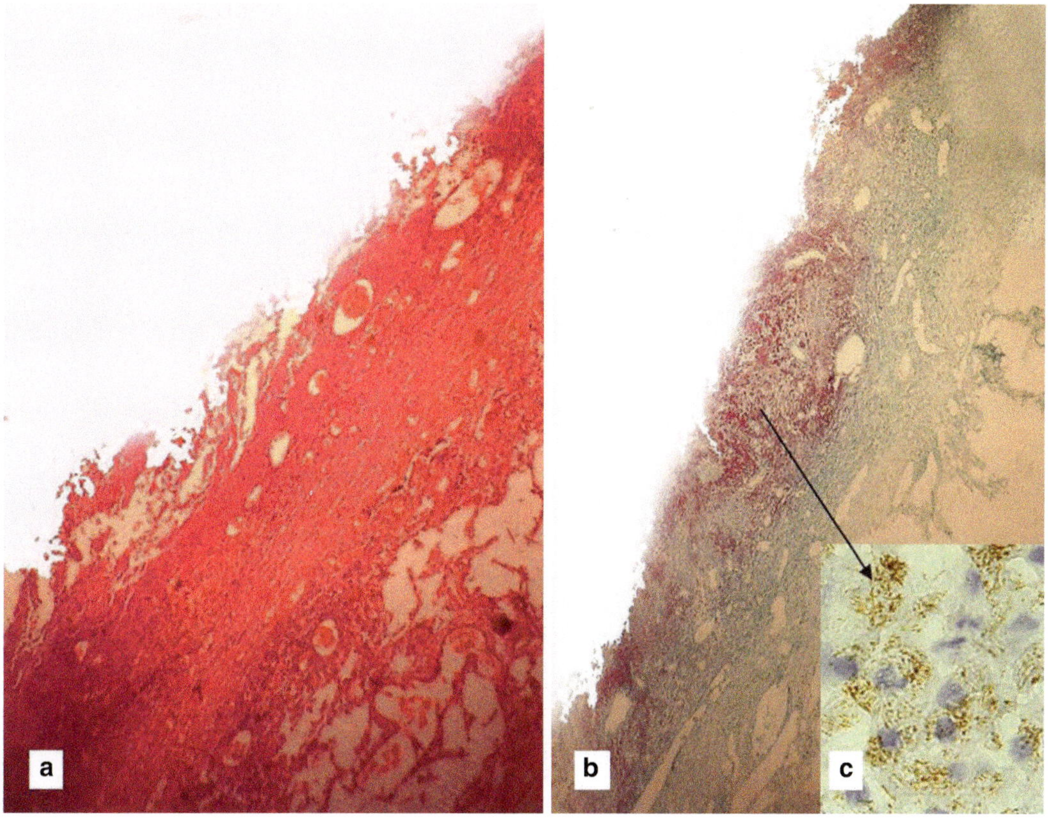

Fig. 13.80 Differential diagnosis of decay cavities in the lungs in HIV-associated infections. (**a–c**) Differential diagnosis of tuberculosis and non-tuberculosis mycobacteriosis MAS; (**d**, **e**) differential diagnosis of tuberculosis and pneumocystis pneumonia; (**f**, **g**) differential diagnosis of tuberculosis and cryptococcosis. (**a**) The wall of the decay cavity in the lung in non-tuberculosis mycobacteriosis MAC; (**b**) the abundance of acid-resistant bacteria in the wall of the decay cavity; (**c**) mycobacteria in an amount that cannot be calculated, localized in the cytoplasm of macrophages. (**d**) the wall of the decay cavity in pneumocystic pneumonia with areas of destruction of the interalveolar partitions and eosinophilic exudate with small calcinates, which gives a similarity to the microscopic picture of tuberculosis; (**e**) positive IHC reaction with pneumocystic antibodies. (**f**) The wall of the decay cavity in the lung in cryptococcosis; (**g**) mycotic cryptococcal structures in necrotic masses. (**a**, **d**, **f**) H.-E.; (**b**) Z-N staining; (**g**) PAS—reaction; (**c**) IHC reaction with Myc. Tuberculosis mouse monoclonal antibody; (**e**) IHC reaction with monoclonal mouse anti-pneumocystis Jiroveci. (**a**, **b**, **d**, **e**) ×100; (**f**) ×200; (**g**) ×400; (**c**) ×1000

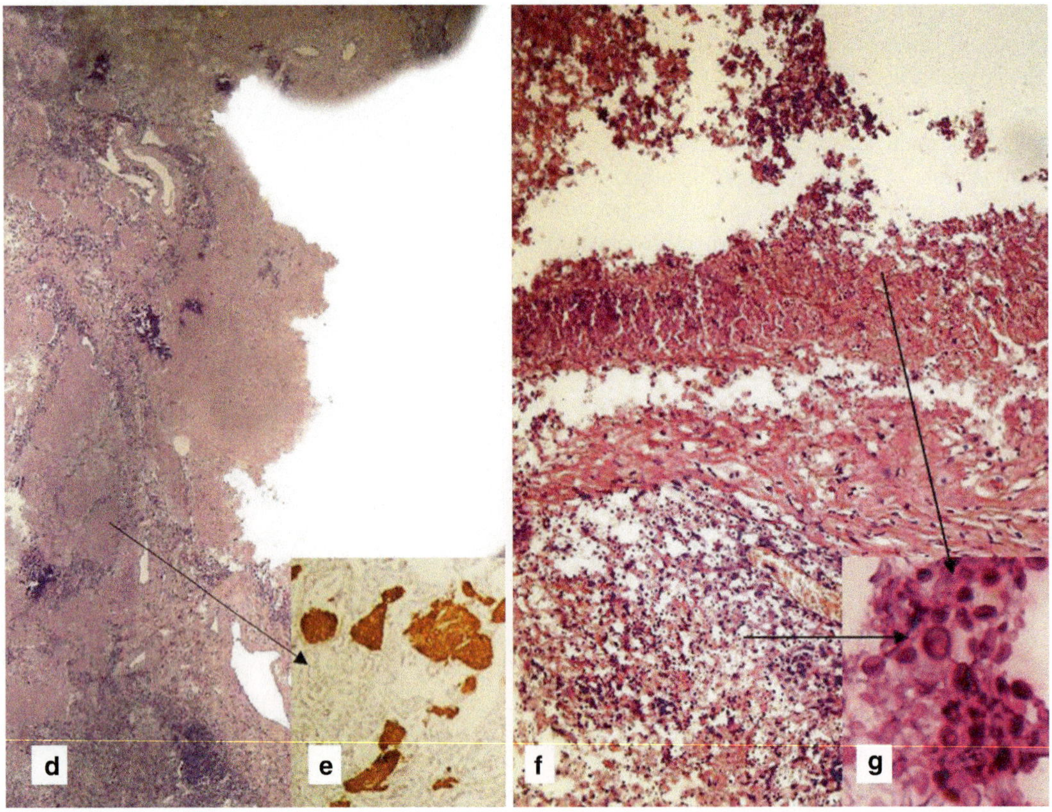

Fig. 13.80 (continued)

Each of the simultaneously developing opportunistic diseases can have erased clinical and morphological signs, atypical microscopic manifestations due to pathomorphism in severe immune deficiency conditions, which makes their morphological verification difficult.

The activity of various infectious inflammatory processes is of the same nature (an actively occurring infection or a combination of diseases with subacute course and organization phenomena), and various severity of course, when one disease progressed sharply, and the other progressed subacutely.

Histologically, in addition to detailing the structure of the foci of inflammation, it was necessary to differentiate perifocal exudative tissue reactions and organization processes while resolving the inflammatory process.

With acute inflammation of the causative agents of infection, in most cases, it can be determined using the histobacterioscopic method of investigation using appropriate histological stains. In the case of organized inflammation, infectious agents are difficult to detect, which requires the use of immunological, IHC, and molecular diagnostic methods for their detection.

The data of a morphological study on the presence of a combined HIV-associated infectious lesion obtained in vivo are important in the clinical aspect since they make it possible to timely correct the therapy. The early appointment of adequate comprehensive treatment to the patient may contribute to a more favorable prognosis for the patient.

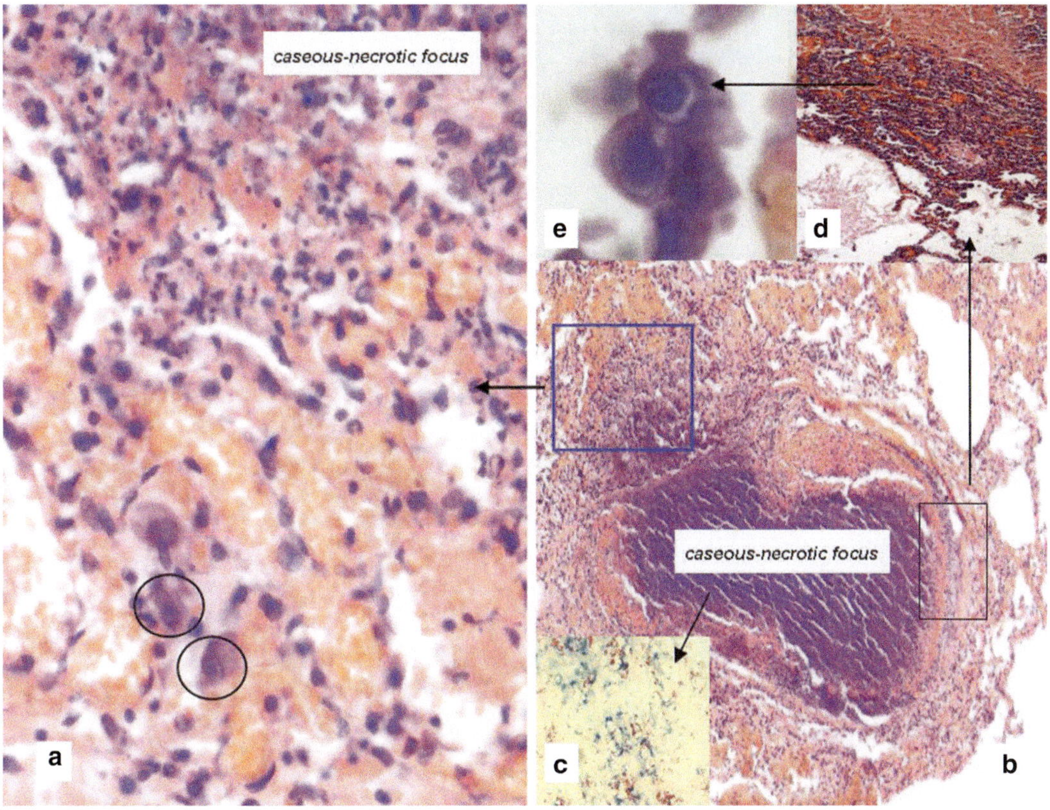

Fig. 13.81 Combined lung damage in HIV infection—tuberculosis and cytomegalovirus infection. (**a**) Caseous necrotic lesion in the lung in HIV-associated tuberculosis in adjacent parts of the cells with cytomegalovirus transformed cells "owl eyes" (see round frames); (**b**) tuberculosis purulent-necrotic focus in the lung and perifocal fibrosis, which creates a false impression about the organization of a tuberculosis outbreak; (**c**) acid-fast bacteria in the focus of tuberculous inflammation; (**d**) plot of perifocal fibrosis (fragment Fig. **b**); (**e**) cells with cytomegalic transformation ("owl's eye" cells in the area of fibrosis around the focus of tuberculosis inflammation). Fibrosing, which develops during cytomegalovirus inflammation, simulated the phenomena of organizing the focus of tuberculosis inflammation, while there was a simultaneous active course of two infectious processes—tuberculosis and CMV. (**a**, **b**, **d**, **e**) H.-E.; (**c**) Z-N staining. (**a**) ×400; (**b**) ×100; (**d**) ×200; (**c**, **e**) ×1000

13.4 Lung Lesions Due to Nontuberculous Mycobacteria Myc. Avium (Mac)

The data presented in this chapter are partly based upon the experiences of Russian phtisiopathology scientific school [26–28], partly own long-term experience of one of the authors (Yu. R. Zyuzya).

Nontuberculous mycobacteriosis is a group of infectious diseases caused by low-virulent pathogenic or conditionally pathogenic mycobacteria that are not amenable to therapy with antituberculosis drugs. In immunocompetent individuals, diseases caused by nontuberculous mycobacteria are rare, and lung lesions are practically not observed. In the case of HIV infection, generalized nontuberculous mycobacteriosis caused by *M. avium* and *M. intracellulare* combined in a complex (*M. avium* intracellulare—MAC) can develop. According to the classification of E.H. Runyon, these NTMBs belong to group 3, these are slowly growing non-chromogenic

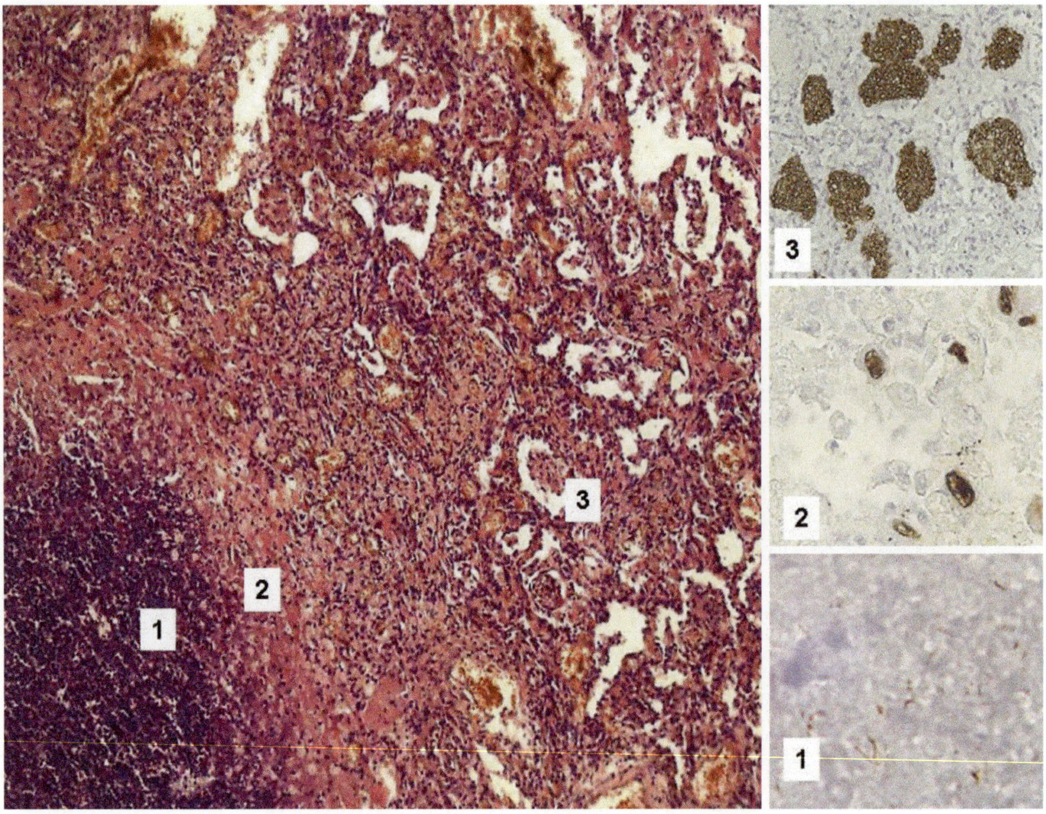

Fig. 13.82 Combined lung damage in HIV infection—tuberculosis, pneumocystic pneumonia, and cytomegalovirus infection. Under review microscopy, the morphological picture of a section of the wall of a subacute lung abscess (1, 2) with organizing pneumonia in adjacent sections of the lung (3). Insets—IHC examination revealed mycobacteria in necrotic masses of the wall of the decay cavity (1), cytomegalovirus lesion in the fibrous layer of the wall of the decay cavity (2), and pneumocysts in the organizing exudate in the lumen of the alveoli of adjacent sections of the lung. IHC study with antibodies: 1—Myc. Tuberculosis mouse monoclonal antibody; 2—monoclonal mouse anti-cytomegalovirus; 3—monoclonal mouse anti-pneumocystis Jiroveci. (1) ×1000; (2) ×400; (3) ×200

mycobacteria [27]. The growth rate on Levenstein–Jensen medium at 37 °C for 10–21 days (average 14 days). They are found on land, mineral springs, seawater, natural reservoirs, tap water, pathogens for humans, wild and domestic birds, and animals. The transmission way is airborne or through the mucous membrane of the gastrointestinal tract (mycobacteria are resistant to the acidic environment of the stomach, penetrate the intestinal epithelium).

Macroscopic picture of mycobacteriosis caused by nontuberculous mycobacteria Myc. avium, identical to generalized tuberculosis with the dissemination of foci of inflammation in almost all organs and the development of total caseous lymphadenitis of all groups of lymph nodes (Fig. 13.84) Microscopically, foci of inflammation were patches of monomorphic histiocyte-like cells, round, sometimes elongated or spindle-shaped, with round and light, slightly dull, sometimes finely vacuolized, cytoplasm, which gave them a resemblance to tumors of histiocytic origin (Fig. 13.85). In addition to the macrophage reaction, fuzzy small forming macrophage–epithelioid granulomas, cases of caseous necrosis, sometimes with leukocyte

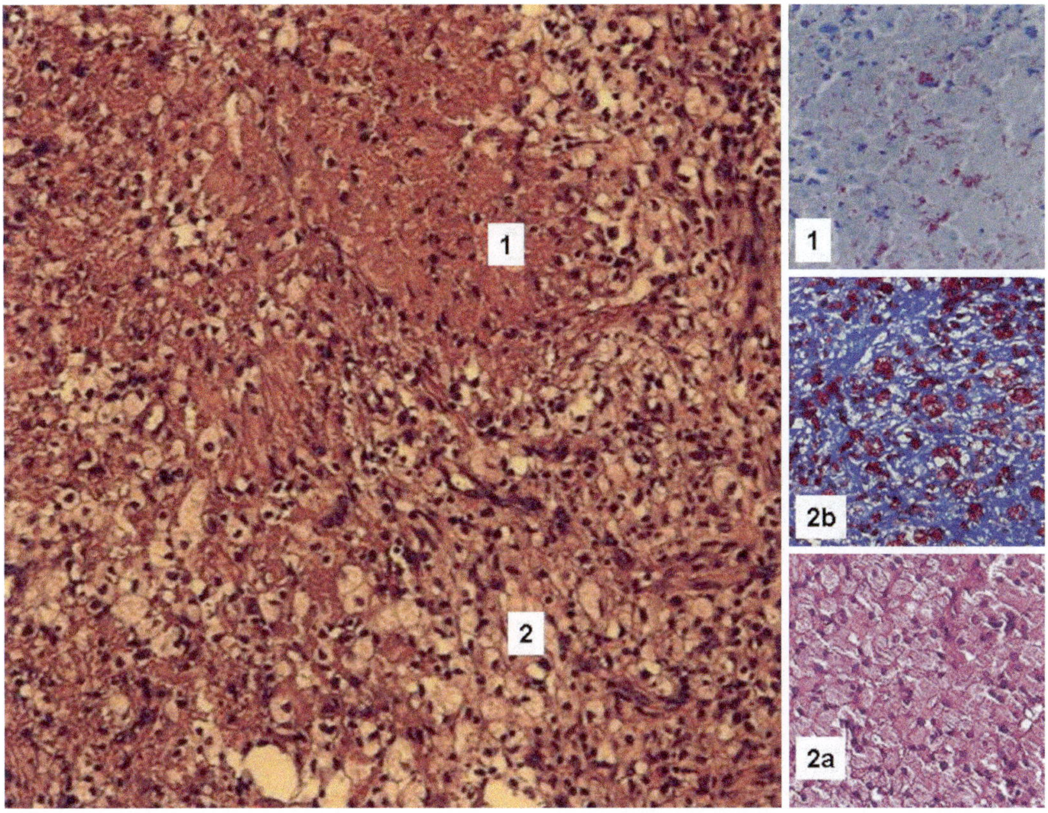

Fig. 13.83 Combined lesion in HIV infection–tuberculosis and non-tuberculosis mycobacteriosis caused by *M. avium* (MAC). Focus of caseous necrosis (1) with macrophage perifocal reaction (2). In the necrosis site (1), acid-resistant bacteria were detected, diffusely dispersed in necrotic masses, and localized in the cytoplasm of neutrophilic leukocytes and outside of destroyed leukocytes. In section 2—monomorphic macrophages with light fine-grained cytoplasm (2a), in the cytoplasm of macrophages acid-resistant bacteria in an amount that cannot be calculated. Plot 1—focus of tuberculosis inflammation; site 2—site of inflammation of the MAS. A PCR study of the material from the paraffin block revealed the DNA of *M. tuberculosis* in the fragment from section 1, and the DNA of *M. avium* in the fragment from section 2. Stained H.-E. ×100. Insets: (1, 2) B-Z-N staining; ×1000. (2b) H.-E.; ×400

infiltration, were found. A histobacterioscopic study according to Z-N revealed a characteristic localization of acid-resistant bacteria in the cytoplasm of macrophages, their number was so large that the pathogens could not be counted (microscopic picture of "stuffed" with bacteria). The localization and number of mycobacteria in non-tuberculous mycobacteriosis was different from those in tuberculous inflammation. In tuberculosis, bacteria are usually visualized in necrotic masses, and even with severe bacterial seeding, they can be counted (Figs. 13.86 and 13.87).

IHC study confirms the assignment of the pathogen to the genus Mycobacterium (Fig. 13.88). More accurate verification of the infection to the species was carried out when the

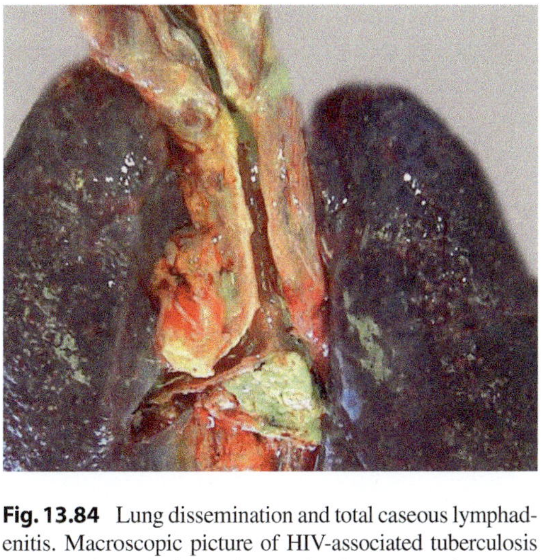

Fig. 13.84 Lung dissemination and total caseous lymphadenitis. Macroscopic picture of HIV-associated tuberculosis and mycobacteriosis MAS. Non-fixed macro specimens

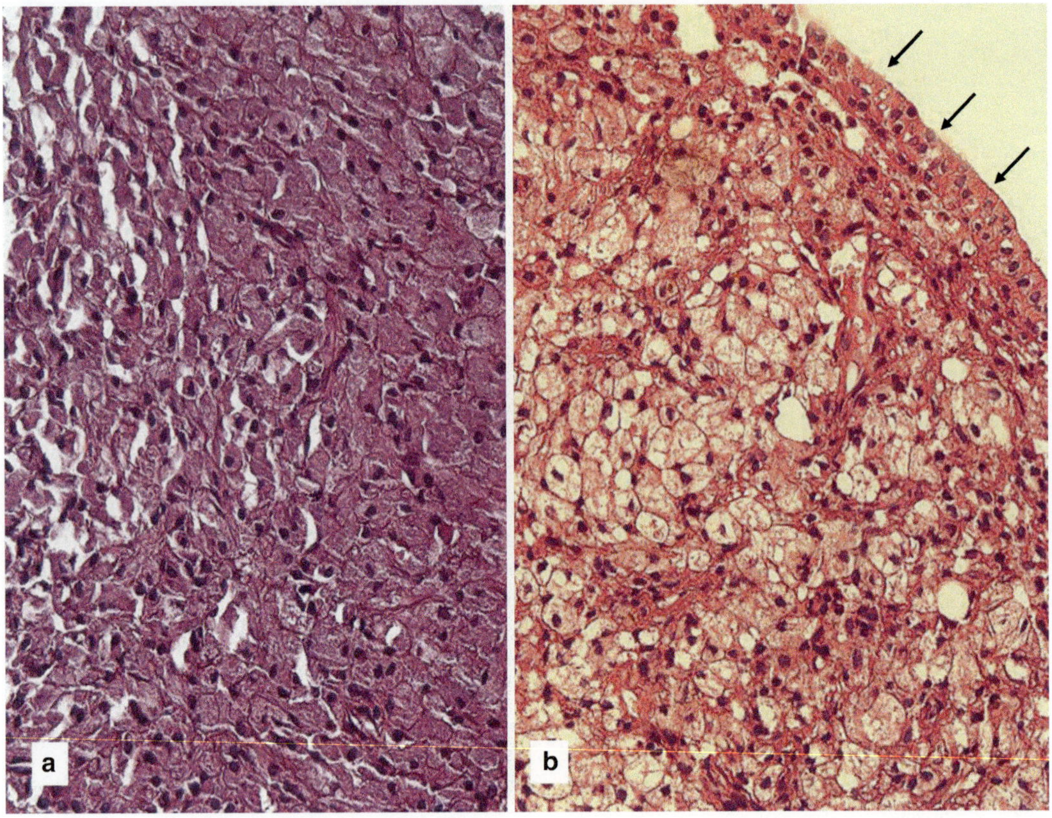

Fig. 13.85 HIV-associated non-tuberculosis mycobacteriosis by MAC. Foci of inflammation of their monomorphic round or polygonal histiocyte-like cells with a light fine-grained cytoplasm and a rounded nucleus. (**a**) The lymph node; (**b**) the bronchial mucosa (respiratory epithelium on the surface of the mucosa indicated by arrows), subepithelial in its own plate, the above histiocyte-like cells. Stained H.-E. ×200

material was sown on special media. In addition, M. avium DNA was detected in material from paraffin blocks through a PCR reaction.

With the localization of the lesion foci in the lungs, the accumulation of histiocyte-like cells under review microscopy created the impression of atelectasis and a focus of pneumosclerosis in it, which caused diagnostic difficulties. Only during an additional histological examination with Z-N staining or IHC examination, it was possible to establish a focus of infectious pneumonia in the lungs, "simulating" changes of a reactive nature, areas of atelectasis, pneumosclerosis (Fig. 13.89). When identifying the single histiocyte-like cells described earlier in the interalveolar septa, in the walls of the bronchi, as part of inflammatory infiltrates, it was also impossible to interpret them as a manifestation of mycobacteriosis without a comprehensive morphological study.

During histobacterioscopic and IHC studies with antibodies to mycobacteria, the development of mycobacterial vasculitis with infiltration of the above-described macrophages of the vascular wall with the detection of the pathogen in the cytoplasm was confirmed (Fig. 13.90).

Nontuberculous mycobacteriosis was accompanied by cavernization in two studied cases. Disintegration cavities of a subacute nature—with thin elastic walls; whitish and in the cavity of decay were determined whitish curdled mass, as in tuberculous lesions. Microscopic examina-

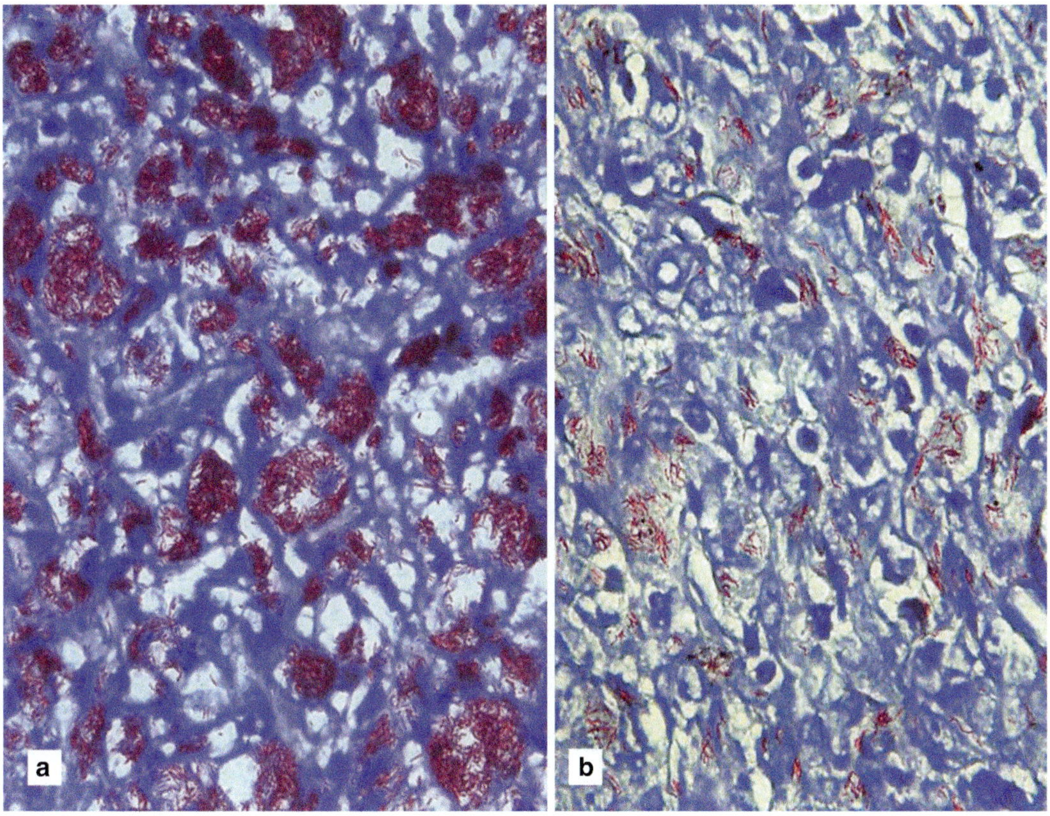

Fig. 13.86 HIV-associated non-tuberculosis mycobacteriosis by MAC. Acid-resistant bacteria are located in the cytoplasm of macrophages, in an amount that cannot be calculated. Stained by Z-N. ×1000

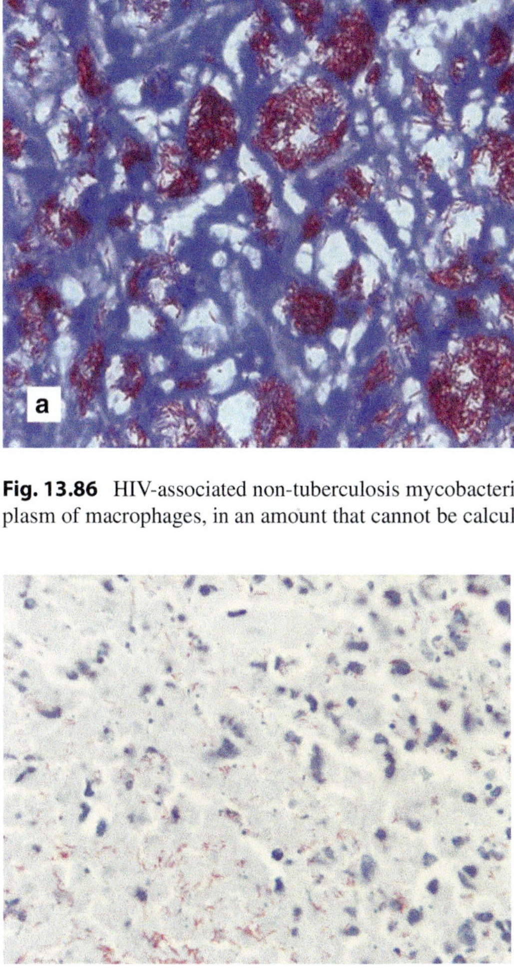

Fig. 13.87 HIV-associated tuberculosis (for comparison with Fig. 13.86). Acid-resistant bacteria are located in caseous-necrotic masses, in the cytoplasm of neutrophilic leukocytes, outside of destroyed leukocytes. Stained by Z-N. ×1000

tion revealed that the inner layer of the caverns consisted of a rather narrow layer of caseous-necrotic masses, among which, at high magnification, clusters of the above-described monomorphic macrophages with a light cytoplasm were found, with the identification of pathogens during histological bacterioscopy according to Z-N. The outer layer of the decay cavities is represented by maturing granulation tissue with adjacent lung tissue with moderate fibrosis and macrophage infiltration (Fig. 13.91).

Thus, taking into account the identical macroscopic picture of HIV-associated tuberculosis and nontuberculous mycobacteriosis caused by M. avium (MAC)—small focal or miliary dissemination in various organs and total caseous lymphadenitis, key morphological differential

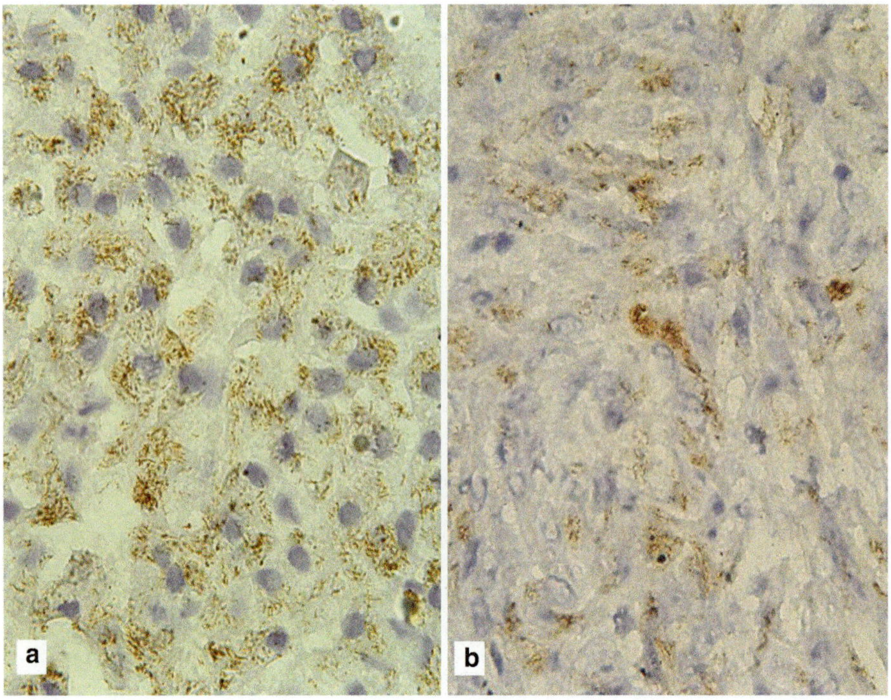

Fig. 13.88 HIV-associated non-tuberculosis mycobacteriosis. Mycobacteria are located in the cytoplasm of macrophages, in an amount that cannot be calculated. IHC reaction with *M. tuberculosis* mouse monoclonal antibody. ×1000

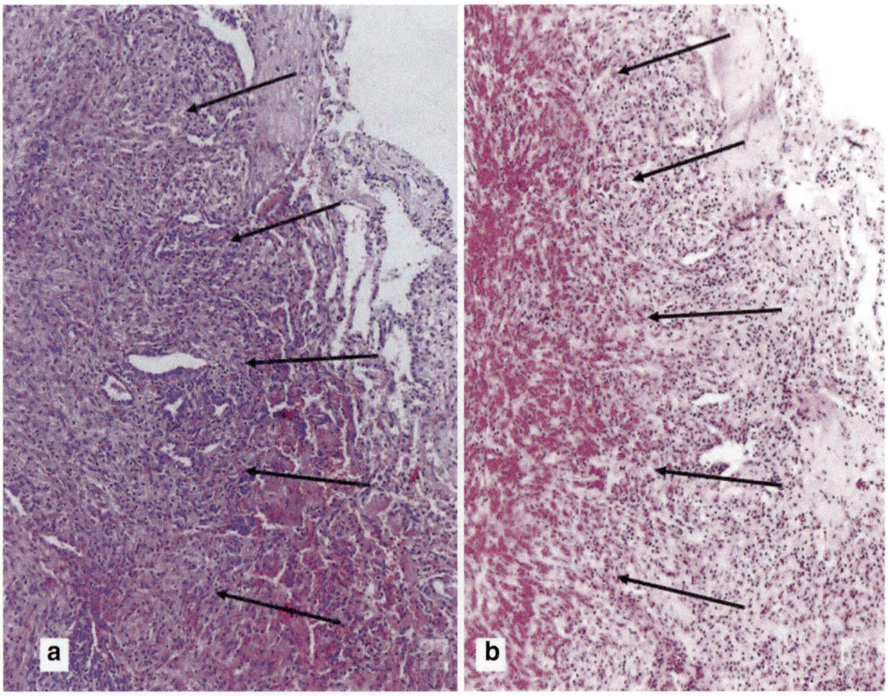

Fig. 13.89 HIV-associated non-tuberculosis mycobacteriosis MAC. (**a**) The site of the lung lesion, which has the form of atelectasis (indicated by arrows). H.-E. ×200; (**b**) a large number of acid-resistant bacteria in macrophages (the same section of the lung, indicated by arrows). Stained by Z-N. ×200

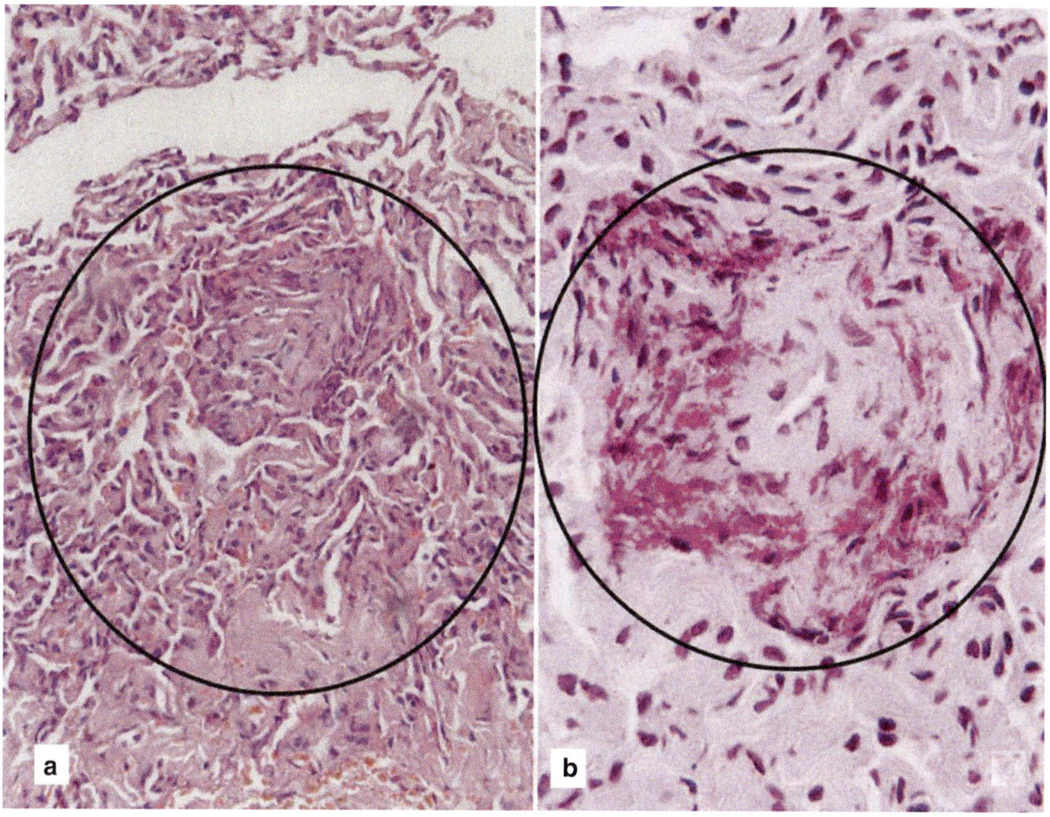

Fig. 13.90 HIV-associated non-tuberculosis mycobacteriosis (MAC) vasculitis. (**a**) Thickened vascular wall. Stained H.-E.; (**b**) multiple macrophages in the vessel wall with the presence of a large number of acid-resistant bacteria in the cytoplasm. Stained by Z-N. ×400

diagnostic signs were revealed during a histological examination. With MAC, the formation of foci of inflammation with a characteristic cellular response from a rounded or polygonal form of macrophages with a clear, opaque, finely vacuumed cytoplasm and a centrally located rounded core was noted. Sites of caseous necrosis and a very erased granulomatous reaction in the form of a small amount of very small fuzzy epithelioid cell granulomas could also form in the foci of inflammation. HIV-associated tuberculosis was characterized by the formation of purulent-necrotic foci with no granulomatous reaction.

In the case of the formation of caseous lymphadenitis during MAC mycobacteriosis, the macrophage reaction described earlier was preserved along the edge of necrosis. In the case of tuberculous caseous lymphadenitis, the entire lymph node tissue was replaced with caseous-necrotic masses with severe leukocyte infiltration in the absence of granulomatous inflammation, sequestration of necrotic masses, abscess formation, and development of lymphogenous caverns.

Given the progressive course of both HIV-associated infections, fibrosis and calcification of the foci of inflammation did not develop. The formation of acute caverns was characteristic of tuberculosis, while the formation of decay cavities in the lungs was atypical for MAC, and isolated cases were described.

The determination of the pathogen during histological studies by Z-N and IHC studies with antibodies to mycobacteria showed the localization of bacteria during MAC in the macrophage cytoplasm, and the number of microorganisms was so great that it could not be counted, while mycobacteria were mostly found in necrotic masses during tuberculosis.

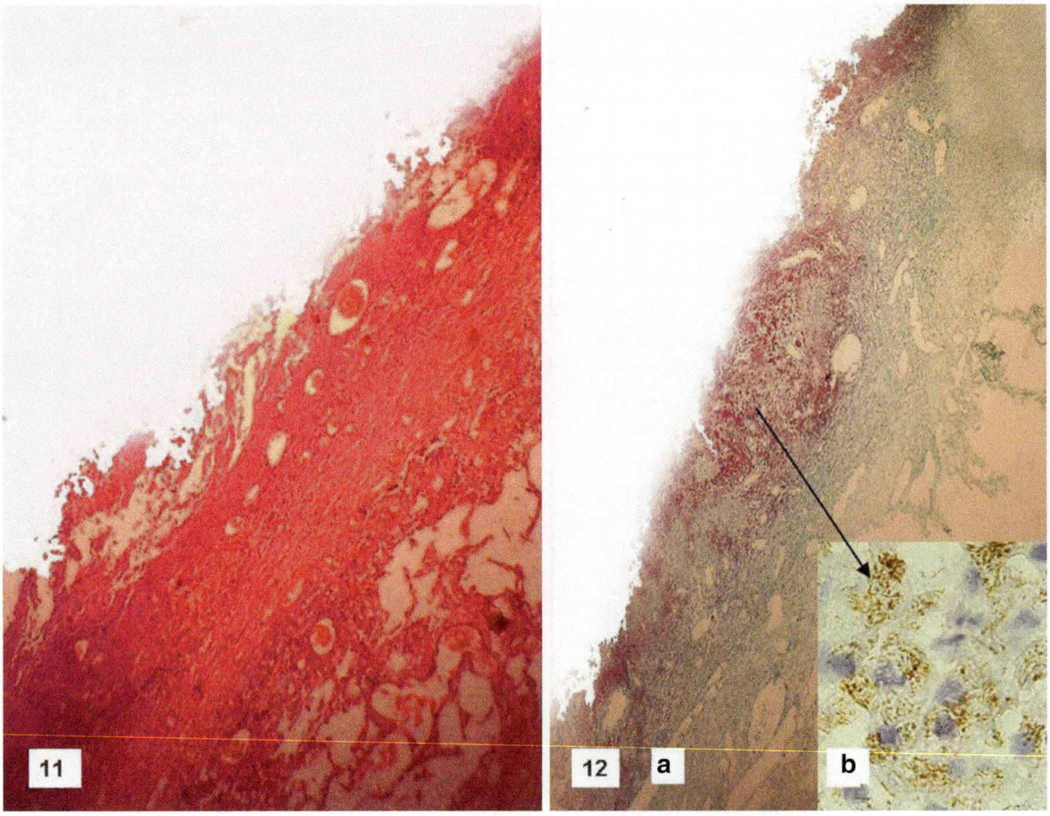

Fig. 13.91 HIV-associated non-tuberculosis mycobacteriosis wall of the decay cavity in the lung. Stained H.-E. ×100. (12a) Abundance of acid-resistant bacteria in the wall of the decay cavity. Color by Z-N. ×100; (12b) mycobacteria in large numbers, localized in the cytoplasm of macrophages. IHC reaction with Myc. tuberculosis mouse monoclonal antibody. ×1000

The confirmation of hematogenous generalization in MAC, as in tuberculosis, was the formation of mycobacterial vasculitis. For MAC, damage to the organs of the abdominal cavity is most characteristic, and in tuberculosis, damage to all organs, including the lungs, is noted in all cases. Confirmation of lymphogenous generalization in mycobacterial infections was the defeat of all groups of lymph nodes.

References

1. Ellinidi VN, Ariel BM, Samusenko IA, Tugolukova LV. Immunohistochemical method in the diagnosis of tuberculosis. Arkh Patol. 2007;69(5):36–8. (In Russian).
2. Agapov MM, Zinserling VA, Semenova NY, et al. Pathological anatomy of tuberculosis in the presence of human immunodeficiency virus infection. Arkhiv Patologii. 2020;82(2):12–9. (In Russian).
3. Zinserling VA, Agapov MM, Orlov AN. The informative value of various methods for identifying acid-fast bacilli in relation to the degree of tuberculosis process activity. Arkh Patologii. 2018;80(3):40–5. (In Russian).
4. Svistunov VV. The molecular biological characteristics of the pathogen of tuberculosis and the pathoanatomic aspects of its fatal outcomes in Irkutsk in 2008-2011. Artkh Patol. 2014;76(1):10–5. (In Russian).
5. Richards JP, Caio W, Zill NA, et al. Adaptation of Mycobacterium tuberculosis to biofilm growth is genetically linked to drug tolerance. Antimicrob Agents Chemother. 2019;63(11):e01213–9. https://doi.org/10.1128/AAC.01213-19.
6. Chistovich AN. Pathological anatomy and pathogenesis of tuberculosis. L.: Medicine; 1973. 175 p. (In Russian).
7. Puzik VI, Uvarova OA, Averbakh MM. Pathomorphology of modern forms of pulmo-

nary tuberculosis. -M.: Medicine; 1973. 215 p. (In Russian).
8. Strukov AI. Forms of pulmonary tuberculosis in morphological light. M.: Publishing House of the USSR Academy of Medical Sciences; 1948. 160 p. (In Russian).
9. Dolgova EA, Alvarez Figueroa MV, Lobashova GP, Halina SN, Zyuzya YR, Fligil DM, Shipulin GA. Application of the PCR method in the diagnosis of respiratory tuberculosis in patients with advanced stages of HIV infection. Mol Diagn. 2014;1:103–4. (In Russian).
10. Babaeva IY, Demikhova OV, Kravchenko AV. Disseminated pulmonary tuberculosis in patients with HIV infection. M.: Newterra; 2010. 164 p. (In Russian).
11. Parkhomenko IG, Ziuzia IR, Fligil DM. Destructive changes of lung in HIV-associated infections: differential diagnosis. Arkh Patologii. 2011;73(5):9–12. (In Russian).
12. Parkhomenko IG, Ziuzia IR, Tishkevich OA. Lung pathology in HIV-associated infection. Arkh Patol. 2007;70(6):44–8. (In Russian).
13. Parkhomenko IG, Erokhin VV, Ziuzia IR, Lepekha LN, Tishkevich OA. Pathomorphological changes in the lung in tuberculosis patients died from HIV infection at the stage of AIDS. Arkh Patol. 2007;69(3):26–8. (In Russian).
14. Parkhomenko YG, Zyuzya YR, Mazus AI. Morphological aspects of HIV infection. M.: Literra; 2016. 168 p. (In Russian).
15. Zimina VN, Kravchenko AV, Zyuzya YR, et al. Analysis of lethal outcomes in patients with newly-diagnosed tuberculosis of the respiratory organs in combination with HIV-infection. Ter Arkh. 2011;83(11):25–31. (In Russian).
16. Zimina VN, Kravchenko AV, Batyrov FA. Features of the course of tuberculosis in the late stages of HIV infection. Tuberc Lung Dis. 2010;3:23–7. (In Russian).
17. Zimina VN, Koshechkin VA, Kravchenko AV. Tuberculosis and HIV infection in adults: a guide. M.: GEOTAR-Media; 2014. 224 p. (In Russian).
18. Kornilova ZH, Ziuzia IR, Alekseeva LP, et al. Clinical and morphological features of the course of tuberculosis in HIV infection. Probl Tuberc Lung Dis. 2008;(10):13–20. (In Russian).
19. Zimina VN, Alvares Figueroa MV, Degtyareva SY, et al. Diagnostics of mycobacteriosis in HIV-positive patients. Infectious diseases. 2016;14(4):63–70. (In Russian).
20. Zimina VN, Kravchenko AV, Zyuzya YR, Vasilyeva IA. Diagnosis and treatment of tuberculosis in combination with HIV infection. -M.: GEOTAR-Media; 2015. 240 p. (In Russian).
21. Zimina VN, Vasilieva IA, Kravchenko AV, Batyrov FA. Generalized tuberculosis in HIV-infected patients with AIDS. J Int AIDS Soc. 2010;8(2):5–8.
22. Zjuzja JR, Kuzina MG, Parhomenko JG. Morphological features of mycobacterioses caused by non-tuberculous mycobacteria. Klinicheskaya i eksperimental'naya morfologiya. 2017;(4):4–14. (In Russian).
23. Zyuzya YR, Barkhina TG, Parkhomenko YG, Chernikov VP. Pulmonary histological and ultrastructural changes in HIV infection concurrent with tuberculosis. Arkh Patologii. 2015;77(1):23–9. (In Russian).
24. Zyuzya YR, Zimina VN, Alvarez Figueroa MV, et al. Morphological characteristics of HIV-associated tuberculosis depending on the number of $CD4^+$ lymphocytes in peripheral blood. Arkh Patologii. 2014;76(5):33–7. (In Russian).
25. Zyuzya YR, Zimina VN, Parkhomenko YG, Alvares Figeroa MV, Dolgova EA. Correlation between the morphological signs of tuberculosis and the immune status in HIV infection. Tuberc Lung Dis. 2014;(11):48–53. (In Russian).
26. Zyuzya YR, Parkhomenko YG, Zimina VN, et al. HIV-associated mycobacteriosis caused by non-tuberculous mycobacterium M. Avium. Features of morphological verification. Tuberc Lung Dis. 2015;(7):56–57. (In Russian).
27. Litvinov VI. Non-tuberculous mycobacteria in "inanimate and living nature", human infection. Tuberculosis and socially significant diseases. 2015;2:28–32. (In Russian).
28. Otten TF, Vasiliev AV. Mycobacteriosis. SPb.: Medical Press; 2005. p. 19. (In Russian).

Respiratory Mycosis 14

14.1 Candidiasis

The causative agent of this disease is yeast-like fungi of the genus Candida. The most frequent and well-studied among them is *Candida albicans* [1]. Recently, there have been isolated reports of a new pathogen, *Candida auris*, with which the catastrophic course of the disease is associated [2]. *C. albicans* cells have the appearance of round or oval bodies with sizes of 2–5 µm. In tissues, their budding and the formation of pseudomycelium filaments of different lengths are usually visible. The latter are elongated cells, with no septs characteristic of a number of other fungi.

Fungi are widespread in nature and quite often can be isolated from various materials obtained from humans without pronounced clinical manifestations of the disease. The historically dominant view is that candidiasis is an autoinfection in which saprophyte activation occurs under conditions of immunodeficiency and/or irrational antibiotic therapy. Recently, there has been evidence that candidiasis may also be a hospital infection caused by more virulent strains of the pathogen [1, 2].

In past decades, pulmonary candidiasis was a relatively common disease and was studied in detail in Leningrad (now St. Petersburg) by A.V. Zinserling [3] and O.K. Khmelnitsky [4]. In recent years, due to unknown reasons, we do not see such lesions frequently.

Macroscopically, changes in the lungs are not very characteristic. In the acute stage of the disease, they are catarrhal bronchitis and pneumonia with small airless foci of a grayish or reddish-gray color, usually quite clearly distinguished from the surrounding tissue. In the later stages of development, small patches of grayish dense granulation tissue are visible. With a microscopic examination, the propagating fungi are determined in the lumen of the respiratory tract and alveoli, occasionally, the bronchial wall can germinate (Fig. 14.1). In places of localization of fungi is noted accumulation of leukocytes, as well as serous fluid and macrophages. Candida cells, despite their relatively large sizes, can be phagocytosed by leukocytes, however, phagocy-

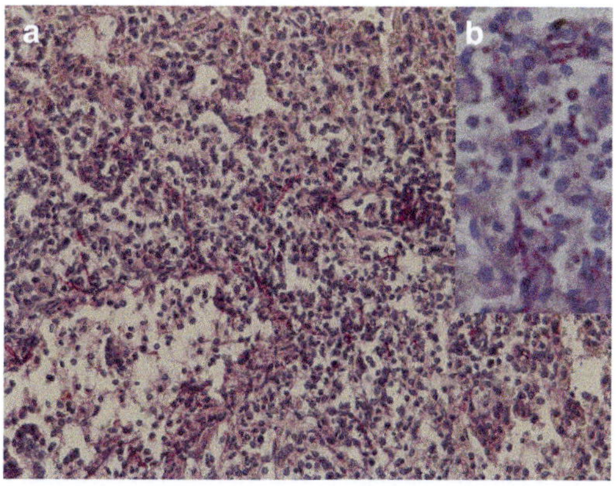

Fig. 14.1 Pneumonia due to *Candida albicans*. PAS (**a**) ×100 and (**b**) ×400

V. Zinserling, *Infectious Pathology of the Respiratory Tract*,
https://doi.org/10.1007/978-3-030-66325-4_14

tosis is incomplete. After a few weeks, with the progression of the disease in the lungs, focal growths of granulation tissue rich in epithelioid, lymphoid, and giant multinucleate cells begin to develop. Fragments of dead fungi can be detected in their cytoplasm, which can only be detected by the PAS reaction. With an even longer duration of the process, distinct granulomas are formed.

In the experimental reproduction of candidiasis, the process is fundamentally similar to that occurring with spontaneous candidiasis of a person. It is important that the introduction of a live causative agent and killed cultures and even polysaccharides and lipids of the fungus to experimental animals, the resulting epithelioid cell reaction is similar. In immunized rabbits, the inflammatory process with candidiasis initially develops more intensively, but it is more quickly delimited. Against the background of the appearance of antibodies 3–4 days after infection, an aggravation of the inflammatory process is noted (up to 9 days) (with an increase in the outbreak in size, hyperemia, and a local increase in temperature) around the already encapsulated area of inflammation in the area of the location of the killed fungal cells introduced at the beginning of the experiment.

14.2 Cryptococcosis

Cryptococcosis is a potentially fatal systemic mycosis caused by *Cryptococcus neoformans*. Causative agent is basidiomycete yeast-like fungus with gelatinous, mucopolysaccharide capsule composed of mannose, xylose, and glucuronic acid. Cells are round-to-oval; their size varies widely and ranges from 3.5 to 8 μm in diameter. *C. neoformans* grows at 37 °C, assimilates inositol, produces urease, and does not produce mycelia on cornmeal agar. Although the genus Cryptococcus contains more than 50 species, only *C. neoformans* and *C. gattii* are considered pathogens in humans. These two species have five serotypes based on antigenic specificity of the capsular polysaccharide; these include serotypes A, D, and AD (*C. neoformans*) and serotypes B and B/C (*C. gattii*) [1].

C. neoformans usually cause infections in persons who have some form of defect in their immune systems; it occurs worldwide and usually presents in soil with main source in pigeon droppings. *C. gattii* is being increasingly recognized as a pathogen in presumptively immunocompetent hosts and it mainly occurs in tropical and subtropical countries. It has been cultured from under the bark and around flowering eucalyptus trees.

The global burden of HIV-associated cryptococcosis approximates one million cases annually worldwide. The annual incidence is 0.2–0.9 cases per 100,000 in the general population and about 13 cases per 100,000 in African countries. According to our data, it is causing about 5–10% of lethal outcomes in AIDS. Other conditions which pose an increased risk include defects in the cell-mediated immunity in patients with lymphomas, sarcoidosis, transplanted organs, malignancies, long-term (cortico-osteroid) corticosteroid therapy, etc. People with CD counts <100 cells/μL are especially susceptible to disseminated cryptococcosis.

It is most prevalent in men, usually those between ages 30 and 60, and is rare in children. *C. gatti* is a little more common in children and young adults than *C. neoformans*. In most studies, cryptococcal disease is more common in men than in women.

The fungus grows asexually as a budding yeast. Under laboratory conditions, it is capable of sexual reproduction between two mating types. After cell fusion, a dikaryotic filament develops, at the tip of which a basidium gives rise to four chains of basidiospores.

The basic way of contamination is the inhalation of the basidiospore from the environment. The initial lesion occurs in the lungs. Yeast spores are deposited into the pulmonary alveoli, where they must survive the neutral-to-alkaline pH and physiologic concentrations of carbon dioxide before they are phagocytized by alveolar macrophages. The essential factor in the survival of *C. neoformans* is the glucosylceramide synthase. The cryptococcal polysaccharide capsule has antiphagocytic properties and encapsulated organisms are more resistant to phagocytosis. The host response to cryptococcal infection includes both cellular and humoral components.

If limited to the lungs, *C. neoformans* infection may cause pneumonia, poorly defined mass lesions, pleural effusion, etc. Those with clinical symptoms complain of cough, sputum, chest pain, loss of weight, and fever.

C. neoformans can cause an asymptomatic pulmonary infection followed later by hematogenous spread, mainly to brain, causing meningoencephalitis, which is often the first indication of disease. Patients have meningeal symptoms, complaining of headache, vomiting, and a stiff neck. In other patients, focal neurological signs, blurred vision and confusion appear.

The laboratory diagnosis of cryptococcal disease includes the direct microscopic examination with India ink staining of clinical specimens, the cultural isolation of cryptococcus on most routine mycological or bacteriological media, the serologic test, the molecular identification of organism's DNA, and also CT and MRI scans.

Culture of CSF, sputum, urine, and blood in heavy infections is considered to be the "gold standard" method of diagnosis for *C. neoformans*, but the latex agglutination test for cryptococcal antigen detection is more rapid.

The treatment of cryptococcal disease, first of all, depends on the immune status of the patient. Most of the cases belong to three specific risk groups: (1) HIV-infected individuals, (2) graft recipients, and (3) non-HIV-infected and non-graft host.

It is important to pay attention to the early diagnostic and treatment of elevated intracranial pressure and immune reconstitution inflammatory syndrome (IRIS). Sometimes on routine H-E sections, the cells of *C. neoformans* are not evident; they have lightly basophilic cell wall surrounded by a clear zone. The organism cell stains with periodic acid–Schiff (PAS) or methenamine–silver. Mucicarmine and alcian blue stains the capsule. Tissue sections can be stained with the Fontana–Masson stain to detect melanin precursors in the yeast cell wall.

In typical cryptococcal granulomas of immunocompetent individual, histiocytes and multinucleated giant cells are positive for HLA-DR and IL-1 beta. Small round CD45RO-positive cells are visible in such granulomas.

In the lesions of AIDS patients, there are no CD45RO-positive cells, and the expression of HLA-DR and IL-1 beta is very weak.

In AIDS patients with HAART, CD45RO-positive cells are present at the periphery of each focus of dense cryptococcal proliferation. Both histiocytes and multinucleated giant cells are positive for HLA-DR as well as IL-1 beta, but their reactivity is relatively weak.

Cryptococcus is known as a fungus that causes granulomatous inflammation, which is considered to be a phenotypic manifestation of normally functioning cellular immunity. Typical granulomas consist of compactly arranged macrophages with features of epithelioid cells and giant multinucleated cells such as "foreign bodies" and Langhans, in the cytoplasm of which there are many yeast-like cells. These cells are positive for both HLA-DR and IL1β. Also in granulomas, CD45-positive small round cells corresponding to CD4+ lymphocytes are found. Despite the fact that necrosis is rarely observed in the center of granulomas, it can be quite extensive. It is explained as a result of ischemia, which occurs with an increase in granuloma, because proliferation of cryptococci alone does not cause necrosis.

In individuals with cellular immunity deficiency, proliferation of yeast-like fungi with histiocytic, minimal lymphocytic, and neutrophilic infiltration is histologically determined; the expression of HLA-DR and IL1β in macrophages and giant multinucleated cells is much weaker. There was an extensive lesion of the capillaries, which is associated with the hematogenous spread of the infection. In experimental cryptococcosis in athymic mice, macrophages were present, but they did not form granulomas; pathogens were localized both internally and extracellularly.

Reactivation of CD4+ cells upon administration of HAART leads to the appearance of granuloma-like formations with the presence of CD4+ cells in them, with the tendency to form giant multinucleated cells.

On histological sections, *C. neoformans* cells often appear collapsed and destroyed. Cases are described when giant forms of cryptococci (up to 50–100 μm) were observed in tissues with their normal sizes in culture. Seven cases of unusual microscopic forms of *C. neoformans* have been described: structures like germ tubes, budding yeast chains, and pseudohyphae. The most detailed literature describes the morphology of lung damage.

McDonnell J.M. and Hutchins G.M [5] proposed four types of pulmonary cryptococcosis: (1) peripheral pulmonary granuloma/granulomas (according to the authors, it is observed in 19% of cases); (2) granulomatous pneumonia—intra-alveolar proliferation of pathogens and various degrees of inflammation: from acute to diffuse intra-alveolar granulomas with giant cells (53%); (3) diffuse intracapillary/interstitial lesion with a large number of cryptococci; inflammation from minimal (almost absent) with many organisms to miliary granulomas with a small number of pathogens (19%); (4) massive pulmonary lesion with a large number of both intra-alveolar and intravascularly located pathogens (8%). In patients with AIDS, lung damage took the form of intracapillary/interstitial or massive; peripheral granulomas or granulomatous pneumonia in them was not observed.

Shibuya K. et al. [6] identified three types of lung lesions in AIDS patients: (1) a small lesion, which is intra-alveolar proliferation of cryptococci with histiocytic infiltration. The histoarchitectonics of the lung are not disturbed, but the affected alveoli are weakly stretched by both proliferating cryptococci and reactive histiocytes. Cryptococci are found in the capillaries. The number of intra-alveolar lesions is different; (2) widespread lesion with focal proliferation of cryptococci and severe histiocytic infiltration. Giant cells of the type of "foreign bodies" with the number of nuclei less than 10. Typical giant Langhans cells are not detected. Pathogens are located both extra- and intracellularly; (3) massive proliferation of cryptococci both in the enlarged alveoli and in the capillaries/interstitium, the septa are destroyed. Histiocytes and giant multinucleated cells are present; focal hemorrhage.

Macroscopically visible changes in the lymph nodes and lungs in HIV infection were identical to those for tuberculosis and the anatomical diagnosis was formulated as "generalized tuberculosis," although some authors note that the foci in cryptococcosis have a gelatinous appearance or a "gelatinous" consistency.

During the autopsy, miliary and small focal bilateral dissemination, necrotic changes of the caseous lymphadenitis type in the intrathoracic lymph nodes were found in the lungs and other organs.

A routine histological examination did not always make it possible to establish an accurate diagnosis, since the inflammation caused by Cryptococcus, in conditions of extremely low immune status, was alternatively exudative in nature with the development of massive necrotic focuses (Fig. 14.2). Occasionally, a pattern of "erased" granulomatous inflammation was observed in the form of small single fuzzy epithelioid cell granulomas with giant multinucleated cells that were detected in separate fields of vision. These changes resembled the microscopic picture of tuberculosis (Fig. 14.3). Subtotal or total necrotic lymphadenitis developed in the lymph nodes.

In severe immunodeficiency conditions and in massive necrotic foci with cryptococcosis, it is rather difficult to recognize the pathogen, which, when stained with H-E, is weakly basophile, subtle, and difficult to detect.

The mushrooms had the shape of rounded, less often oval cells with a diameter of 2–20 nm, with one slightly elongated capsule in the form of

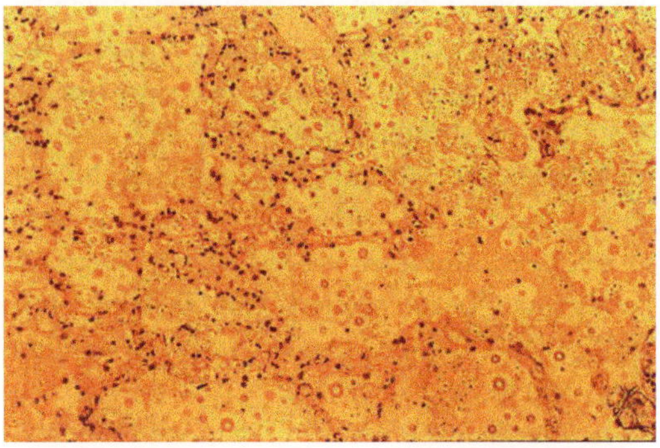

Fig. 14.2 Cryptococcal pneumonia in a patient with AIDS. H.E. ×100

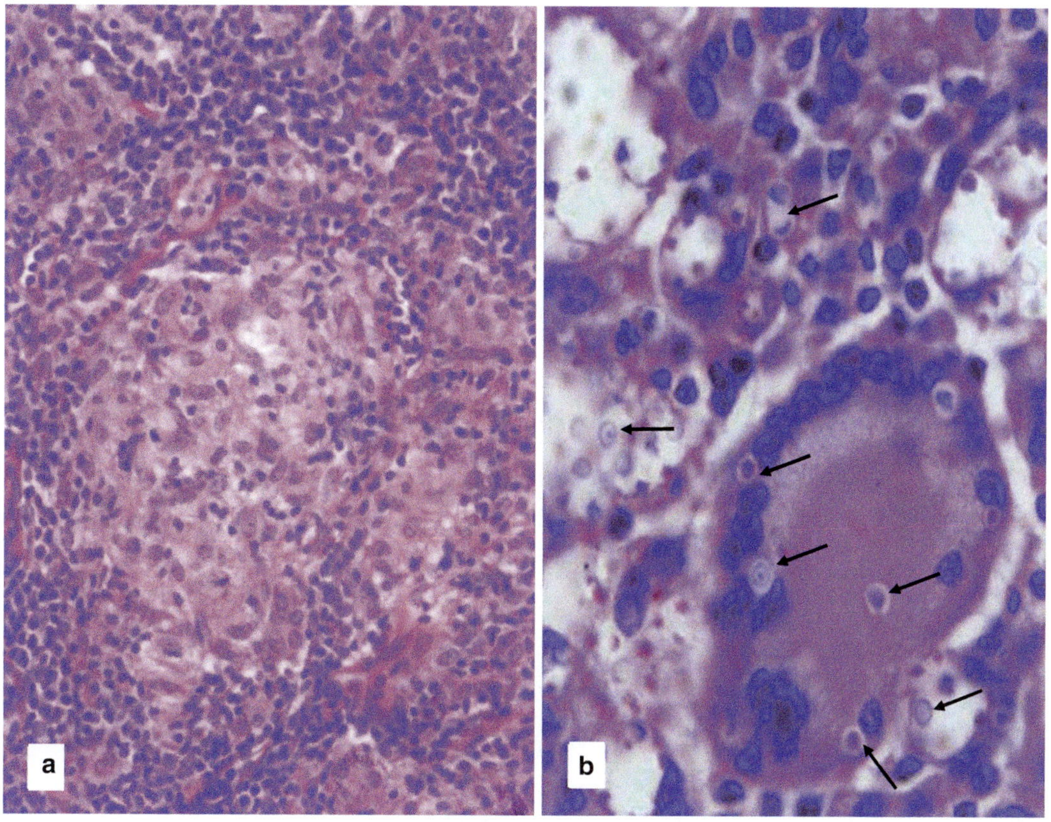

Fig. 14.3 HIV-associated cryptococcosis. (**a**) Erased granulomatous inflammation in the lung—forming macrophage–epithelioid granulomas; (**b**) a giant multicellular cell of the Langhans type in the focus of cryptococcal inflammation (cryptococci are indicated by arrows). H.-E. (**a**) ×200 and (**b**) ×400

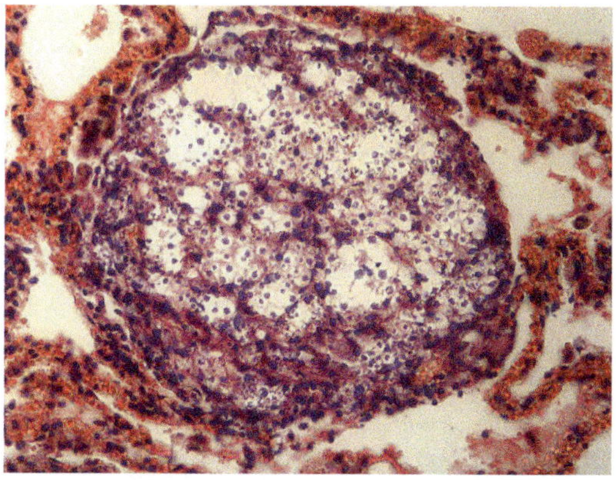

Fig. 14.4 Cryptococci in the lung. H.-E. ×200

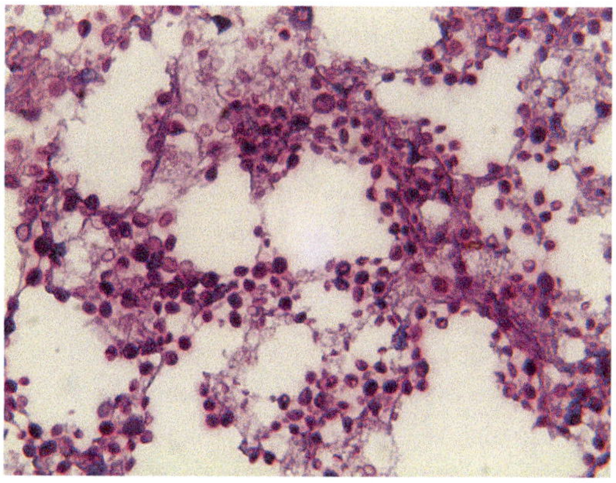

Fig. 14.5 Cryptococci in the lung. PAS ×1000

a light halo (Fig. 14.4). There were also elongated or filamentous forms of fungal cells. In the process of infection, the pathogen can increase in size, its capsule—thicken or collapse. The PAS reaction revealed cryptococci whose capsule was colored pink or raspberry red (Fig. 14.5). One can use other stains, for example, according to Gram, Gram-Weigert, Grokkott. Z-N histobacte-

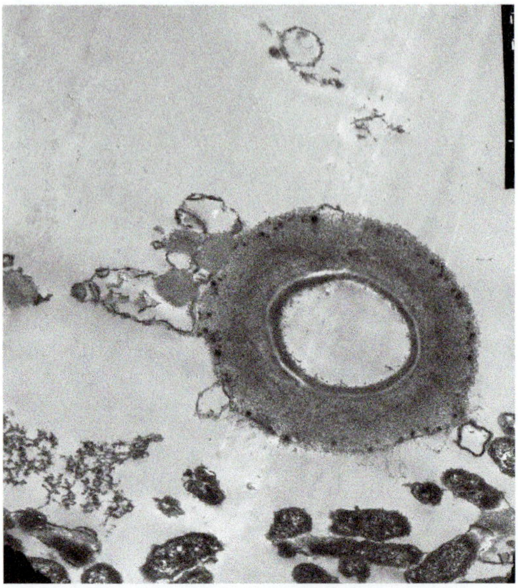

Fig. 14.6 Free laying Cryptococcus. EM ×60,000

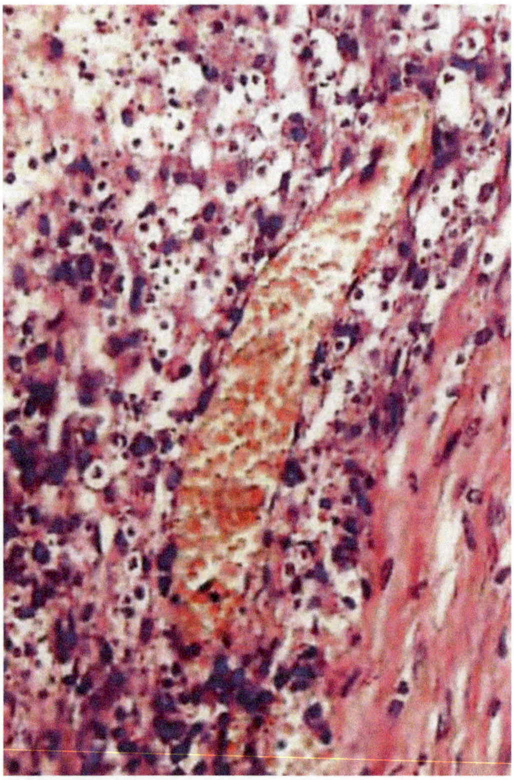

Fig. 14.7 Cryptococcal vasculitis. Edema in the vessel wall, diffuse inflammatory infiltration; cryptococci in the vessel wall and perivascular. H.-E. ×200

rioscopy in these cases was negative. During EM study, we succeeded first of all to reveal the typical capsule (Fig. 14.6).

Cryptococcosis was characterized by a minimal inflammatory reaction in the form of a small, small-focal lymphoid-histiocytic infiltration. In tuberculosis, perifocal and pericavitary exudative changes, mononuclear infiltration, and edema of the alveolar septa were usually observed.

Vascular cells with cellular infiltration, mainly from lymphocytes and eosinophilic leukocytes, with signs of invasion of cryptococci into the vascular wall, i.e., the formation of cryptococcal vasculitis, which is evidence of hematogenous generalization (Fig. 14.7). Involvement in the pathological process of all groups of lymph nodes that macroscopically looked like total caseous lymphadenitis, and histological examination showed accumulations of cryptococci in the foci of necrosis, consistent with the presence and lymphogenous form of generalization of the infectious process.

In one case, a decay cavity (cryptococcal abscess) was identified. Morphological manifestations of cryptococcosis with the development of a decay cavity in the lung during macroscopic examination were similar to the tuberculosis process. Macroscopically, the decay cavity had thin elastic walls; their inner surface was represented by whitish structureless masses. During histological examination, the inner layer of the mycotic abscess consisted of necrotic masses and an abundance of cryptococci, which are quite clearly distinguishable at high magnification. During the PAS reaction, mycotic structures acquired a bright pink or crimson blue and were clearly visible among tissue detritus; acid-resistant bacteria were not detected during Z-N staining. The outer layer of the decay cavity was represented by areas of granulation tissue and areas of the lung with moderate exudative changes (Fig. 14.8).

A bacteriological study of autopsy material with growth in culture from the contents of the decay cavity of cryptococci made it possible to establish the etiology of the destructive process of the lungs.

Identity of the macroscopic picture of HIV-associated tuberculosis and cryptococcosis with

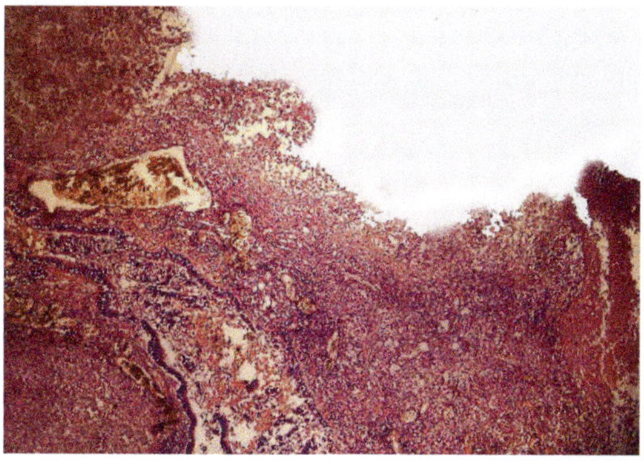

Fig. 14.8 The wall of a cryptococcal abscess in the lung. H.-E. ×100 (see Fig. 13.80f, g)

the detection of predominantly small focal dissemination in the lungs and other organs, the presence of lymphadenitis (including caseous) with the lesion of all groups of lymph nodes, as well as the similarity of the histological picture with panoramic microscopy with the definition of necrosis sites, fuzzy elements of granulomatous inflammation caused difficulties in identifying the infectious process.

In HIV-associated cryptococcosis, granulomas are fuzzy, macrophage–epithelioid–giant cell, with an admixture of eosinophilic leukocytes, the formation of sites of necrosis, and the detection of cryptococci with panoramic microscopy in the foci of granulomatous-necrotic inflammation. For tuberculosis associated with HIV, the detection of purulent necrotic foci without signs of granulomatous inflammation was more characteristic, with the rare occurrence of scanty numbers of epithelioid and giant Langhans cells.

In both cases, the lesions were localized mainly perivascular, fibrosis and calcification were not characteristic. The development of decay cavities (acute caverns) was characteristic of tuberculosis, while with cryptococcosis, the development of mycotic abscesses was noted in isolated cases.

A positive result of a histochemical study using the PAS reaction, Grokkott staining and detection of cryptococci with negative results of the detection of *Mycobacterium tuberculosis* with Z-N histobacterioscopy, an IHC study with antibodies to mycobacteria, and PCR testified in favor of cryptococcosis and made it possible to differentiate HIV tuberculosis and cryptococcosis.

The involvement of many organs in the pathological process with HIV-associated cryptococcosis, the presence of cryptococcal lymphadenitis of all groups of lymph nodes, and the development of mycotic vasculitis testified, as with HIV-associated tuberculosis, to a mixed lymphohematogenous form of generalization.

Infection can be reproduced by intravenous challenge of mice. The histological features of experimental infection are comparable with those observed in men and allow to study the morphological peculiarities of cryptococcus strains and tissue reactions in different organs in dynamics.

14.3 Histoplasmosis

The causative agent of histoplasmosis is *Histoplasma capsulatum* [1]. In tissues, it is found in the form of rounded, less often pear-shaped cells with sizes of 1–5 nm. Their budding is noted. The nucleus of the fungus is well stained with hematoxylin. In tissues, fungi are most naturally detected intracellularly. With a large number of histoplasmas that have entered the lungs, there is serous, hemorrhagic, or desquamative focal pneumonia, with an unfavorable course with necrosis in the center. When the process calms down, encapsulation occurs with a pronounced calcification. Large foci in the lungs with a diameter of 0.5–3.5 cm, surrounded by a capsule sometimes denote the term histoplasmoma. Caverns in the chronic stage have a three-layer wall structure: necrotic 2, granulation, and fibroblastic layers. The tissue response arises, rather, not on the pathogen itself, but on the soluble antigen. With a moderate amount of histoplasms, a macrophage reaction predominates from the very beginning, then a tubercle consisting of epithelioid as well as giant cells and the peripheral zone of lymphocytes and fibroblasts form. In the center of such a focus, coagulation necrosis often occurs; in the future, leukocyte emigration is possible here.

14.4 Aspergillosis

The causative agent is various species belonging to the genus Aspergillus (*A. niger*, *A. fumigatus*, *A. flavus*, *A. nidulans*, etc.), which in the tissues have an almost identical structure—uniformly septated filaments (hyphae) with a thickness of 1.5–5 μm. They can dichotomously divide at an acute angle, sometimes the mycelium forms tangles. With the death of the fungus, the mycelium, especially in the peripheral areas, as it swells. Fruiting organs. On the surface of a spherical swelling in the form of a wreath, more often cylindrical or pin-shaped cells are located radially—sterigms, from which chains of round or oval spores—conidia—are unfastened. These structures are clearly visible during cultivation of the fungus, but they are practically not detected in the tissues. Fungi stain well with hematoxylin, with PAS reactions only young forms of the fungus are weakly stained [1, 7].

In the clinic, it is customary to distinguish between delimited lesions—aspergilloma and a disseminated process—invasive aspergillosis. In addition, aspergillus sometimes settles on the inner surface of the tuberculous cavity. The development of pulmonary aspergillosis is usually associated with immunodeficiency, especially arising in hematological patients during cytostatic therapy. Aspergillosis as a complication of HIV infection in the AIDS stage is relatively rare. The occurrence of aspergillosis in people having contact with mold plants (grain, hay), rags, and wool is also described. Aspergillus infection is also possible with fungal infections of the premises, as they are one of the most important biodestructors.

A microscopic examination reveals the structures of the fungus and alterative changes in the surrounding tissues (Figs. 14.9 and 14.10). It should be noted that with prolonged treatment with antimycotics, the morphology of the fungus can significantly change (Fig. 14.11). We also noticed that in different organs during the generalized process, the elements of the fungus can significantly differ from each other.

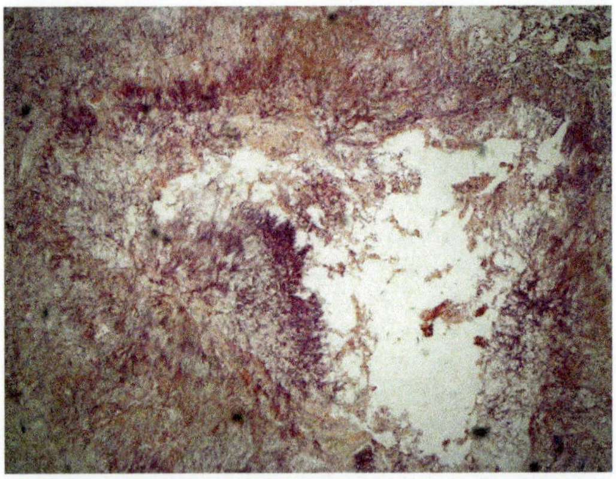

Fig. 14.9 Aspergilloma of the lung. H.-E. ×100

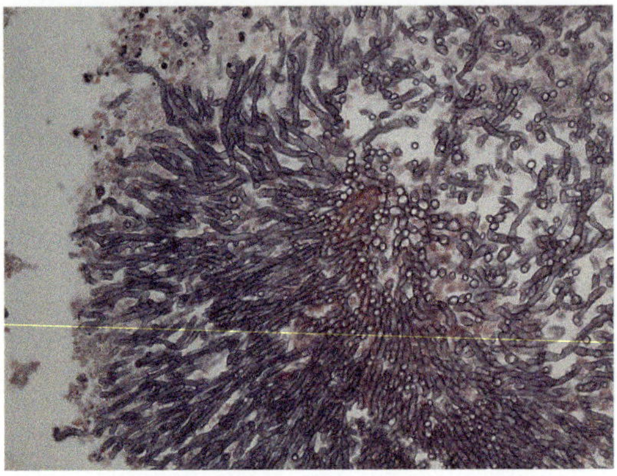

Fig. 14.10 Accumulation of typical Aspergillus. H.-E. ×400

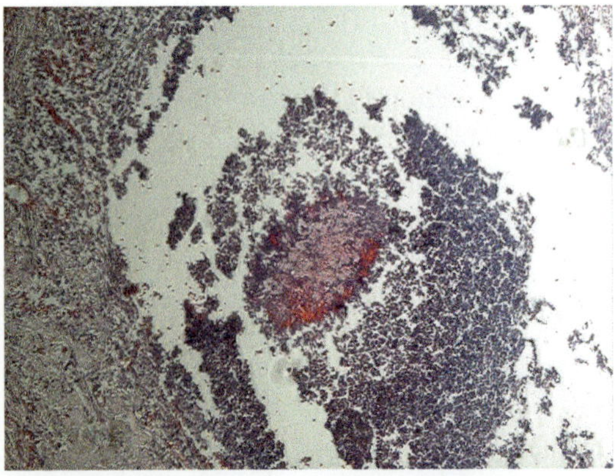

Fig. 14.11 Aspergillus of atypical morhology after long-term antimycotic treatment in the bronchial lumen. H.-E. ×100

In the experiment, aspergillosis can be reproduced in animals only under conditions of immunosuppression.

14.5 Mucormycosis (Former Zygomycosis, Phycomycosis)

Currently, a number of mold mycoses (due to Rhizopus, Mucor, Rhizomucor, Cunningamella, Absidia, Saksenaea, Apophysomyces, etc.), which cannot be differentiated by morphological features, are generally designated now as mucormycosis [1]. In the tissues, hyphae of the fungus with a thickness of 3–20 μm are detected, and it can vary in different parts of the hypha. Unsepted filaments with a double-circuit sheath, they can dichotomously cling, more often at an obtuse angle. The hyphae of zygomycete are often described as twisting or ribbon-like. Older texts described zygomycete hyphae as aseptate, but the term "pauciseptate" is more accurate (Fig. 14.12).

Accumulations of mycelium are sometimes random. The fruiting organs at the ends of the mycelium in the form of large sporangia of a round or pear-shaped form in the tissues, as a rule, are not determined. Mycelium is slightly stained with hematoxylin, somewhat better according to Grokkot.

Mushrooms are widespread in countries with different climatic conditions; the infection is mainly aerogenic with dust. Various organs may be affected. The disease is rare, most often against an unfavorable background; however, it is uncharacteristic for HIV infection in the AIDS stage. Clinical diagnosis is difficult; fungi do not grow well on artificial nutrient media, poorly sensitive to the most common antimycotics.

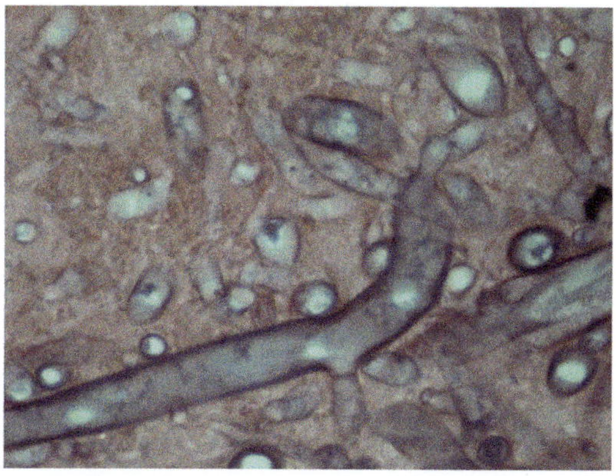

Fig. 14.12 Typical structures for zygomycetes H.-E. ×200

Alterative inflammation and a mild serous-leukocyte reaction occur at the locations of the fungi. Mushrooms very often sprout blood vessels, which leads to infarctions. In the later stages, granulation tissue can grow with a few multinuclear giant cells of foreign bodies. The most important is bronchopulmonary zygomycosis, which can occur as an isolated lesion. Possible combinations with lesions of the paranasal sinuses, pharynx, palate, and digestive tract.

14.6 Pneumocystosis

Pneumocystosis is one of the most common secondary infections in AIDS, but can be associated with immunodeficiencies of other origin as well. Mortality in pneumocystis pneumonia is 10–60%. In previous years, patients often died from this infection after kidney transplantation and with malignant neoplasms. It has also been noted in immature infants with probable primary immunodeficiency. Pneumocystis have a pronounced tropism for lung tissue. However, there are extremely rare cases of extrapulmonary pneumocystis infection, which occurs, as a rule, against the background of severe lung damage, and rarely in the form of local extrapulmonary foci.

14.6.1 The Causative Agent

The causative agent of pneumocystosis is *Pneumocystis carinii* (*Pneumocystis jiroveci*). In 1909, a Brazilian researcher C. Changes, first discovered the pathogen in the lungs of guinea pigs and mistakenly considered it as schizogen form *Trypanosoma cruzi*, because he reproduced an experimental model of trypanasomiasis in these animals. In 1910, A. Carini found pneumocysts in the lungs of uninfected rats. When carefully studied and compared with other parasites in 1926, they were classified as the simplest classes of Sporozoa, a subclass of Coccidiomorpha.

The protozoal nature of pneumocysts was first questioned in 1952 (W. Giese). In the future, with the development of electron microscopy in the study of the ultrastructural features of the microorganism, many researchers put forward assumptions about the possible relationship of pneumocysts with protozoa, spore protozoa, yeast, virus-infected yeast, structurally altered host cells. Over the past decades, the most significant evidence of their fungal nature has appeared. Irrefutable facts were obtained in the study of phylogenetic relations of pneumocysts, fungi, and protozoa. Comparison of the macromolecular sequences of ribosomal RNAs showed an 80–90% identity between *Pneumocystis carinii* and Saccharomyces and only 10% between *P. carinii* and Plasmodium trypanosoma, which indicates a close evolutionary relationship between pneumocystis and fungi. There was also a proposal to classify pneumocystis as separate unicellular microorganisms.

Great difficulties in the study of pneumocystis are associated with their extreme sensitivity to environmental factors and the inability to cultivate them on artificial nutrient media. Successful attempts have been made to cultivate pneumocystis in a pulmonary tissue culture of a chicken embryo, as well as in a fibroblast culture of human embryonic lung tissue.

In practice, at present, only tissue forms of the pathogen obtained from pathological material (biopsy samples, bronchoalveolar lavage, sputum) are available for study.

With routine staining methods (hematoxylin and eosin, van Gieson, etc.), the accumulation of the pathogen in the tissues is defined as uniform cellular masses—diagnostically significant mature forms of pneumocystis remain invisible. According to the Gram, the pneumocystis stains inconsistently. Tissue forms of the pathogen are well detected by impregnation according to Gomori–Grokkot, when staining the PAS reaction according to the Romanovsky–Giemsa method, when staining with toluidine blue, thionine.

Morphologically mature pneumocystis are rounded cells in the form of cysts up to 10 nm in diameter with a dense multilayer cell wall of a polysaccharide nature. The wall of the pneumocystis contains chitin, which indicates their similarity with true mushrooms. In mature pneumocystis, basophilic intracellular bodies (ascospores) are visible—the number is 2.4.8. Around the ripeness of the pneumocystis, a large number of young forms are usually concentrated—trophozoids with labile outlines, as well as intermediate forms—precysts with a thin polysaccharide-containing wall. An electron microscopic study revealed that the cytoplasm of mature cysts contains a rough endoplasmic reticulum, poorly developed mitochondria with a small number of cristae, vacuoles, glycogen, and lipoid inclusions. Many researchers especially point out the absence in the cytoplasm of lysosomes, phagosomes, the Golgi apparatus, and motor organelles—structures so characteristic of protozoa. The ability of pneumocystis to phagocytosis and self-movement is completely rejected. Nuclear material is not always well differentiated from cytoplasm—nuclear zones are sometimes defined without clear membranes, or nuclear membranes develop without sufficient chromatin organization.

The life cycle of a pneumocystis consists of successive stages, including the process of spore formation within mature cysts and the processes of direct division and/or copulation of trophozoids (Fig. 14.13). Ascospore formation begins after differentiation of an even number of daughter nuclei in the cyst cytoplasm. Then a membrane forms that surround the nucleus with part of the maternal cytoplasm and some of its components.

The maximum number of intracellular bodies up to 8 is described, which in the early stages have a rounded shape up to 1 μm in size. As they mature, they completely fill the cyst, its membrane breaks, and intracellular bodies are pushed out. Maternal cells acquire cup-shaped or lunate outlines and gradually degenerate.

After leaving the mother cell, the intracellular bodies turn into young forms—trophozoid—oval or amoeba-shaped cells, up to 5 μm in size, with one nucleus. The shell is thin (pellicle), collected in folds, which are presented in sections as a branched tubular system or protru-

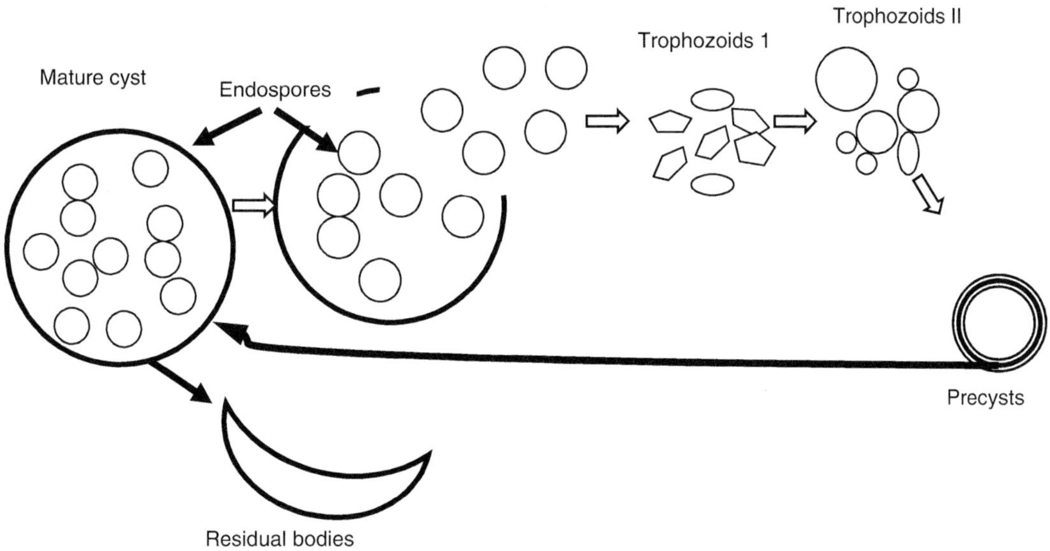

Fig. 14.13 Scheme of *P. carini* development in human tissues

sion. It is assumed that by means of the tubular system, trophozoids are fed with low molecular weight substances from intra-alveolar fluid, and possibly from cells of the alveolar epithelium. Young trophozoids having a haploid set of chromosomes, after leaving the mother cell, are capable of copulation. As a result, a diploid trophozoid is formed, which, as it ripens, turns into precysta. The formation of intracystic bodies in ripened precysta is associated with the processes of meiosis and mitosis that flow sequentially. The similarity of the mechanisms of the formation of intracystic bodies with ascospore formation with a large base of the subclass Hemiascomycetides.

14.6.2 Clinic

In previous years, pneumocystosis was well known to pediatric pathologists causing severe pneumonia in preterm babies with probable immunodeficiency as sporadic disease or in small hospital outbreaks. In isolated cases, it has been described in adults, especially military personnel, in whom the presence of secondary immunodeficiency of an exogenous nature could not be ruled out.

The disease has a long, gradual development, in some cases with a wave-like course. Patients have nonspecific symptoms of intoxication, rapid breathing, shortness of breath, cyanosis at subfebrile, or normal temperature. Later, after 10–14 days, against the background of increasing shortness of breath, a dry, intrusive cough appears. Progressing respiratory acidosis, symptoms of respiratory failure. At this stage, serious complications can occur in the form of dry sickle-shaped pneumothorax, mediastinal emphysema, the formation of pulmonary caverns, and lung necrosis. With an unfavorable prognosis, patients die from asphyxia. The duration of the disease varies widely and depends on the severity of the course, timely diagnosis, and specific therapy. In cases where pneumocystis pneumonia occurs against the background of AIDS, an even longer development of the disease is observed for several months. Clinical symptoms are more erased, relapses and disseminated forms often occur.

The X-ray picture is characterized by bilateral basal or lower lobe infiltration, which turns into a total decrease in lung transparency with the appearance of a spotty pattern due to the alternation of the areas of infiltration and emphysema. Perhaps the formation of cysts with the subsequent development of pneumothorax.

An X-ray examination of AIDS patients with pneumocystosis revealed the presence of atypical manifestations on the radiograph of the lungs, in particular, in the form of local infiltrates in the lung tissue, the presence of a mesh pattern in the zones of infiltration; intrathoracic adenopathy and pleural effusion. Similar changes are also observed in the case of joining other infectious processes to pneumocystis pneumonia. At the same time, there are observations that in some patients with proven pneumocystis pneumonia, radiological changes in the lungs are not detected. In the case of a prolonged recurrent course of the disease in the peripheral blood, moderate anemia, lymphopenia, and leukocytosis are noted.

In the acute period, eosinophilia is possible. ESR increases in the presence of microbial superinfection. It is noted that pneumocystis pneumonia is characterized by high serum lactate dehydrogenase activity. A decrease in LDH level has a favorable prognostic value, indicating the clinical resolution of pneumatic foci caused by pneumocystis. When studying the functional ability of the lungs, a decrease in the saturation of arterial blood with oxygen in patients with pneumocystis pneumonia was revealed. Sharp manifestations of hypoxemia can be early signs of the disease. However, the detection of the pathogen in pathological material is crucial in the diagnosis. Empirical diagnosis of pneumocystosis is unacceptable due to the absence of specific clinical symptoms and laboratory examination methods. In order to detect the pathogen, sputum, bronchoalveolar fluid, and biopsy specimens obtained by transbronchial biopsy of peripheral lung regions are examined. Pathological changes in the lungs explain the severe degree of respiratory failure, which develops with pneumocystis pneumonia and is often the cause of death of patients.

Despite the fact that the occurrence of pneumocystis pneumonia is supposed to be the result of activation of a latent infection, the mechanisms of the damaging effect of the pathogen remain largely implicit. The generally accepted view explaining the pathological effect of pneumocystis is a violation of alveolar–capillary gas exchange due to the accumulation in the airways of the lungs of "foamy" masses containing the pathogen. However, there are observations indicating the possibility of a direct damaging effect of the pneumocystis. Electron microscopic studies have shown that pneumocystis attaches to the alveolar epithelium, and selectively to 1 type pneumocytes. It was shown that the consequence of the attachment of pneumocystis and their multiplication in close connection with alveolar epithelium was an increase in alveolar–capillary permeability, leading to intracellular edema of first-order pneumocytes with subsequent degeneration. It has been suggested that pneumocystis secrete substances that affect the permeability of host cells. Some authors pay special attention to the importance of surfactant (a component of the surface-active lining of the pulmonary alveoli) in the pathogenesis of pneumocystis pneumonia. Vital activity and reproduction of pneumocystis occur in a layer of surfactant, which is secreted by cells of the alveolar epithelium of the second order. The ability of pneumocystis to absorb surfactant was revealed, which explains the reduced amount of it in the lungs: with pneumocystis pneumonia, which may be one of the causes of respiratory failure.

14.6.3 Pathology

Currently, pneumocystis pneumonia is one of the most frequent AIDS-associated infections, including a combined etiology [8]. Its frequency in different years and different regions can vary significantly [9].

Macroscopic examination attracted attention to the "rubber-like" density of the airless lungs, with a smooth shiny, so-called vitreous section surface, with which, with pressure, the mucous-bloody masses flow down (Fig. 14.14). The mucous membrane of the trachea and bronchi is pale, in the lumen-foamy liquid. There are three stages of the development of the pathological process in the lungs: edematous, atelectatic, and emphysematous.

Diagnosis of the disease in the edematous stage did not cause difficulties due to the typical morphological picture with the presence of a homogeneous

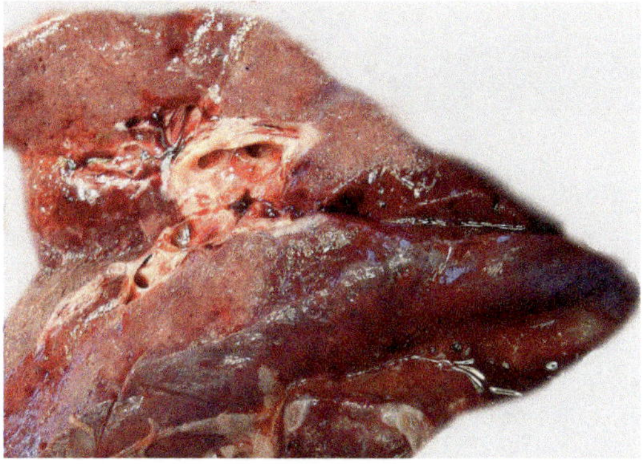

Fig. 14.14 Pneumocystic pneumonia. The surface of the lung incision is grayish–pinkish, smooth, shiny, glassy. Unfixed macropreparation

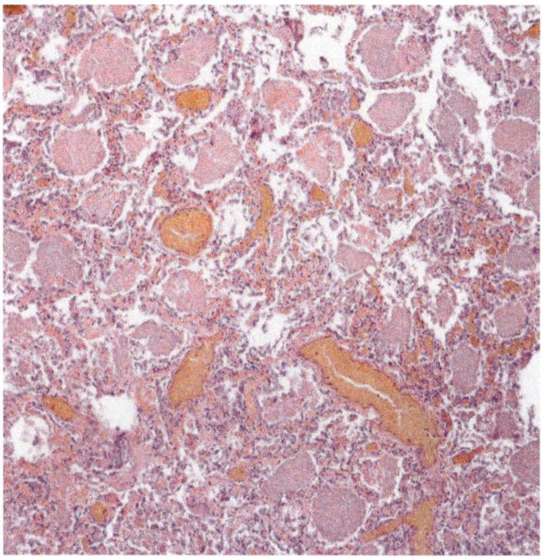

Fig. 14.15 Pneumocystic pneumonia, edematous stage. In the lumen of the alveolus is a homogeneous foamy eosinophilic exudate with very small weakly basophilic inclusions. H.-E. ×100

foamy eosinophilic exudate containing small rounded weakly basophilic cysts with daughter forms, and being a pathognomonic for pneumocystic pneumonia (Fig. 14.15). When staining histological sections of the lungs according to Gram-Weigert, Brown–Hopps, fibrin was not detected in the lumen of the alveoli, and cysts and intracystic bodies were stained basophilic. In PAS reaction, the pathogen was painted in raspberry color, when stained according to Romanovsky–Giemsa, it was blue (Figs. 14.16 and 14.17).

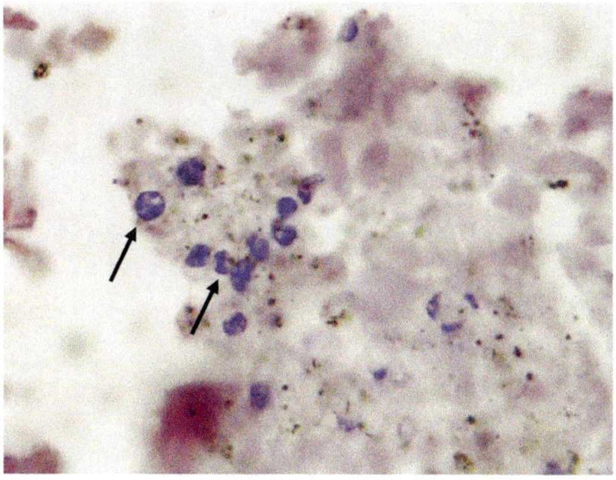

Fig. 14.16 Pneumocysts (indicated by an arrow). Stained by Gram-Weigert; ×1000

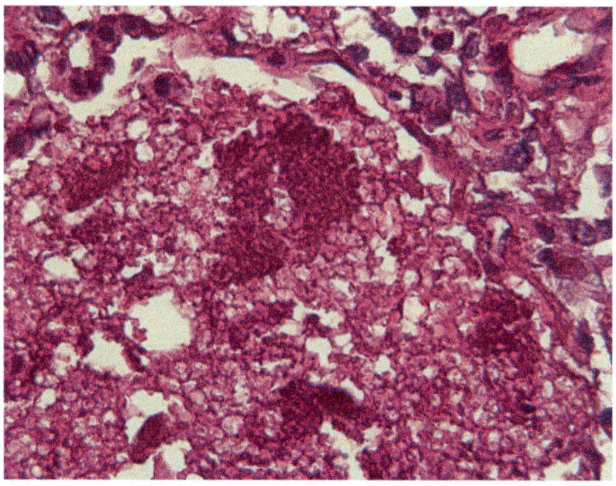

Fig. 14.17 Pneumocysts. PAS-positive reaction of the alveolar contents; ×400

In the cytological preparations of smears from the lung or content of the respiratory tract with Romanovsky–Giemsa staining, the cytoplasm of the pathogen acquired a blue color, and the nucleus became red–violet (Fig. 14.18).

An immunohistocytochemical study with monoclonal antibodies to *Pneumocystis jiroveci* revealed accumulations of a large number of pneumocysts in the lumen of the alveoli (Fig. 14.19).

Pneumocystis pneumonia is more difficult for morphological diagnosis in the atelectatic stage that develops further for 1–4 weeks. It was characterized by the addition of inflammatory interstitial infiltration with possible subsequent destruction of the alveolar septa, which was

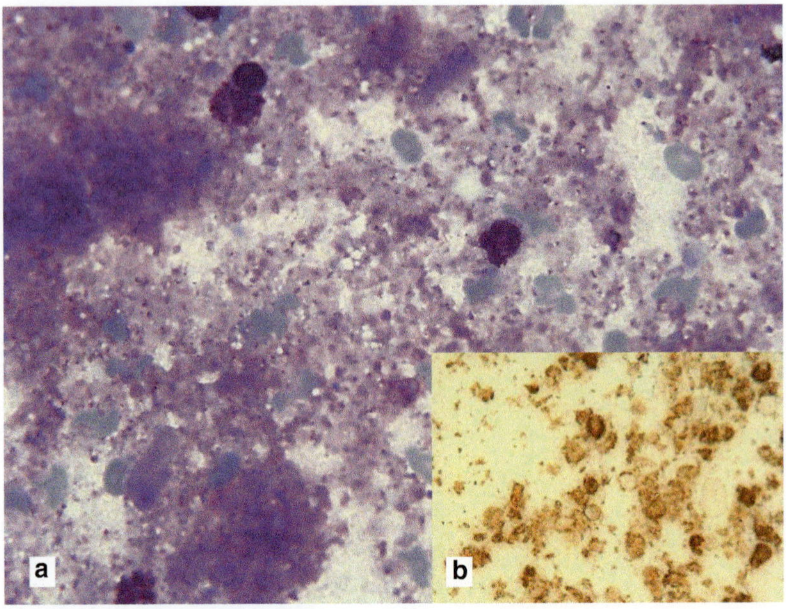

Fig. 14.18 Pneumocystic pneumonia. Smear—the imprint of a lung. Cytological preparation. (**a**)—Romanovsky–Gimza; (**b**)—positive immunocytochemical reaction with monoclonal mouse anti-*Pneumocystis jiroveci*. ×1000 antibodies

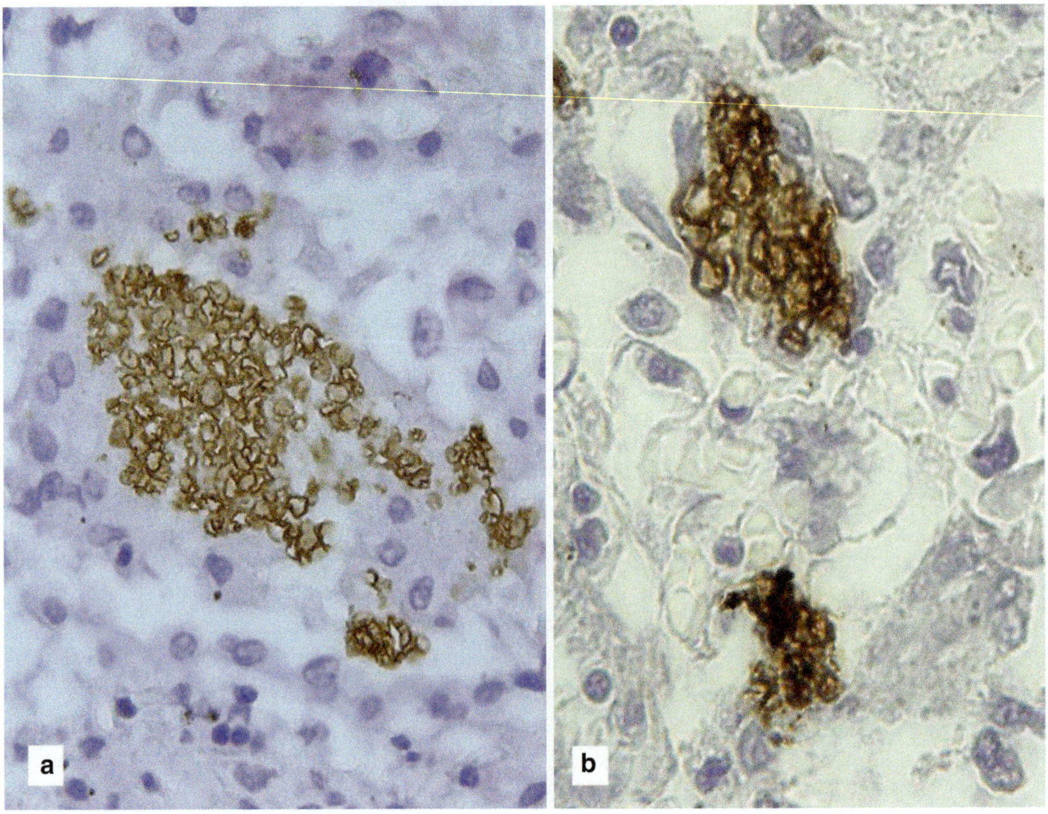

Fig. 14.19 Pneumocysts. Different variants of positive IHC reaction in the lung when using monoclonal antibodies monoclonal mouse anti-*Pneumocystis jiroveci* (**a**, **b**). ×400

usually found in the recurrent course of the disease and the formation of larger focuses of pneumocystosis. Such vast areas of damage, especially in the presence of giant multinucleated cells, can be mistaken for focal lesion due to tuberculosis while panoramic microscopy. Organization phenomena in the above focuses of pneumocystosis were accompanied by small focal deposits of calcium salts, which imitated petrification in the healing foci of tuberculous inflammation (Fig. 14.20). Koss's staining confirmed the presence of calcifications. However, taking into account the immune status of the studied deceased with AIDS, the presence of organized tuberculosis with calcification was unlikely. Z-N histobacterioscopy, IHC, and PCR for causative agent of tuberculosis were negative. At the same time, the PAS reaction showed a positive result when staining the contents of the alveoli in raspberry red, which is typical for pneumocystosis (with tuberculosis, foci of caseous necrosis are PAS-negative). During a Grokkott histochemical study, pneumocystis was stained black and was clearly visible on a pale green background of protein exudate in the alveoli. In an immunohistochemical study with antibodies to *Pneumocystis jiroveci*, the reaction was sharply positive, with a large number of pneumocystis detected (Fig. 14.21).

Occasionally, we have described lung decay cavities with pneumocystis pneumonia. The cavities had fuzzy contours and a rough whitish–grayish or yellowish–grayish inner surface and, upon macroscopic examination, it was impossi-

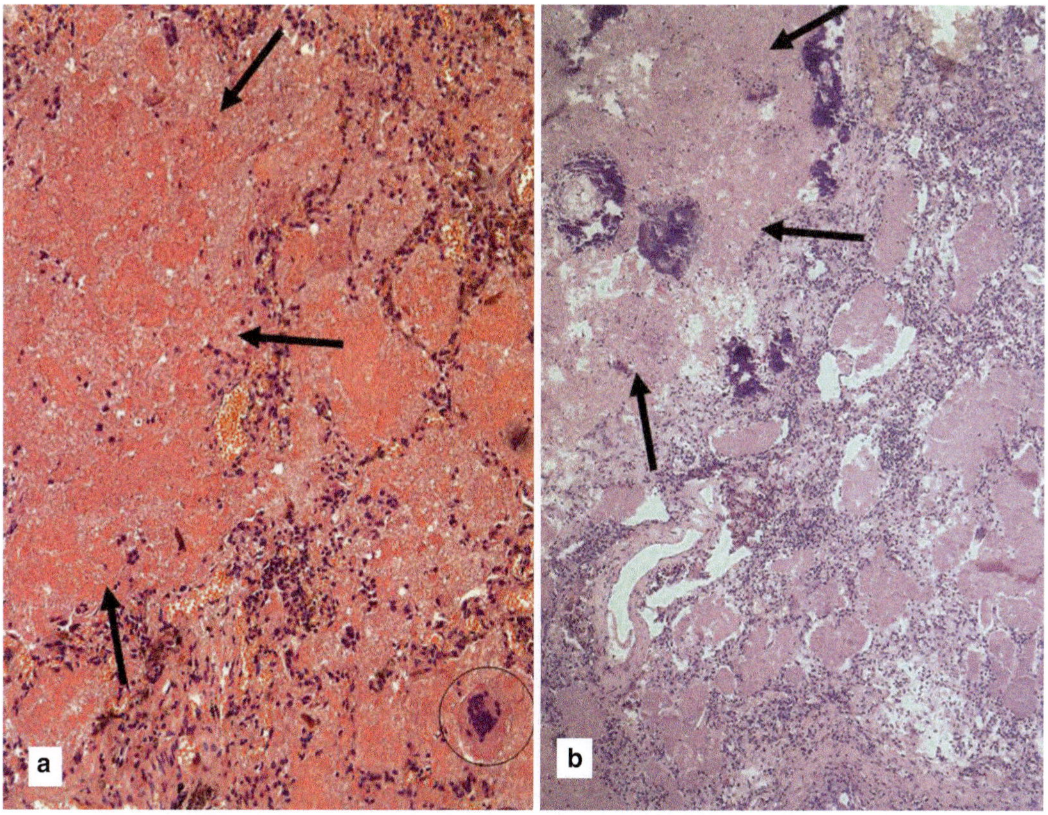

Fig. 14.20 Pneumocystic pneumonia, atelectatic stage. (**a**) degradation interalveolar partitions in focus Pneumocystis (indicated by arrows), multinucleated giant cell in the exudate (in circular frame); (**b**) land degradation interalveolar partitions in focus Pneumocystis (indicated by arrows) with microcalcifications. Stained with hematoxylin and eosin. ×100

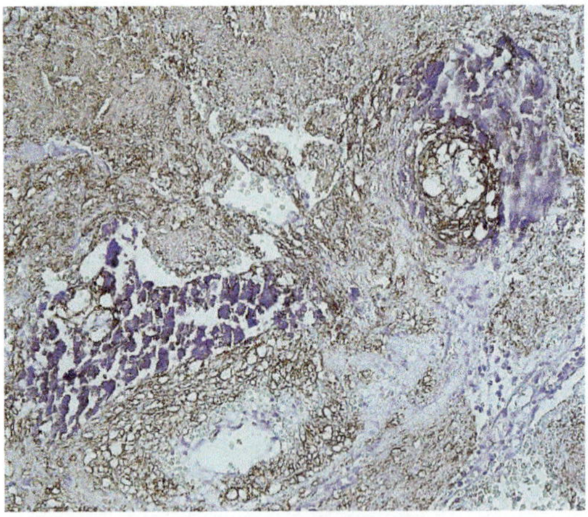

Fig. 14.21 Pneumocystic pneumonia, atelectatic stage. The abundance of pneumocysts in the area of destruction of interalveolar partitions in the focus of pneumocystic pneumonia with microcalcinates (see Fig. 14.20b). Positive IHC reaction in the lung when using monoclonal antibodies monoclonal mouse anti-*Pneumocystis jiroveci*. ×200

ble to exclude the presence of an acute or subacute tuberculous cavity. The macroscopic picture of these decay cavities with tuberculosis and with pneumocystosis had an almost identical appearance—thin-walled rounded small caverns with elastic soft walls and a whitish–yellowish inner surface. However, with pneumocystis pneumonia, the parietal masses were very scarce; there was no content in the lumen of the cavity. The cavern with tuberculosis usually had more abundant yellowish pus-like overlays, sometimes with fine-grained whitish curd-like inclusions, the same semiliquid content was also found in the lumen.

Microscopically, the walls of the caverns with pneumocystis pneumonia were represented by eosinophilic masses identical in morphological and histobacterioscopy picture to the contents of the alveoli; however, with a review microscopy at low magnification, this could "simulate" caseous masses. In the process of organizing protein masses, small calcifications are formed in the walls of the cavities, which make it even more similar to the decay cavity during tuberculosis (Fig. 14.22). Morphological verification of the destructive process in the lungs was carried out according to given algorithm.

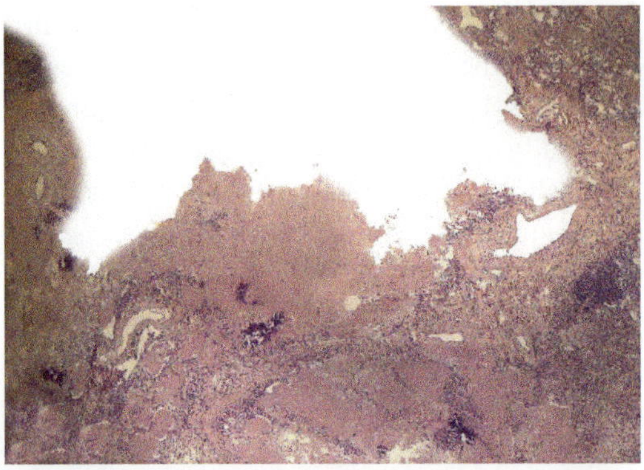

Fig. 14.22 Cavity in the lung in pneumocystic pneumonia. H.-E. ×100

The greatest difficulties in the morphological verification of PCP arose during the reverse development of the process, in the so-called emphysematous stage, the duration of which is quite variable. It was characterized by the formation of fibrocystic changes resembling a fibrosing alveolitis, with obliteration of the bronchioles, alternation of atelectic areas with emphysematous dilated alveoli. With the development of sclerotic changes in the outcome of PCP, the microscopic picture in the lungs was similar not only to organized carnified bacterial pneumonia but also to the organization of perifocal exudative phenomena in healing tuberculosis, with interstitial fibrosis due to cytomegalovirus infection. The alveolar septa are moderately thickened due to fibrosis, with diffuse moderately pronounced mononuclear infiltration. The alveoli were filled with exudate with phenomena of organization of varying severity—stained by van Gieson; the exudate was yellow–green, containing collagen fibers, in some areas, they completely filled the lumen of the alveoli with the formation of small zones of lung carnification (Fig. 14.23). During morphological study (IHC reaction with antibodies to cytomegaloviruses and mycobacteria, Z-N histobacterioscopy), CMV and tuberculosis pathogens were not detected. Detection of small accumulations of pneumocystis in the exudate being organized during the PAS reaction and IHC study using monoclonal antibodies monoclonal mouse anti-*Pneumocystis jiroveci* (clone 3F6, DAKO) made it possible to differentiate pneumo-

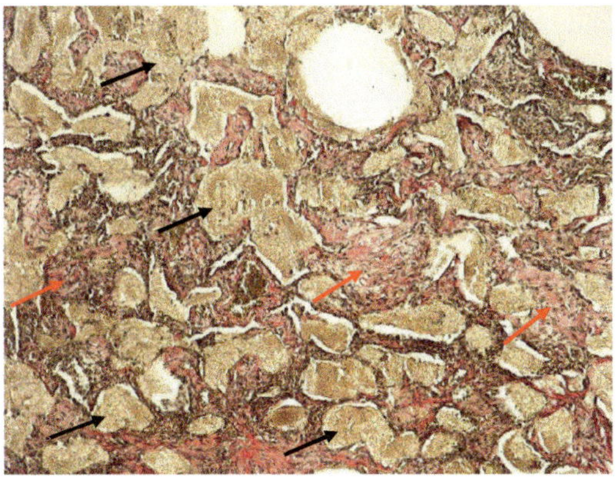

Fig. 14.23 Pneumocystic pneumonia, emphysematous stage. Organization of exudate in the lumen of the alveoli and fibrosis of the intervertebral partitions. Organized and organizing exudate is colored red (indicated by red arrows in several alveoli), preserved protein exudate is colored green–yellow (indicated by black arrows in several alveoli). Stained by van Gieson. ×100

cystis pneumonia and other infectious processes and changes of a reactive nature (Fig. 14.24).

In rare cases, signs of generalization of pneumocystosis with the development of lesions of blood vessels, lymph nodes, and various organs were detected. In a relatively small part of cases, pneumocystis pneumonia was complicated by the development of diffuse alveolar damage (DAD) and it has not been clinically diagnosed in any case. In most studies, an acute (exudative) stage of DAD was noted, which was morphologically expressed by hemorrhage, pronounced plethora of capillaries of the alveolar septa with their small mononuclear infiltration, focal proliferation and desquamation of the alveolar epithelium, and the formation of alveolar membranes (Fig. 14.25). In two cases, the late (proliferative) phase of DAD was revealed, which was charac-

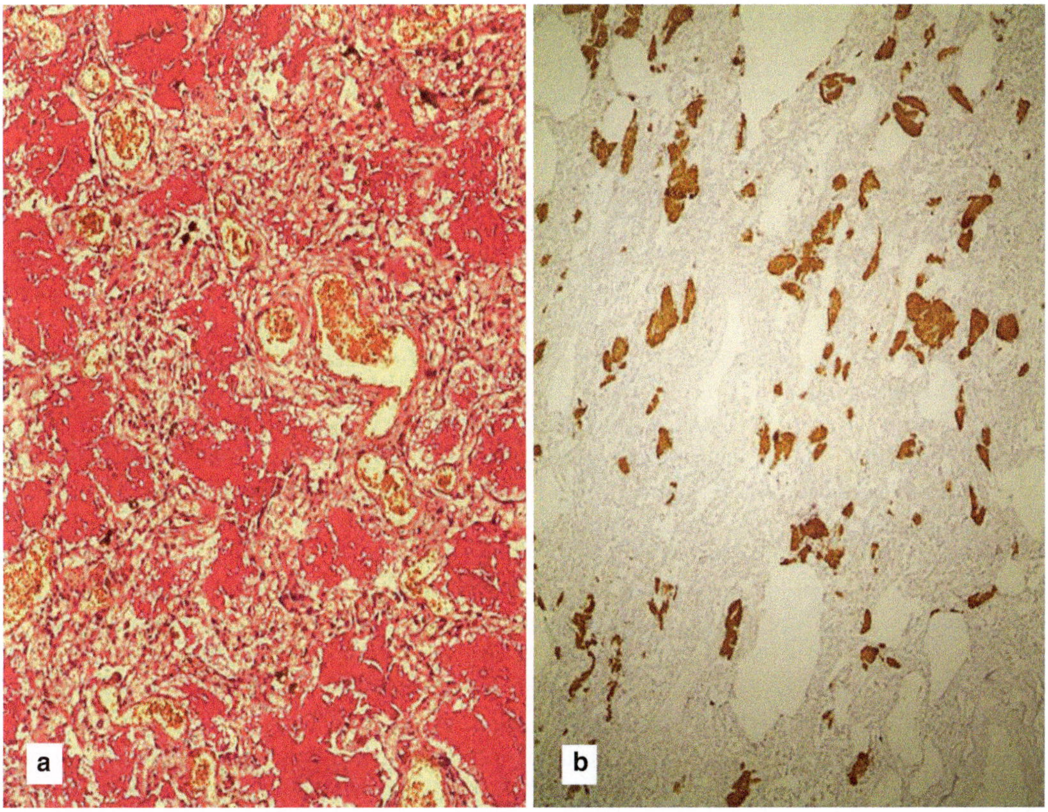

Fig. 14.24 Pneumocystic pneumonia, emphysematous stage. A section of the lung with the organizing exudate and the formation of lung carnification (see Fig. 14.23). (**a**) PAS-positive masses in the organizing exudate in the alveolus lumen; (**b**) small clusters of pneumocysts in the organizing exudate in the alveolus lumen. (**a**) PAS-reaction. ×100 and (**b**) IHC reaction with monoclonal mouse anti-*Pneumocystis jirovecii* antibodies. ×100

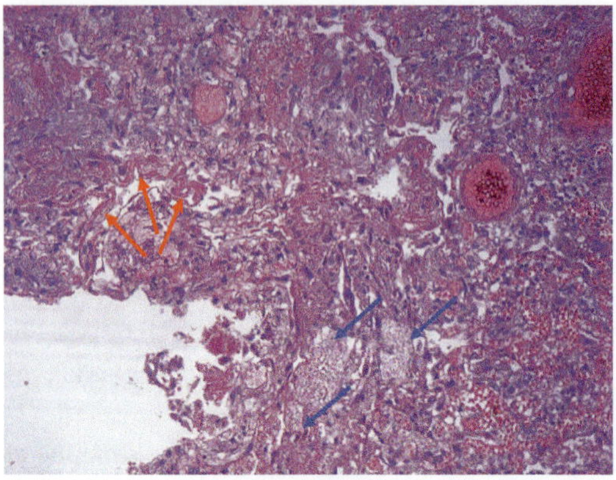

Fig. 14.25 Diffuse alveolar lung injury (respiratory distress syndrome) in pneumocystic pneumonia (pneumocystic exudate in the lumen of the alveoli is indicated by blue arrows; hyaline membranes—by red arrows). H.-E. ×100

terized by the development of fibrosis of the interalveolar septa, the presence of granulation tissue in the lumen of the alveoli, and squamous metaplasia of the alveolar epithelium. These changes were leveled by sclerotic changes during the reverse development of pneumocystis pneumonia, and only the detection of hyaline membranes in individual alveoli made it possible to judge about the presence of DAD. It can be assumed that the late phase of DAD with the emphysematous stage of pneumocystis pneumonia is much more common, but a similar microscopic picture complicates the morphological diagnosis of the latter.

Thus, the greatest difficulties in the differential diagnosis of tuberculosis and pneumocystosis were cases of pneumocystis pneumonia in its atelectatic and emphysematous stages, reminiscent of a macroscopic picture of organized tuberculosis, as well as destructive forms of pneumocystis pneumonia with the development of a decay cavity in the lung, a generalized form of pneumocystis disease with small miliary with tuberculosis. With pneumocystosis in the vast majority of cases, the lungs are involved in the process. Generalized forms of pneumocystosis, unlike tuberculosis, develop quite rarely.

In the atelectatic stage of pneumocystis pneumonia, during destruction of the alveoli and the formation of large areas with an eosinophilic exudate that is microscopically reminiscent of foci of caseous necrosis, especially in the presence of giant multinucleate cells (granulomatous inflammation was not detected) and small calcifications in the exudate, the morphological picture could be mistaken for tuberculosis. However, with HIV-associated tuberculosis, marked leukocyte infiltration of necrotic masses was noted, which was not observed with pneumocystis pneumonia, in which a small leukocyte infiltration in the contents of the alveoli was occasionally observed. Calcifications in acute tuberculosis progression did not form.

In the emphysematous stage of pneumocystis pneumonia with fibrocystic changes, areas of emphysema, histological changes were identical to various organized infectious lesions of the lungs (tuberculosis, cytomegalovirus infection, bacterial pneumonia with carnification). The main point of morphological differential diagnosis in these cases was the determination of the pathogen of the process.

The formation of lung decay cavities with pneumocystis pneumonia, unlike tuberculosis, is not a typical sign of it. However, the structure of the wall of the decay cavity performed by protein eosinophilic exudate with small calcifications under review microscopy was similar to acute tuberculosis or subacute cavern. The presence of pneumocystis was confirmed by the identification of pneumocystis using the histochemical method (PAS reaction, Gram-Weigert, Brown–Hopps, Grokkott stain) and immunohistochemical reaction with antibodies to pneumocystis with negative results of a complex morphological study to detect *M. tuberculosis* (cytological and histopathological methods Z-N stain, IHC analysis with antibodies to mycobacteria, molecular genetic PCR method with a negative result for the detection of MBT DNA).

A feature of the pathology of pneumocystosis in AIDS compared with cases in childhood is the almost complete absence of plasmacytic infiltrates and less expressed hypertrophy of the interalveolar septa.

14.7 Other Mycoses

Fusarium is relatively common, nondimorphic hyaline pathogen. It is often implicated in ocular infections, but can cause lesions of any organ system including respiratory. Possible blood cultures are possible. Definitive identification without visualization of characteristic conidia (very rarely detected in tissues) is impossible. Macroconidia are canoe-shaped and septate.

Another fungus with septate hyphae with acute angle branching, thus impossible to distinguish from Aspergillus species without studies of fungal culture is *Scopulariopsis brevicaulis*.

Most pathogenic fungi classified as dimorphic (usually yeast forms in human tissues and mold in environmental conditions) are geographically restricted, thus we have no own experience. Pulmonary infections (with many being subclinical) are common for several Blastomyces species most frequently diagnosed in Ohio and Mississippi river valleys. Histologically is a described mixture of predominantly acute and both necrotizing and non-necrotizing granulomatous inflammation. The pathogen can be revealed even by H.E. staining as a round yeast with thick walls, but better highlighted by impregnation according to Gomori–Grokkot.

Coccidiodes immitis and *C. passadena* are dimorphic fungi as well; their areal is restricted in North and South America. On histopathologic examination, the hallmark feature is the presence of large (20–120 nm) spherules that contain numerous endospores. Growing spherules eventually rupture, releasing the endospores which begin to develop into spherules themselves. Histologically is seen granulomatous inflammation intermixed with areas of acute inflammation. Older granulomas with necrotic center can be circumscribed by fibrotic capsule and lymphocytic infiltrate. Splendore–Hoeppli phenomenon is possible with "starburst" pattern of eosinophilic material, representing deposition of immunoglobulin surrounding a spherule.

References

1. Guarner J, Brandt ME. Histopathologic diagnosis of fungal infections in the 21st century. Clin Microbiol Rev. 2011;24(4):247–80. https://doi.org/10.1128/CMR.000.
2. Spivak ES, Hanson KE. Candida auris: an emerging fungal pathogen. J Clin Microbiol. 2017;56:e01588–17. https://doi.org/10.1128/JCV.01588-17.
3. Zinserling AV. Lung Candidosis (pathologic anatomy and pathogenesis). Leningrad. "Meditsina"; 1964. 155 p. (In Russian).
4. Khmelnitsky OK, Araviysky RA, Exemplarov ON. Candidosis Leningrad. "Meditsina"; 1984. 200 p. (In Russian).
5. Mc Donnel JM, Hutchins GM. Pulmonary cryptococcosis. Hum Pathol. 1985;16(2):121–8. https://doi.org/10.1016/s0046-8177(85)80060-5.
6. Shibuya K, Coulson WF, Wolman JS, et al. Histopathology of cryptococcosis and other fungal infections with acquired immunodeficiency syndrome. Int J Infect Dis. 2001;5(2):78–85. https://doi.org/10.1016/s1201-9712(01)90030-x.
7. Korablina IM, Zinserling VA, Aravijskij RA. Aspergillosis according autopsy data in Leningrad regional clinical hospital (2001-2010). Probl Med Mycol. 2011;13(2):45–9. (In Russian).
8. Zyuzya YR, Parkhomenko YG, Zimina VN, Tishkevich OA. Morphological features of pneumonia caused by Pneumocystis in HIV-infected patients. Pulmonologiya. 2012;(5):56–61. (In Russian).
9. Lepekha LN, Barhina TG, Parhomenko YG. Lung pneumocystosis in experiment and clinic. Arkh Patol. 1998;46(5):46–52. (In Russian).

15 Lesions Due to Protozoa and Helminthes

In this chapter, we tried to present first of all the lesions which we were able to observe in our climate, taking account of the excellent manuals [1–4].

15.1 Echinococcosis

15.1.1 Introduction

There are four forms of human Echinococcosis. The most common form is caused by hydatid larvae of the canine tapeworm, *E. granulosus*. Its cycle exists worldwide, alternating between shepherd dogs and sheep. Its more virulent arctic strain alternates between wolves and deer and is found mainly in far northern regions. A separate echinococcal species: *E. multilobularis* exists in Alaska, Siberia, and central Europe; in nature, it cycles between moles and wild canines; in man, it gives rise to a multilocular alveolar hydatid, a rare but highly malignant condition. Similar, multilocular hydatids are found in South America, caused by *E. vogeli*, a parasite of wild dogs and pacas. All forms of human echinococcosis are thus zoonotic and the role of man is that of intermediate host; the tiny, adult tapeworms (2–6 mm) prosper only canines.

Unilocular hydatid disease has its greatest impact among sheep-raising populations. Because hydatids grow very slowly, human infections can rarely be traced to a specific source.

15.1.2 Pathology

Many patients have only a single cyst. Over half are located in the liver and 10–15% in the lung. Initially, cysts are microscopic in size and elicit fleeting eosinophil-enriched acute inflammatory responses, leading to the formation of nonspecific infiltrates surrounding the hydatids as they grow to sizes visible to the naked eye. After several years, cysts not uncommonly get diameter of >10 cm, but even large cysts may not cause significant clinical symptoms till the rupture occurs. Thin-walled round-shaped formations of various sizes filled with a light transparent liquid containing "daughter" and "granddaughter" bubbles are revealed macroscopically in the lung (Figs. 15.1 and 15.2). Lung tissue around the periphery of the cavities is sealed.

Mature hydatids are filled with opalescent fluid enclosed by ban inner nucleated germinative membrane and an outer acellular gelatinous membrane which is about 1 mm thick and on histology shows multilayer structure called the laminated membrane. The parasite membrane is surrounded by a thin fibrous host capsule containing mononuclear inflammatory cells and/or eosinophils. As the hydatid grows, its germinative membrane generates short-stalked brood capsules, which later are transformed into daughter cysts. Inside these cysts, multiple scolices are formed by budding, each having four sucker cups and shark tooth-shaped hooklets. Later on, the

V. Zinserling, *Infectious Pathology of the Respiratory Tract*,
https://doi.org/10.1007/978-3-030-66325-4_15

scolices come loose and form hydatid sand at the bottom of the cyst. Even small fragments of laminated membrane or even single hooklet are sufficient for diagnostics. As hydatids grow and age, they tend to become leaky, even without any traumatic event.

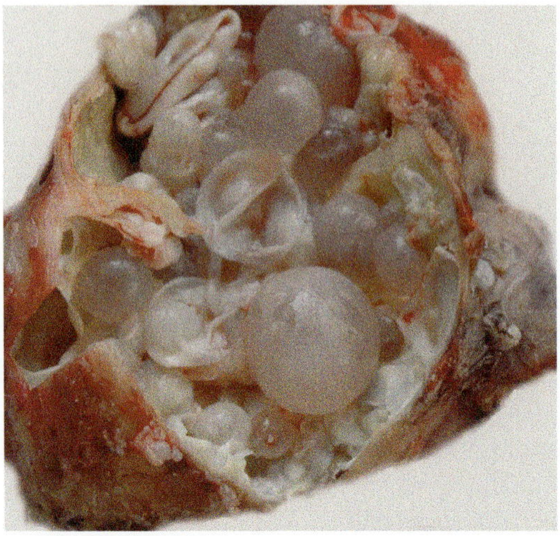

Fig. 15.1 Echinococcosis of the lung. An echinococcal cyst with many "daughter" blisters. Non-fixed specimen

Hydatids of the lung are relatively thin-walled (in comparison to those in the liver) erosion of such a cyst into a large bronchus may result in coughing up the entire cyst and all. More commonly parasite material is retained in the airways resulting in bronchial obstruction and/or pneumonitis, followed by bacterial superinfection and pulmonary abscess. Invasion of a large vessel may lead to embolism of daughter cysts. Additionally, absorption of cyst fluid by alveoli or pleural serosae can cause severe asthma or even anaphylactic shock.

Microscopic examination of the chitin membrane of the echinococcal cyst (both maternal and daughter) had a characteristic multilayer structure, as well as Finns (Figs. 15.3 and 15.4). The wall of the cavity can be represented by fibrous tissue, a shaft of epithelioid cells of various severity and a layer of necrosis with focal leukocyte (including eosinophilic) infiltration were revealed

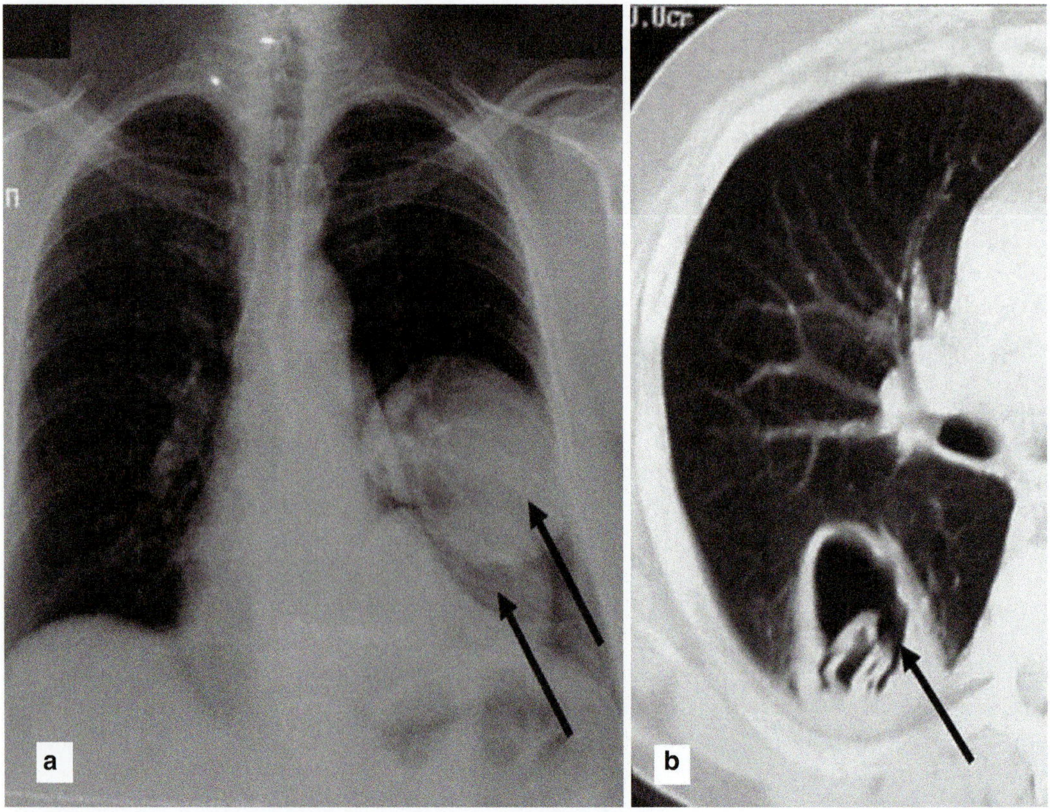

Fig. 15.2 Hydatid disease of the lung. Echinococcal cysts (indicated by arrows). (**a**) Overview radiography of the lungs and (**b**) computed tomography of the lungs

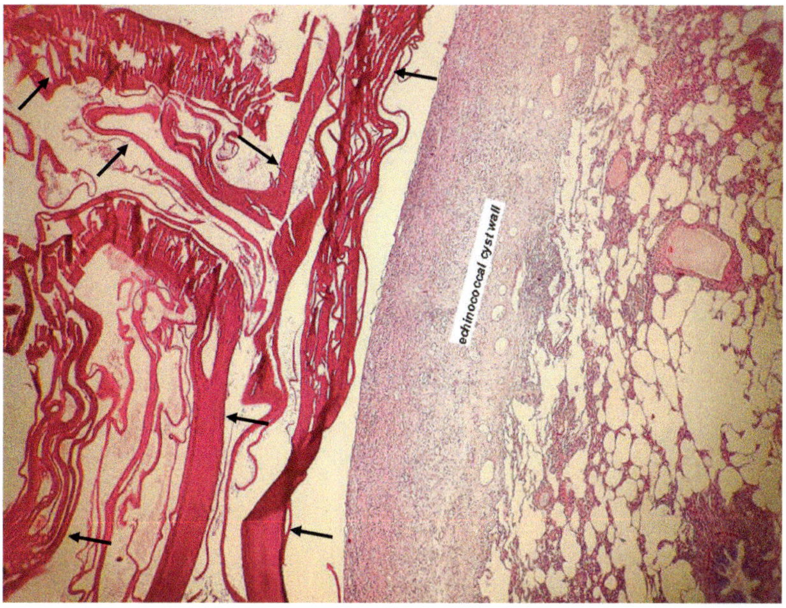

Fig. 15.3
Echinococcosis of the lung. Echinococcal cyst. Echinococcal shells, PAS-positive (indicated by an arrow). PAS reaction. ×100

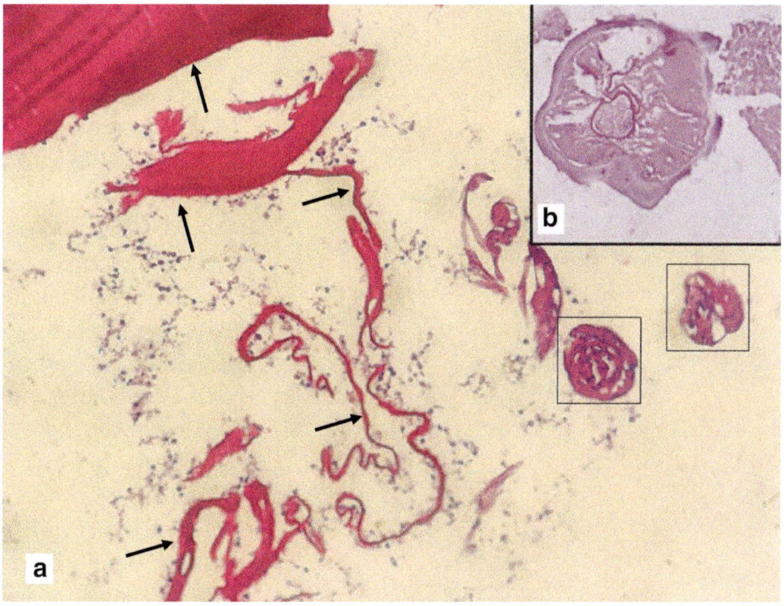

Fig. 15.4
Echinococcosis of the lung. (**a**) Echinococcus shells, PAS-positive (indicated by an arrow), finns (circled); (**b**) Echinococcus finns. PAS-reaction. (**a**) ×200 and (**b**) ×400

subcapsularly. The necrotic layer is of varying severity, with extensive necrotic masses; it is not always possible to microscopically reveal the wall elements of the echinococcal cyst, which can lead to morphological overdiagnosis of tuberculosis. In this situation, it is advisable to conduct a serial deep cut of paraffin blocks to identify the elements of the parasite shells. Atelectasis or exudative areas are determined perifocal (Fig. 15.5). Large number of eosinophilic leukocytes and plasma cells in the inflammatory infiltrate are noteworthy. There are also giant multicore (Fig. 15.6) cells with the predominance of giant cells such as foreign bodies, as well as granulomas, mainly macrophage–giant cell (Fig. 15.7) that with undiagnosed parasitic structures can also lead to an erroneous conclusion about the presence of tuberculosis. In the nearby bronchi, signs of productive or subacute inflammation, an eosinophilic reaction, goblet

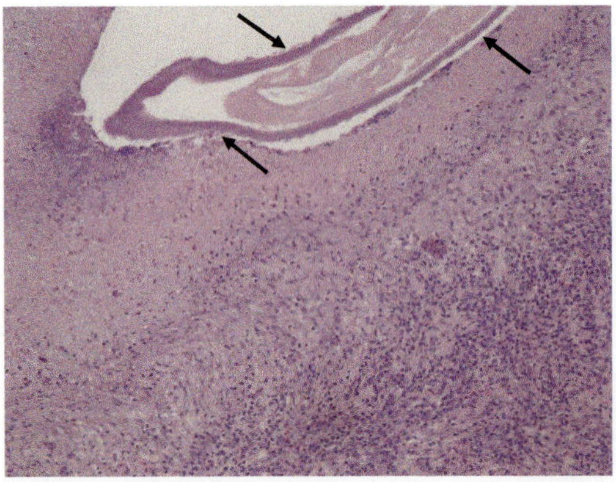

Fig. 15.5 Hydatid disease of the lung. In the necrosis site, a fragment of the echinococcal bladder wall (indicated by arrows). Stained H.-E. ×200

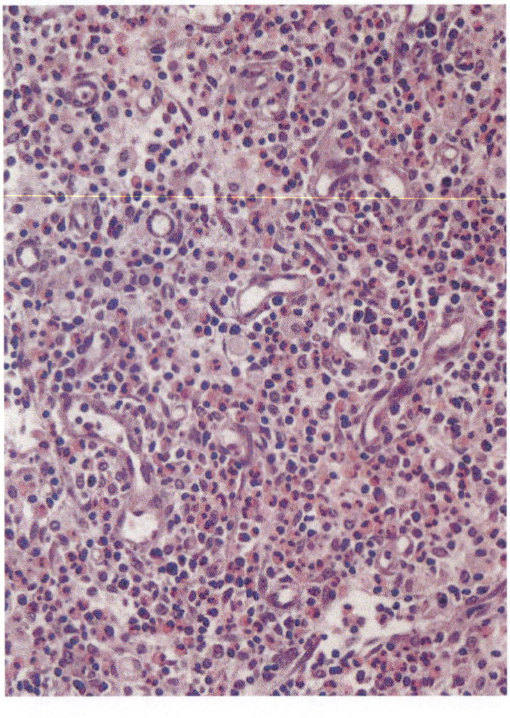

Fig. 15.6 Echinococcosis of the lung. In the area of echinococcal lesion, there is a pronounced reaction from eosinophilic leukocytes. Stained with H.-E. ×200

cell hyperplasia of the respiratory epithelium with hypersecretion of mucus were found.

In the regional bronchopulmonary lymph nodes, the follicular structure was preserved, the follicles are large, with wide reactive centers, a significant macrophage reaction of the sinuses.

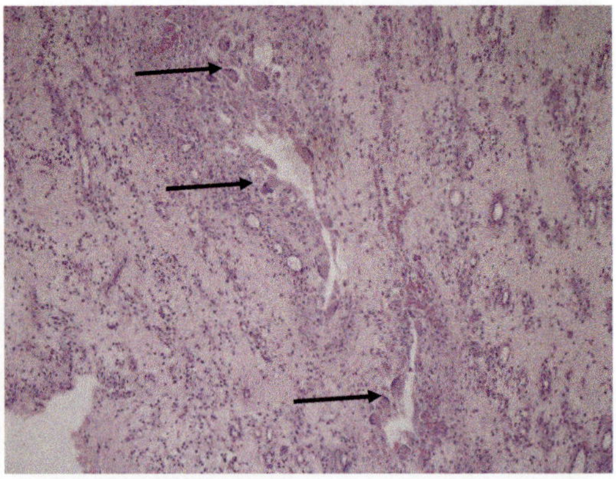

Fig. 15.7 Echinococcosis of the lung. In the area of echinococcal lesion, there is an indistinct granulomatous reaction (mainly macrophage-giant cell granulomas (indicated by arrows)). Stained H.-E. ×200

In the process of organization, the fibrous walls of the parasitic cyst are compacted, hyalinized, and the structure of the parasite is calcified (Fig. 15.8).

15.2 Lung Lesions by Toxoplasma in HIV in AIDS Stage

With HIV infection, toxoplasmosis develops with a predominant damage to the brain. Damage to other organs, in particular the lungs, is rare, usually with a generalized toxoplasma process. The intravital blood test reveals a high titer of toxoplasma antibodies, and *Toxoplasmae gondii* DNA was detected in the cerebrospinal fluid by PCR.

Macroscopic examination against the background of pronounced venous congestion and pulmonary edema did not identify foci of toxoplasma lesion.

Microscopic examination revealed small necrotic foci in the lung. Plots of necrosis in the lungs with toxoplasmosis were histologically more consistent with changes in the type of heart attack. No leukocyte infiltration and abscess formation were observed, as with HIV-associated tuberculosis. On the periphery of necrosis, a macrophage reaction and moderate exudative phenomena were formed. Macrophages phagocytosed parasites, forming pseudocysts, in which there were clusters of rounded small basophilic

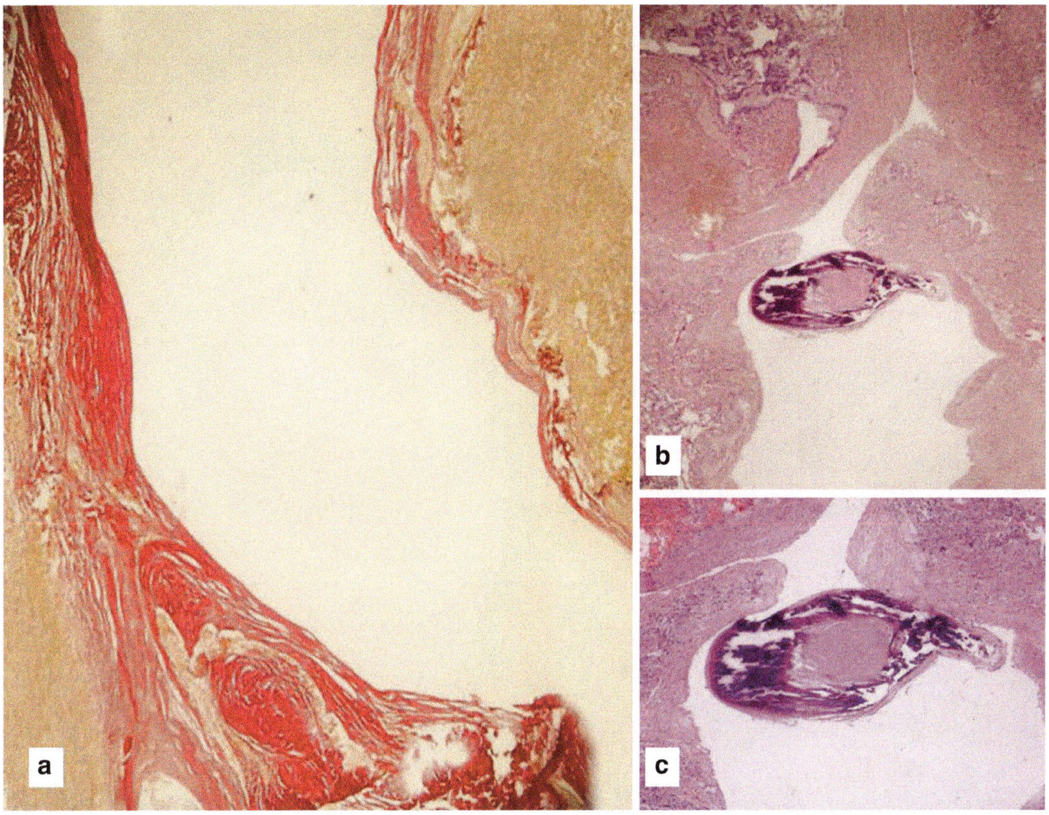

Fig. 15.8 echinococcosis of the lung. Phenomena of the organization. (**a**) Hyalinosis of the echinococcal cyst wall; (**b**) calcified structure of the parasite; (**c**) fragment of Fig. "**b.**" (**a**) van Gieson stain; (**b**, **c**) H.-E. (**a**, **c**) ×200; (**b**) ×100

structures of the pathogen, stained red during the PAS reaction. Toxoplasma was also determined in tissues by means of an immunohistochemical study with antibodies to *T. gondii* (Figs. 15.9 and 15.10).

15.3 Other Parasites

Amebiases. The pathogen is *Entamoeba histolytica*, usually causing dysentery-like gastrointestinal infections usually in warmer areas. Extraintestinal lesions are also possible. Most frequent are liver abscesses, but occasionally they are encountered in the lung, heart, kidney, and brain. Such abscesses remain long after the acute intestinal illness has passed. Main diagnostics is based upon detection in feces or tissues of the pathogen, which can exist in two forms: non motile cysts and motile trophozoites. Peculiarities of lung lesions were not described in the literature and we have no own experience.

Cryptosporidiosis is a human parasitic infection occurring worldwide, especially in children and immunocompromised people, especially with HIV infection. Main pathogen is *Cryptosporidium parvum.* Usually, cryptosporidiosis presents as gastroenteritis with the involvement of small intestine and large bowel, but other sites including lungs are possible.

Pathological diagnosis upon detection of the parasite by PCR and IHC and its detection in tissues using Giemsa, Z-N stains, and toluidine blue. Peculiarities of lung lesions remain unknown; we have no own experience either.

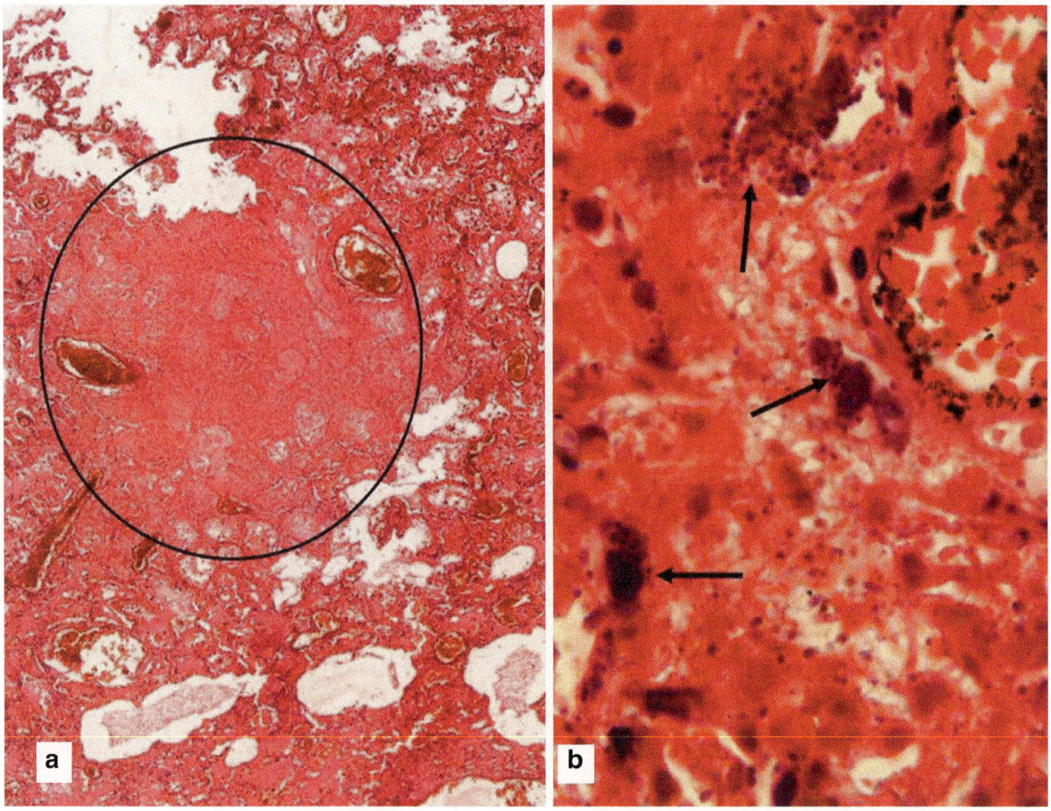

Fig. 15.9 HIV-associated lung toxoplasmosis. (**a**) The site of Toxoplasma lesion of the lung (focus of necrosis); (**b**) Toxoplasma cysts (indicated by arrows) on the periphery of the necrotic focus. Stained H.-E. (**a**) ×100; (**b**) ×1000

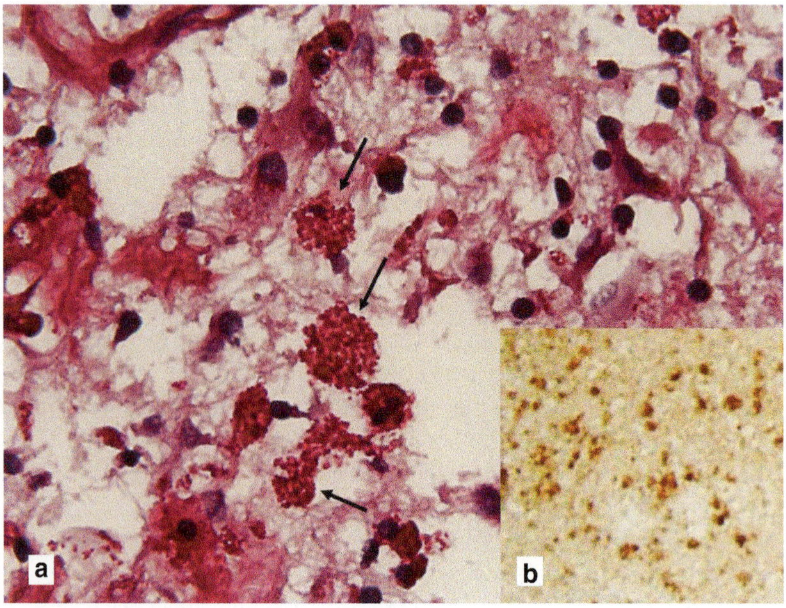

Fig. 15.10 HIV-associated lung toxoplasmosis. (**a**) Toxoplasma cysts (indicated by arrows) with multiple toxoplasmas, toxoplasmas PAS-positive; (**b**) positive IHC reaction with Toxoplasma antibodies. (**a**) Staining H.-E.; (**b**) IHC reaction with *Toxoplasma gondii* antibodies. (**a**) ×1000; (**b**) ×100

Among helminths in lungs certain nematodes can be detected—larva of *Ascaris lumbricoides*, *Dirofilaria immitis* (male and female), *Angiostrongylus cantonensis* (male and female). Among helminth, eggs in the lungs can be detected those of *Paragonimus westermani*, *Schistosoma haematobium*, and *Schistosoma mansoni*. All these helmithiases are extremely rare in many countries with moderate climate and we have no own experience in this field. For special interest in such pathology, special manuals can be recommended [1].

References

1. Meyers WM, editor. Pathology of infectious diseases. Vol. 1. Helminthiases. Armed Forces Institute of Pathology. American Registry of Pathology; 2000. 530 p. ISBN: 1-881041-65-4.
2. Kradin RL, editor. Diagnostic pathology of infectious diseases. Elsevier; 2018. 698 p.
3. Procop GW, Pritt BS, editors. Pathology of infectious diseases. Elsevier; 2015. 706 p.
4. Leslie KO, Wick MR, editors. Practical pulmonary pathology. A diagnostic approach. 2nd ed. 2011. 828 p.

16 Mixed Infectious Lesions. Pathogenesis and Morphological Diagnostics

Mixed infections are a serious but poorly understood problem. Their occurrence can be associated with sequential infection by several pathogens, including with the activation of preexisting chronic latent infections. As part of a mixed infection, there can be either two or a greater number (in our experience up to 10) of infectious processes. Various interactions between individual processes within the framework of a combined infection are possible: (1) they do not significantly affect each other; (2) each infection contributes to the development of another; and (3) one infection inhibits the development of others.

Spatial localization of the pathogens can be different. In many cases, their hallmarks can be present in the same field of view (Figs. 16.1, 16.2, and 16.3); otherwise, one has to detect them in differ-

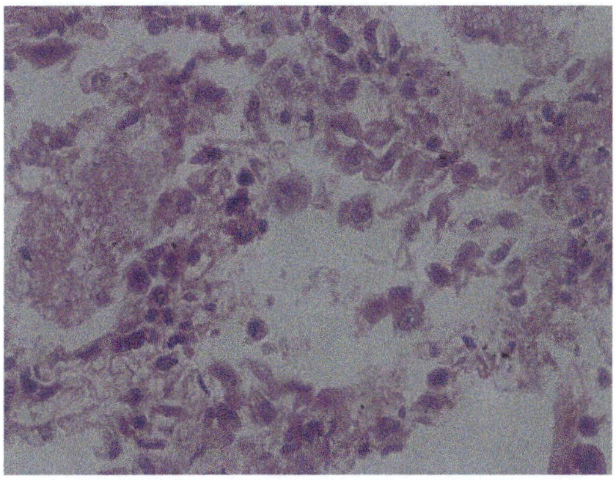

Fig. 16.1 Simultaneous lesions due to HIV and pneumocystis in the lung. H.-E. ×400

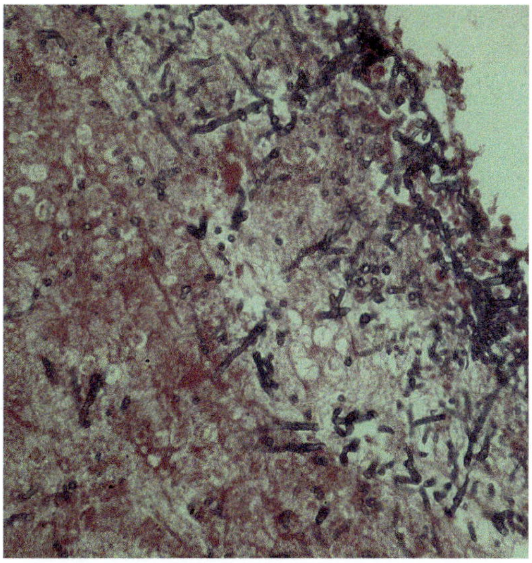

Fig. 16.2 Simultaneous lesions due to Aspergillus and pneumocystis in a patient with HIV infection H.-E. ×400

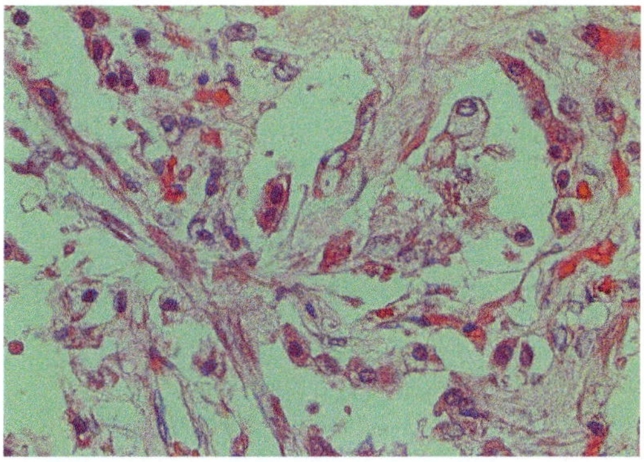

Fig. 16.3 Simultaneous lesions due to SARS-coVi-2 and probable Chlamydia

V. Zinserling, *Infectious Pathology of the Respiratory Tract*,
https://doi.org/10.1007/978-3-030-66325-4_16

ent parts of the respiratory system. In real practice, there are all the options. See also Sect. 13.3.

In certain situations, more severe lesions such as neutrophilic infiltration due to bacterial pathogens can veil more delicate associated with viruses, mycoplasmas, and chlamydia. Most pathologists are satisfied when revealed one most prominent etiology of the pathological process.

Direct contact between different pathogens has been also described, but in practice, it is extremely difficult to verify it in tissue slices. We can also assume that different microorganisms being "neighbors" in host tissues as a part of microenvironment can influence upon each other expression of pathogenic factors and even morphology. We do not possess any direct evidences of this kind.

However, many aspects of mixed infections are still not well understood.

The results of long-term studies of acute respiratory infections (pneumonia) in both children and adults indicate that mono-infections with a fairly complete examination are relatively rare. Among the most well-known and somewhat better studied are bacterial–viral associations. The severity of the disease in different deceased in some cases can be determined by viral (including mixed), and in others by bacterial/bacterial infections.

The best studied are virus–bacterial associations [1]. Many studies have shown that the complicated course of any viral respiratory infections is associated with the attachment of a bacterial microbiota. On the other hand, a detailed study of focal bacterial pneumonia has shown that in most cases, both in children and adults, the viral component is also determined. In some cases, the formation of such viral–bacterial associations can be relatively simply explained. Clinically, a manifest viral infection, such as influenza, leads to the defeat of the ciliated epithelium of the respiratory tract with subsequent desquamation, which facilitates the entry of bacteria into the respiratory parts of the lungs due to a violation of its protective functions. It should be noted, however, that in many cases of previous viral infection, there is no marked desquamation of the ciliated epithelium. Consequently, other mechanisms that have not yet been sufficiently studied are probably connected.

In the 1970s of the 20th in St. Petersburg (then Leningrad) in the period of the A2 Hong Kong influenza epidemic among adults, there were dozens of deaths. In the vast majority of cases, postmortem examination revealed necrotic tracheobronchitis and purulent-necrotic, sometimes abscessed pneumonia; *Staphylococcus aureus* was isolated during bacteriological examination. In connection with this, the term "complicated influenza" was proposed by some researchers, and criteria for diagnosing influenza were developed primarily for characteristic changes in the trachea. From our point of view, this is fundamentally wrong, since although at that time the indicated changes were very characteristic, they testified to the presence of only, albeit a typical, but by no means obligate complication. In subsequent years, deaths from influenza, although they continued to occur occasionally (before the epidemic rise of 2009), such influenza–staphylococcal associations became much rarer. How can one explain the regularity of the appearance of such combinations in that period of time? On the one hand, the mutual tropism of the influenza virus and staphylococcus strains circulating at that time period cannot be ruled out, but reliable facts in support of this version were not obtained then. On the other hand, it can be assumed that the flu epidemic simply coincided with an increase in the incidence of staphylococcal infections caused by a highly virulent antibiotic-resistant *S. aureus* strain, for which effective drugs were not widely available at that time. It should also be noted that the sharp predominance of staphylococci with secondary bacterial layering among pathogens compared with pneumococci can be partially explained by their lower demand for nutrient media, especially those introduced into the practice of bacteriological laboratories at that time.

Under the guidance of A.V. Zinserling [1], experiments were carried out with infection of mice with influenza virus (Hong Kong, 68) and *S. aureus* in different sequences. It turned out that a mixed infection with a primary infection with the influenza virus and simultaneous infection with both pathogens was more difficult than with the initial infection with *S. aureus*. It has been suggested that the influenza virus suppressed local defense mechanisms, in particular the production of interferon, and staphylococcus, on the contrary, was able to activate them. Similar results, but analyzing the activity of NK cells and their production of TNF-α were published 40 years later [2].

Currently, many researchers note that mixed HIV infections are naturally detected in the lungs with HIV infection. There are reviews proving that HIV infection differently influences lung microbiome due to clinical stage, treatment, and investigated cohort; however, no correlation between molecular–biological and pathological data has been provided [3]. Moreover, morphological signs of many infections may be present in the lung. A study of the frequency of various combinations showed that some combinations are more typical: pneumocystosis + cytomegaly, tuberculosis + cryptococcosis, etc. There are no explanations for this phenomenon in the literature. It should be noted that the frequency of lung lesions of mixed etiology largely depends on the qualifications of the pathologist conducting the study and the number of slices studied. Often, true ideas about the etiology of the process can only be obtained with a full and careful study of many microscopic preparations. Signs of some infections can be mild and detected only to a limited extent.

Another extremely important question in practical terms is the need to determine the clinical significance of certain changes and, therefore, the need for their treatment. There are no clear recommendations on this subject, but it can be assumed that the pathological processes represented only by single infected cells do not have to undergo massive specific therapy.

We are quite sure that the problem of mixed infections is underestimated, but has not only extraordinary theoretical interest. In many cases, they have also practical importance in optimization of treatment strategies and for epidemiological analysis.

References

1. Zinserling AV. Mixed infections in human pathology. Arkh Patol. 1991;(9):8–13.
2. Small CT, Shaler CR, McCormick S, et al. Influenza infection leads to increased susceptibility to subsequent bacterial superinfection by impairing NK cell responses in the lung. J Immunol. 2010;184:5558–68. https://doi.org/10.4049/j.immunol.0902772.
3. Twigg HL III, Weinstock GM, Knox KS. Lung microbiome in HIV infection. Transl Res. 2017;179:97–107. https://doi.org/10.1016/j.trsl.2016.07.008.

17 Lung Lesions in Intrauterine Infections

17.1 General Considerations

Intrauterine infections are very significant and certainly require a separate special presentation [1].

It is impossible to count the number of intrauterine infections. Nearby the "classical" ones (such as syphilis, toxoplasmosis, cytomegaly, listeriosis, herpes, hepatitis, rubella), certain attention is paid to the new ones, such as HIV. In certain infections, the possibility of intra- or antepartum challenge has been proved, but usually considered either as extremely rare or clinically unimportant (influenza, mycoplasmosis, etc.). Nowadays, it is obvious that practically all known pathogens, including newly appeared (such as SARS-covid2 [2]) are, at least theoretically, able to course intrauterine infection. One can find in the literature sceptic opinions about possibility of intrauterine infections due to respiratory viruses [3]. Unfortunately, the authors had no possibility to get acquaintance with the studies, in which it has been proved. There is a serious lack of information, especially related to histopathology, in majority of etiological forms. However, it should be noted that for all variants of infection, lung lesions are among the most frequent and clinically significant. A detailed analysis of the lethal outcomes in infants reveals that the etiology of pneumonia is often mixed and includes both lesions that have developed in utero and those that have joined later, including in the framework of nosocomial infection.

Intrauterine lesions can have a long course with minimal clinical and macroscopic manifestations and often remain out of sight of both pediatricians and pathologists. Their diagnosis must necessarily include an analysis of all information relating to the health status of the mother (and, in some cases, the father), as well as an in-depth study of the placenta and other internal organs, especially the liver and brain. A prolonged low-grade course of intrauterine infections with respiratory damage can periodically lead to exacerbations, which are often interpreted as a new infection and allow the child to be classified as "frequently ill."

A detailed presentation of these data is supposed to be depicted in the next issue of our manual, but we considered it appropriate to provide selected data on such lesions in this issue as well.

During the autopsy, it is impossible to find any signs which can allow to suspect the concrete etiology of lung lesion in intrauterine infection, with exception of listeriosis. As the rule, the lungs appear slightly firm, reddish. Hallmarks of aspiration may be present. We possess only several own cases with typical necrotic granulomas in several organs including lungs.

V. Zinserling, *Infectious Pathology of the Respiratory Tract*,
https://doi.org/10.1007/978-3-030-66325-4_17

17.2 Intrauterine Influenza

Possibility of transplacental passage of different strains of influenza A has been proved several decades ago [1], more recently it was demonstrated that H1N1 virus has special tropism to placenta and fetal tissues [4].

Microscopic examination of the lungs of premature babies who died in the first 1.5–2 days of life, despite mechanical ventilation, in all cases revealed the phenomenon of distelectasis. The morphological picture is dominated by pronounced signs of increased permeability of the vessel walls. The capillaries of the interalveolar septa are significantly expanded, stasis is observed in some of them. Multiple perivascular hemorrhages are determined, and in some cases, extensive intra-alveolar and intrabronchial hemorrhages. In some observations, a typical transformation of alveolar epithelial cells is noted, similar to that observed at an older age [1]. Alveolocytes swelled, increased in size, their nuclei became enlightened, the cytoplasm was slightly basophilic, part of the cell lost contact with the wall of the alveoli. Among the desquamated alveolocytes and alveolar macrophages in the lumens of the alveoli, a small number of stab and segmented leukocytes was also determined. The described changes were regarded as viral pneumonia. On the part of the bronchial epithelium, the changes were less significant. In a number of cases, enlightenment of its cells, focal proliferation, and metaplasia were noted.

When EM lungs of children with intrauterine influenza A N.R. Shabunina-Basok et al. [5] describe the most pronounced destructive changes in type 2 alveolocytes. The cytoplasmic membrane of the alveolocytes looked discontinuous, sometimes fuzzy, and blurry. On the surface of the cells, processes and invaginations were traced. A large number of vesicles of various shapes and sizes were found in the cytoplasm, plasmolemma, and nucleolemma of alveolocytes. In the nuclei—the uneven distribution of chromatin. The nuclei are dense, located eccentrically. In type 2 alveolocytes, due to the disappearance of free ribosomes, polysomes, and the granular endoplasmic reticulum, a sharp clarification of the cytoplasm was observed. An extension of the preserved cisterns and tubules of the granular and agranular endoplasmic reticulum was noted. Mitochondria—hypertrophic, swollen. Their matrix is sharply enlightened, bypass membrane and cristae are broken. In the cytoplasm of type 2 alveolocytes, lamellar formations of various shapes and sizes were found. In places, they had blurry contours and merged with each other, forming bodies of gigantic proportions. In the cytoplasmic matrix of the endoplasmic reticulum of type 2 alveolocytes, osmiophilic structures of a spherical shape with a dense nucleotide about 100 nm in size with outgrowths uniformly located on the surface were found. According to the shape, size, and nature of localization, the above formations corresponded to influenza A virus. Ultrastructural changes were also detected in the walls of the capillaries. The endothelial cells looked swollen. In the presence of a large number of pinocytotic vesicles and vesicles, cytoplasm clearing was observed due to a violation of the cell organelle structures. The basement membrane of the capillaries in places looked loosened, uneven thickness.

In cases of influenza B, the picture of the lesion was similar.

In an EM study of various parts of the brain (trunk, periventricular zones of the lateral ventricles, cerebral cortex), performed by N.R. Shabunina-Basok et al. [5] is described the accumulation of viruses in the periventricular zones. Virions of influenza A and B viruses had a characteristic structure and did not differ in morphology from virions of similar viruses in the lungs of infants. They were located freely in edematous intercellular spaces and on cell membranes with signs of dystrophic changes.

17.3 Intrauterine Parainfluenza

The possibility of intrauterine infection due to parainfluenza viruses with trans-placental passage has been proved decades ago, basing upon comparative serological studies of maternal and fetal (from umbilical cord) blood and amniotic fluid [1]. Morphological characteristics of parainfluenza in aerosol infection were presented in Sect. 5.1.

There are practically no data on the clinical and morphological manifestations of the intrauterine parainfluenza in the literature.

During our clinicopathological studies, it was shown that in majority of observations, this infection has a light or even symptomless course [1], but rare lethal outcomes were noted as well.

On our material, in the study of the lungs of the dead preterm and fetuses, distelectases and manifestations of edematous–hemorrhagic syndrome were noted, expressed more weakly than with influenza infection. Hyaline membranes were common. Often there were signs of aspiration of uninfected amniotic fluid. In the alveolar epithelium, swelling of the cytoplasm, its enlightenment, the appearance of fine granularity, and a decrease in the size of the nucleus were noted. A homogeneous exudate with an admixture of desquamated alveolocytes and a small number of macrophage and lymphoid cells were noted in the lumens of the alveoli.

With EM, N.R. Shabunina-Basok et al. [5] describe pronounced changes in type 2 alveolocytes. They sharply bulge into the lumen of the alveoli, possibly due to the expansion of cisterns and tubules of the endoplasmic reticulum. In separate sections of the cytoplasm, ribonucleoproteins appeared in the form of granules, which resembled flocculent clusters, worm-shaped structures, as well as strands and threads. These structures correspond to the stages of formation of parainfluenza virions. At the same time, ribosomes and polysomes disappear in the cytoplasm. The sharp vacuolization of the cytoplasm does not allow to differentiate organelles. Mitochondria are sharply expanded; there is a violation of the bypass of the membranes. Fragments of crista and delicate flaky material are visible. In vacuolated cytoplasm, is noted a lot of lipids. Lamellar bodies of a rather dense form are located in vacuoles. The nuclei are hyperchromic, pycnotic. The outer nuclear membrane forms cavities. There are areas with complete destruction of alveolocytes. In place of dead cells in the lumen of the alveoli—scraps of membranes, flocculent material. The capillary endothelium is swollen, in the cytoplasm, there are a lot of pinocytotic vesicles. The basement membrane of uneven thickness, loosened.

Changes in the brain during intrauterine parainfluenza are usually localized.

17.4 Intrauterine RS Infection

The possibility of intrauterine infection due to RS virus with transplacental passage has been proved decades ago, basing upon comparative serological studies of maternal and fetal (from umbilical cord) blood and amniotic fluid [1]. Morphological characteristics of RS-infection are presented in Sect. 5.2.

The main morphological manifestations of this infection are considered specific proliferative changes in the bronchial and alveolar epithelium.

During our clinicopathological studies, it was shown that in majority of observations, this infection has a light or even symptomless course [1], but rare lethal outcomes were noted as well.

There are practically no data on the clinical and morphological manifestations of intrauterine RS infection in the literature.

On our material, during histological examination of the lungs of premature newborns, distelectases and manifestations of edematous hemorrhagic syndrome were constantly met. The severity of these changes was moderate. Hyaline membranes appeared in the first hours of a child's life. Proliferative changes on the part of the alveolar epithelium were unstable; in single observations, they had symplastic structures. There are few desquamated alveolocytes and mononuclear cells in the lumen of the alveoli. With the addition of a bacterial infection, segmented neutrophils appeared in the exudate.

When EM N.R. Shabunina-Basok et al. [5] noted the destruction of type 2 alveolocytes. The cytoplasmic membrane is intermittent, in places blurred. The tubules and cisterns are expanded, with flocculent material inside. The cytoplasm is sharply clarified due to the disappearance of free ribosomes and polysomes and the granular endoplasmic reticulum. The destruction of mitochondria with a violation of the bypass of the membranes and deformation of the cristae was noted. Lamellar bodies are rather dense, homogeneous. There were violations of the outer nuclear membrane with the formation of cavities in it. In the nucleus, chromatin is unevenly distributed.

In the cytoplasm of type 2 alveolocytes, various types of viral particles were found. In shape and size (120–150 nm), they corresponded to the RS virus. Some particles seemed to bud from the cytoplasmic membrane with flocculent contents inside; others were located on the membranes of the endoplasmic reticulum or lay freely. Virions had a shell and a dense center. Around them was a bright zone. Particles were also encountered without a dense center. It can be assumed that these viral particles were at different stages of formation. Endothelial cells looked swollen, with many pinocytotic vesicles. The basement membrane is loosened. In type 1 alveolocytes, minor destructive changes were detected that were not accompanied by virus reproduction.

17.5 Intrauterine Herpes

Intrauterine herpes infection, predominately due to HSV-2 virus has been intensively studied for a long time. Most evident (but nowadays extremely rare) are the cases of infant's intrapartum challenge due to expressed maternal genital herpes with development of skin, eye, and visceral lesions, including pneumonia with typical for herpes cell changes [1]. The possibility of intrauterine herpes infection due to virus transplacental passage was also proved decades ago. Clinical course differs significantly from subclinical till severe generalized infection with multiple necrotic lesions.

Among other locations, we also often observed lung damage–focal pneumonia [1]. In the early stages of the development of the disease, the lumen of the alveoli contains serous fluid, small accumulations of mononuclear cells and desquamated, enlarged alveolocytes with metamorphosis characteristic of herpes. Possible addition to the exudate of red blood cells marked areas of decay of the alveoli. With the greatest severity of the lesion, pronounced alterative changes occur with the formation of coagulation necrosis fields of the lung tissue.

The most complete information about the results of an EM study of the lungs of newborns who died from herpetic infection is provided by N.R. Shabunina-Basok et al. [5]. As with other infections, type 2 alveolocytes were subjected to the most destructive changes, where virus reproduction was intensive. In the expanded cisterns of the endoplasmic reticulum, the author found a large number of nucleocapsids of the herpes simplex virus, around which numerous lysosomes were localized. In these cells, the cytoplasmic membrane was fuzzy; in some places, its ruptures and the release of organelles into the lumen of the alveoli were noted. Mitochondria looked swollen, hypertrophied, with tearing of cristae and violation of membrane bypass. An expansion of the tubules and cisterns of the endoplasmic reticulum was noted. The cytoplasm at the sites of virus reproduction acquired an osmiophilic appearance. The number of viral particles detected in various cells of the alveolar epithelium was different. So, in some cells, single virions with a supercapsid membrane were found. In others, nucleocapsids were located in groups of two to eight or more, surrounded by a membrane. Changes also occurred in the nuclei of cells. The chromatin in them was located unevenly: either along the edge of the nuclear membrane or in the form of clumpy clusters in the nucleoplasm. Changes in capillaries were expressed in the swelling of endothelial cells, their enlightenment, and thinning of the basement membrane.

17.6 Intrauterine Cytomegaly

Cytomegaly has been described in the early 50th of the XX century is one of best known intrauterine infections, characterized by famous diagnostic intranuclear "owl eye" inclusions in the cells of different origin [6].

Characteristic cytomegalic changes can be detected both in many organs, which is denoted by the term "generalized cytomegaly," or in some of them, "localized cytomegaly." The latter refers to the salivary glands (cytomegalic sialadenitis).

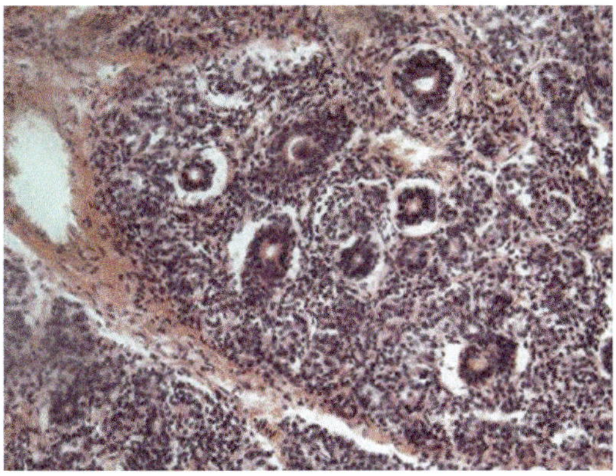

Fig. 17.1 Typical salivary gland lesion in CMV infection H.-E. ×100

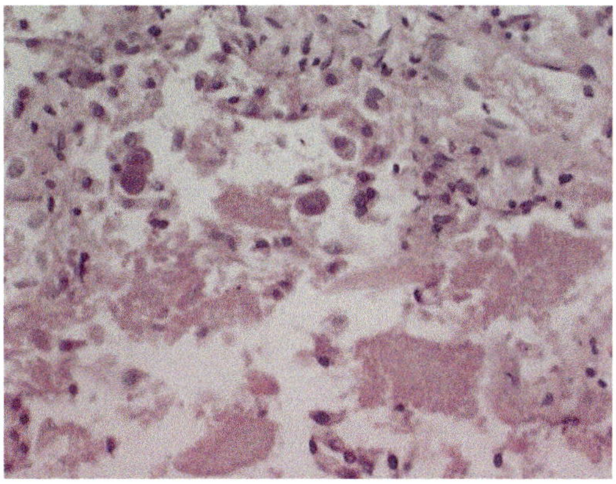

Fig. 17.2 Lung lesion in generalized intrauterine CMV infection H.-E. ×400

There is reason to believe that cytomegaly always or almost always develops as a generalized infection with a chronic course. As inflammatory changes subside, in most of the organs, cytomegalic cells first form and then disappear, although focal interstitial mononuclear infiltrates still persist. Later in these areas, only focal sclerotic changes are detected. The changes in the salivary glands last longer and even progress. The very high frequency of this localization of the lesion was the reason that previously the cytomegalovirus was called the salivary gland virus. It is in this organ that the most pronounced characteristic giant cell metamorphosis of cells, primarily the epithelium of the excretory ducts, is revealed (Fig. 17.1). It is combined with mononuclear infiltration of the interstitial tissue. The severity and ratio of giant cell metamorphosis and infiltrates may vary significantly in different patients.

According to the frequency of damage in the first place, after the salivary glands is the respiratory system. They can be detected in about 60% of all cases of generalized cytomegaly. True, there is apparently no information about the defeat of the nasopharynx, but typical changes in the larynx and trachea are detected only occasionally. Alveolocytes and cells of the ciliated epithelium of the bronchi, bronchioles, bronchial, and tracheal glands undergo a characteristic metamorphosis (Fig. 17.2). Affected cells are subsequently desquamated. Along with this, mononuclear infiltration with varying severity and moderate fibrosis is easily detected in interstitial tissue. In the same areas, chronic inflammatory changes with adenomatous reconstruction of the lung tissue, alveolar collapse, and the formation of a lining of the cubic epithelium in these areas are often found. Often there is vasculitis, sometimes with a cytomegalic transformation of endothelium. The materials at our disposal suggest that CMV lung lesions can be a significant factor in the development of immunopathology in a child, including bronchial asthma [7].

17.7 Intrauterine Mycoplasmosis

The ability of mycoplasmas (*M. hominis*, *M. genitalium*, *U. urealyticum*, and probable other species) to cause intrauterine infection was proved by numerous researchers in the descriptions of individual observations in the late 1960s and early 1970s of the XX century. The most complete information about intrauterine mycoplasmosis was obtained in Soviet Union in the 70th of XX century by various teams in Leningrad (A. V. Zinserling et al.), Moscow (B. S. Guzman et al.), Kishinev (I. G. Schroit and A. S. Kozlyuk) as a result of studying various autopsy and experimental materials using light; luminescent; and electron microscopy and cultural; serological; and autoradiography methods [8].

Unfortunately, later on, due to a number of objective and subjective reasons, researchers began to pay less attention to this pathology. The small number of similar publications has led a number of experts to express doubts about the practical significance of this problem. At the same time, our data allow us, to speak about the preservation of this infection's important role in the etiology of intrauterine infections at the present time.

The question of the location of mycoplasmas is currently being discussed. Many authors consider mycoplasmas as an extracellular pathogen located on the surface of cellular membranes. In numerous studies performed in former USSR and Russia, including those using EM, the ability of mycoplasmas to both intracellular (in the most severe course of the disease) and extracellular location (in mild forms) has been repeatedly proved.

According to our data, the most characteristic feature of intrauterine mycoplasmosis is the multiplication of mycoplasmas in epithelial cells. Changes in alveolocytes are particularly typical in the respiratory organs, along with protein masses, red blood cells, and sometimes a small number of leucocytes are found in the lumen of the alveoli and small bronchi (Fig. 17.3). There are also circulatory disorders in the form of increased blood filling of vessels of all calibers, hemorrhages in the alveoli, and sometimes thrombosis of blood vessels. Moderate mononuclear infiltration is often detected, as well as fibrosis of peribronchial and, to a lesser extent, perivascularic and interalveolar interstitial tissue. Macroscopic changes are moderate and nonspecific.

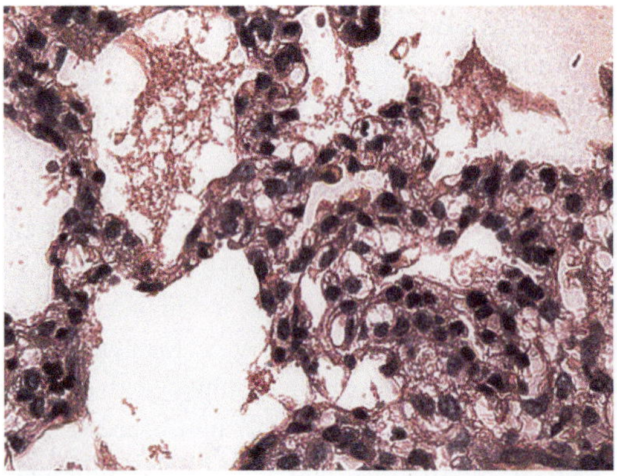

Fig. 17.3 Lung in intrauterine infection due to *Mycoplasma hominis* H.-E. ×200

EM studies of the lungs with mycoplasma infection were performed by N.R. Shabunina-Basok et al. [5]. They found marked changes in type 2 alveolocytes and structures of the airborne barrier. A sharp vacuolization of the cytoplasm of alveolocytes was observed. Vacuoles were of the most varied sizes, from small to large. There were cells where the cytoplasm resembled a "honeycomb." More often this vacuolization was observed at the periphery of the cell. At the same time, ribosomes were preserved in the matrix. The cisterns and tubules of the endoplasmic reticulum were expanded. Mitochondria are swollen, with a violation of the cristae. Lamellar bodies are deformed, ragged, sealed. The cytoplasmic membrane is fuzzy, intermittent. The nuclei are lobed, chromatin margination was noted. Often met pycnosis of the nuclei. Alveolocytes with empty cytoplasm, i.e. transparent, without organelles (cell lysis). The capillary endothelium looked bright, the basal layer was thickened.

17.8 Intrauterine Chlamydiosis

The frequency and great clinical significance of intrauterine chlamydia are currently recognized by many researchers discussing perinatal infections. There is evidence that at least 6–7% of children already at birth may be infected with chlamydia. In the clinic of intrauterine chlamydiosis, it is customary to distinguish between local (conjunctivitis, gastroenterocolitis, atypical pneumonia) and generalized forms of infection. The most important manifestations of generalized chlamydial infection are meningoencephalitis, cardiomyopathy, pneumonia, gastroenteritis, hepatitis, lymphadenitis, which are often complicated by the development of DIC. A significant part of the infected (up to 22%) has no clinical manifestations of the disease in the early neonatal period, an exacerbation of the process can occur throughout the first year of life, and even later, when the connection with intrauterine infection may no longer be traced.

It is important to note that at present, urogenital and intrauterine chlamydia is a very important problem in veterinary, especially in cattle [9]. In bulls with genital chlamydia, testicular lesions are observed in 100% of cases (in the form of small focal necrotic or chronic sclerosing orchitis), in 96%—serous-fibrinous or adhesive periorchitis, in 86%—catarrhal urethritis, less commonly chronic prostatitis, vesiculitis. In calves with intrauterine chlamydia, gastroenteritis, pneumonia, hepatitis, nephritis, meningoencephalitis, polyarthritis, and bursitis are considered the most typical. With many localizations, the intracellular location of the pathogen is shown.

Morphological changes in the tissues of the fetus/child are either not discussed at all in the literature or are considered to be nonspecific and described in total without taking into account the probable mixed infectious lesions. The foregoing served as the basis for the analysis of our own materials [10].

The diagnosis of chlamydia was made on the basis of a comparison of clinical and anamnestic data (in many cases, the detection of chlamydia in the mother), the results of a morphological study, and IF of the detection of extra- and intracellular forms of chlamydia in smears from different organs. The results of the analysis of one of the perinatal departments of St. Petersburg for the year are presented. As a result of the analysis of 104 autopsies of fetuses and newborns, intrauterine chlamydia was detected in 43 (41.3%), including as the main disease, which was the direct cause of death in 12 cases.

The morphological manifestations of chlamydia consisted in a peculiar transformation of cells of various origins, which were determined in various affected organs (Fig. 17.4). The cytoplasm increased quite significantly in size, becoming finely vacuolated. At the same time, fine granularity was determined in it, which is better visible when stained with azure–eosin and Schiff's reagent.

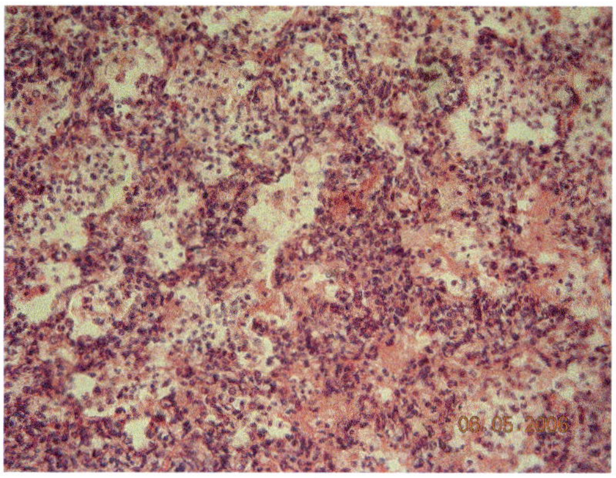

Fig. 17.4 Lung in intrauterine infection due to *Chlamydia trachomatis* H.-E. ×200

17.9 Intrauterine Syphilis

Intrauterine syphilis has been studied and described morphologically long before other infections and has an honorary position in short list of many manuals. According to our data, intrauterine syphilis is uncommon and we practically do not see "classical" changes, including those of lungs [1].

There are two "classical" types of changes in the lungs: this is the so-called "white pneumonia" (focal catarrh-desquamative pneumonia), or "white carnification" (interstitial lymphoplasmacytic infiltration with desquamation of the alveolocytes and accumulation of neutrophilic granulocytes in the alveoli). In the foci of inflammation, a large number of treponemas are found.

17.10 Intrauterine Tuberculosis

Intrauterine tuberculosis can occur if a pregnant woman is sick with progressive tuberculosis. In this case, specific placentitis occurs with subsequent damage to the embryo. For this disease, the most characteristic foci of cheesy necrosis containing a huge number of mycobacteria. Specific granulation tissue in the deceased in the perinatal period, as a rule, is absent.

Several forms of intrauterine tuberculosis are distinguished, depending on the route of infection

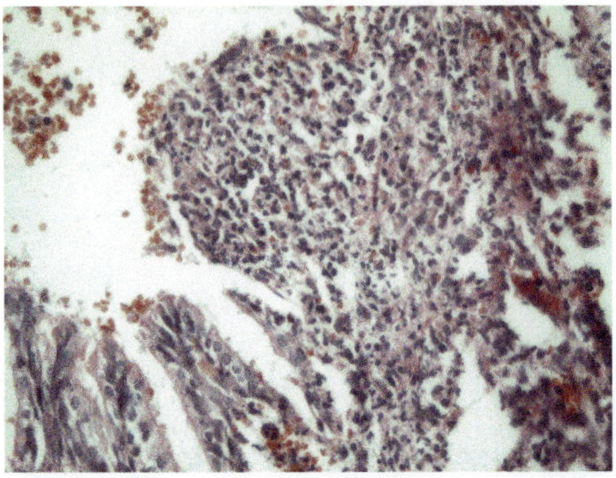

Fig. 17.5 Lung lesion in intrauterine tuberculosis H.-E. ×200

of the embryo. With hematogenous infection, primary generalization is possible. In this case, foci occur in the liver, spleen, lungs, lymph nodes, kidneys, adrenal glands, bone marrow, meninges, and other organs.

The sizes and number of foci in different organs vary to a large extent. With enteral infection, as a result of ingestion of infected amniotic fluid, foci of cheesy necrosis appear in the mucous membrane of the digestive tract, followed by the development of regional tuberculous lymphadenitis. With the aspiration form, numerous small tuberculous lesions are found in the lungs with a secondary lesion of the regional lymph nodes.

Intrauterine tuberculosis is rare (Fig. 17.5). There are only several case reports [11]. At the autopsy material of St. Petersburg, it currently almost never occurs [1].

References

1. Zinserling VA, Melnikova VF. Perinatal Infections: questions of pathogenesis, morphological diagnostic and clinic-pathological correlations. Manual for doctors. “Elbi-SPb”; 2002. 351 p. (In Russian).
2. Vashukova MA, Zinserling VA, Semenova NY. Is perinatal COVID-19 possible: first results. Jurnal Infektologii. 2020;12(3):51–5. https://doi.org/10.22625/2072-6732-2020-12-3-51-55.
3. Schwartz DA, Dhaliwal A. Infections in pregnancy with Covid19 and other respiratory RNA virus diseases are rarely, if ever, transmitted to the fetus: experiences with coronavirus, HPIV, hMPV RSV, and influenza. Arch Pathol Lab Med. 2020. https://doi.org/10.5858/arpa.2020-0211-SA on line ahead of print.
4. Silasi M, Cardenas I, Racicot K, et al. Viral infections during pregnancy. Am J Reprod Immunol. 2015;73(3):199–213. https://doi.org/10.1111/aji12355.
5. Shabunina-Basok NR. Ultrastructural pathology of perinatal viral infections. Atlas. Ekaterinburg: UrORAN; 2003. ISBN 5-7691-1369-3. 132 p. (In Russian).
6. Samokhin PA. Cytomegalovirus infection in children: clinic-morphological aspects. Moskva, “Meditsina”; 1987. 159 p. (In Russian).
7. Zinserling AV, Zinserling VA. Modern infections: pathologic anatomy and issues of pathogenesis: a guide. SPb: Sotis; 2002. 346 p. (In Russian).
8. Zinserling AV, Shastina GV, Melnikova VF. Changes in fetal organs and placenta in cases of intrauterine mycoplasma infection. Zentralbl Allg Pathol. 1986;132:109–17.
9. Tsinzerling AV. Chlamydiosis: diagnosis and its role in human pathology. Arkh Patol. 1989;51(1):3–9.
10. Gorbunov EF, Tsinzerling VA, Semenov NV. Characteristics of perinatal visceral lesions caused by Chlamydia trachomatis. Arkh Patol. 2007;69(3):33–6. (In Russian).
11. Bogdanova EV, Kiselevich OK, Yusubova AN, Sevostyanova TA, Shirshov IV, Klimov GV, Zyuzya YR, Alvarez Figueroa MV, Dolgova EA. Congenital tuberculosis. Tuberc Lung Dis. 2012;98(7):6–13.

18 Morphological Differential Diagnosis of Some Focal and Diffuse Granulomatous and Necrotic Processes in the Lungs

18.1 General Aspects

One of the most important tasks that the clinic poses for pathologists is to clarify the nature of focal and diffuse changes in the lungs. Despite the significant capabilities of modern methods of radiology imaging and the introduction into clinical practice of modern molecular biological technologies, in many cases, the main contribution to the diagnosis is made by morphological studies of surgical and biopsy material. It should be noted that this section of clinical pathology is one of the most difficult. Granulomatous and granulomatous necrotic processes quite often have a similar microscopic picture, despite a different etiology of the processes, which can lead to diagnostic errors. Given that the treatment of granulomatous diseases can be completely different and mutually exclusive, their accurate verification is required.

By granulomas, it is customary to understand the focal accumulation of cells of mononuclear origin that have arisen as a result of proliferation and transformation. Over the past century, their numerous classifications have been proposed, which are based on the etiology, pathogenetic mechanisms, and structural features. Despite numerous studies that have shown that delayed-type hypersensitivity and impaired intercellular interactions are playing a prominent role among the mechanisms of granulomatosis, we cannot talk about their complete decoding. From a clinical point of view, granulomatosis in the vast majority of cases is a pathological process but still plays a certain protective role.

The most comprehensive guidelines provide information that granulomas can appear in 150 diseases of a very different nature. Perhaps there is some exaggeration since we have not seen detailed morphological descriptions for all such numerous nosologies.

At the same time, one often has to deal with a situation where phthisatricians, pulmonologists, and thoracic surgeons pose a question to a pathologist examining surgical or biopsy material: tuberculosis or sarcoidosis? Often there is a need to exclude a tumor. Differential diagnosis of numerous lung tumors is beyond the scope of this manual.

The possibilities of morphological diagnostics largely depend on the material obtained for the study, which is especially important for endobronchial, transbronchial, and transthoracic biopsies. In the study of surgical material, of course, the possibilities for morphological research are expanding. When diagnosing pulmonary granulomatous processes, it is advisable for the pathologist to obtain the maximum possible amount of material for morphological examination—lung, pleura, and intrathoracic lymph node. This makes it possible to more fully assess the changes and with a greater degree of probability speak out about the etiology of the process. In addition, it is often necessary to conduct a wide range of

V. Zinserling, *Infectious Pathology of the Respiratory Tract*,
https://doi.org/10.1007/978-3-030-66325-4_18

morphological studies—histochemical, histobacterioscopic, IHC, and molecular biological, which requires a sufficient amount of surgical and biopsy material. Unfortunately, one often has to deal with uninformative material that does not allow to come to an unambiguous diagnosis and confine to a descriptive conclusion. However, even the final opinion of the pathologist in the form of a differential diagnostic series assists the clinician in further research and the formation of the correct diagnostic tactics. In some institutions, thoracic surgeons practice the systematic sending of specimens for an urgent intraoperative study. Obviously, it has an absolute sense if it is necessary to differentiate focal processes of a tumor and non-tumor nature, but trying to find out the nature of granulomatous inflammation and necrotic changes in such a study is not justified.

A new chapter in the clinical pathology of the lungs is fluid biopsies, which in some cases allow the morphologist to come to a certain clinically important conclusion.

Unfortunately, sometimes differential diagnosis of granulomatosis has to be carried out on autopsy material.

In this chapter, we present a comparatively small number of nosological forms for which we have our own diagnostic experience during many years of practice in specialized thoracic clinics. In addition, we briefly mention those forms that are fully described in the literature but were not diagnosed for various reasons on our material.

In the present chapter, we took into account excellent reviews of lung surgical pathology [1–3] but tried to present our long-term practical experience, including our publications [4].

18.2 Tuberculosis

18.2.1 Tuberculosis in Immunocompetent Individuals

Most often, a clinical pathologist examining biopsy and surgical material from the respiratory system is asked by clinicians about the presence of tuberculosis. For tuberculosis, the main characteristics are different-sized fused epithelioid–giant cell granulomas, with a lymphoid reaction along the periphery in the form of a rim in the absence of annular fibrosis. With an active process in the center of granulomas, neutrophilic leukocytes and cases of caseous necrosis can be detected (Figs. 18.1, 18.2, and 18.3).

A tissue reaction is formed perifocal with exudate in the alveoli, thickening of the interalveolar septa due to edema, lymphoid histiocytic infiltration with an admixture of neutrophilic leukocytes, fibrosis (Figs. 18.4 and 18.5).

When granulomas are localized in the mucous membrane of the bronchus, squamous metaplasia of the respiratory epithelium, pronounced lymphoid or lymphoid–histiocytic infiltration of the lamina propria is observed (Fig. 18.6). Lamina propria of the mucous membrane can be replaced by granulation tissue, including elements of granulomatous inflammation. In the foci of caseous necrosis with tuberculosis, a frame of elastic fibers of the interalveolar septa remains for a rather long time. This is manifested by the fact that in the necrotic masses one can see the outlines of the alveoli (Fig. 18.7). This symptom is not typical for areas of abscess formation in destructive pneumonia, for necrosis with rheumatoid lesions of the lungs, for necrosis with granulo-

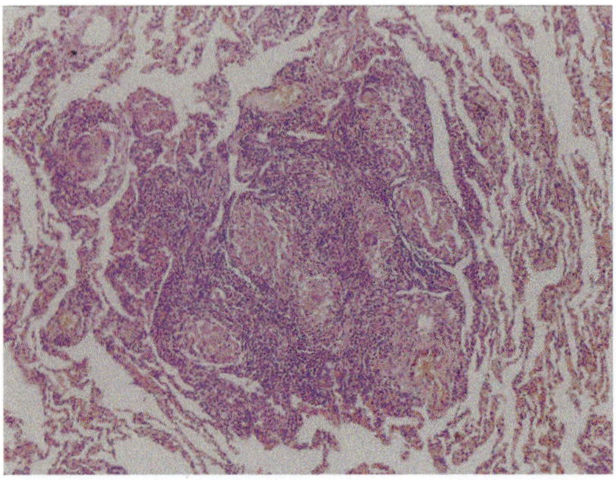

Fig. 18.1 Tuberculosis of the lungs. Merging epithelioid–giant cell granulomas, with perifocal lymphoid reaction. Stained with hematoxylin and eosin. ×100

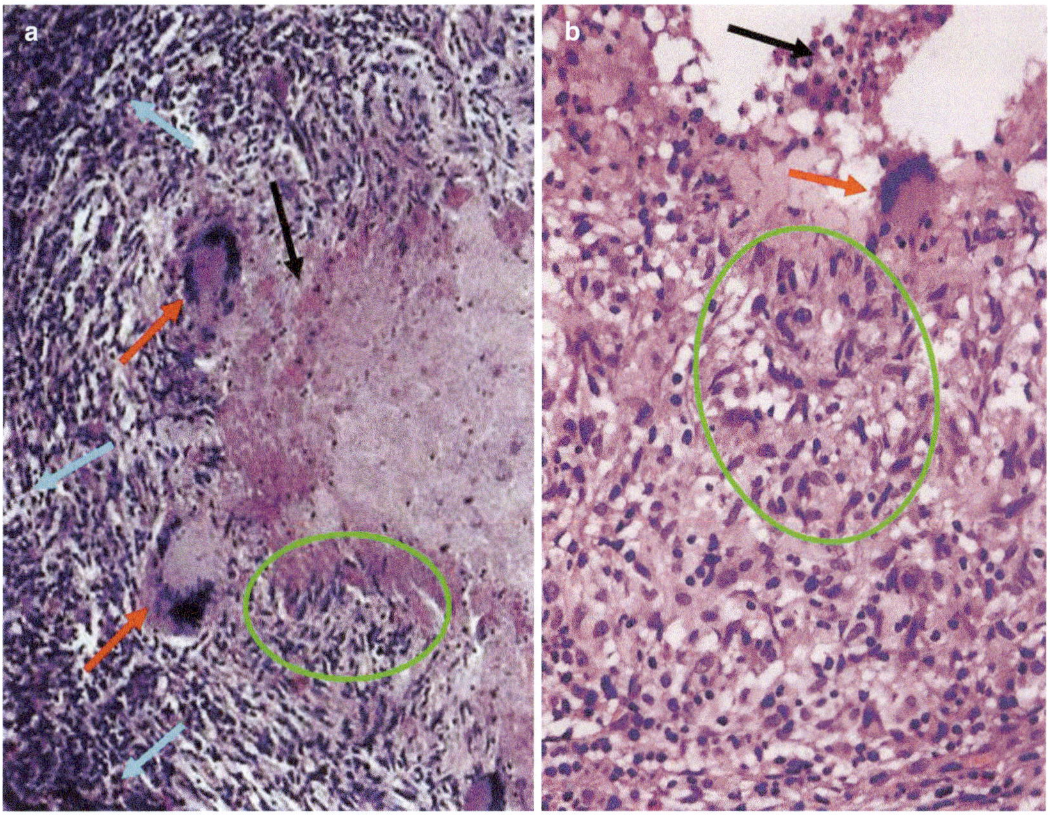

Fig. 18.2 Tuberculosis of the lungs. Fragments of granulomas. Necrosis with white blood cells in the center of the granuloma is indicated by black arrows, giant Langhans cells—by red arrows, epithelial cells—by a round frame, lymphoid cells on the periphery of the granuloma—by blue arrows. (**a**, **b**) stained with hematoxylin and eosin. ×400

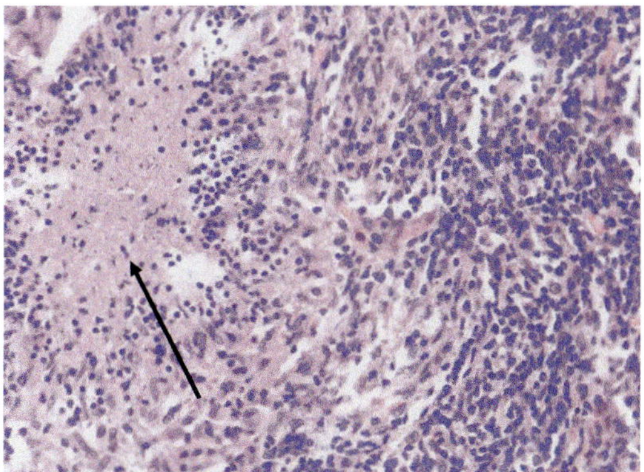

Fig. 18.3 Tuberculosis of the lungs. Granuloma fragment with necrosis and white blood cells in the center (indicated by an arrow). Stained with hematoxylin and eosin. ×400

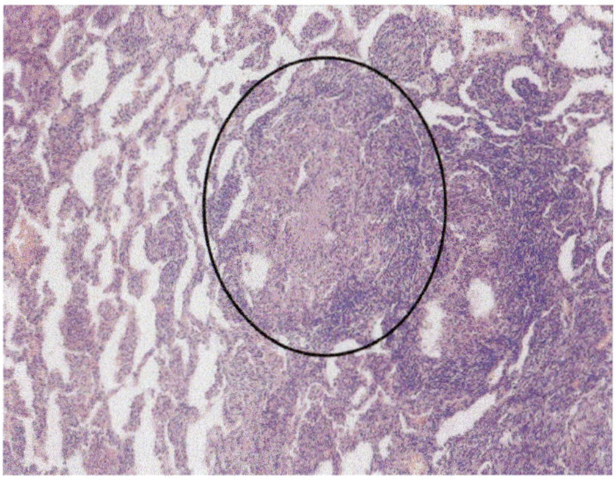

Fig. 18.4 Tuberculosis of the lungs. Merging granulomas with necrosis in the center and lymphoid reaction on the periphery (circled by a round frame). In the adjacent alveoli, exudate, interalveolar partitions are thickened due to edema and fibrosis, with mononuclear (mainly lymphoid) infiltration. Stained with hematoxylin and eosin. ×100

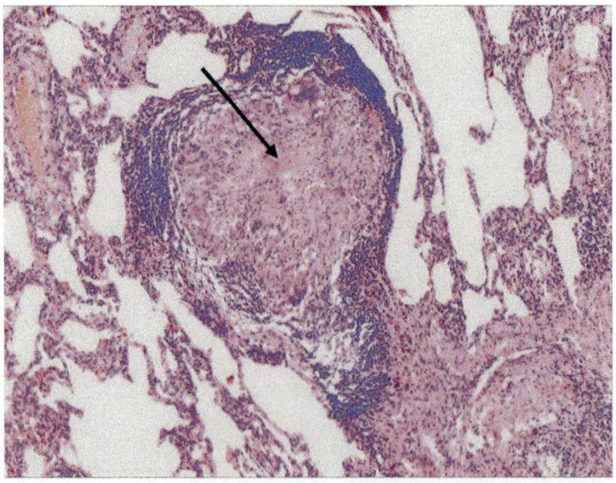

Fig. 18.5 Tuberculosis of the lungs. Merging granulomas with forming necrosis in the center (indicated by an arrow) and a lymphoid shaft on the periphery. The interalveolar partitions are thickened due to edema, fibrosis, and lymphoid infiltration. In the lower right corner, there is a section of pneumofibrosis. Stained with hematoxylin and eosin. ×200

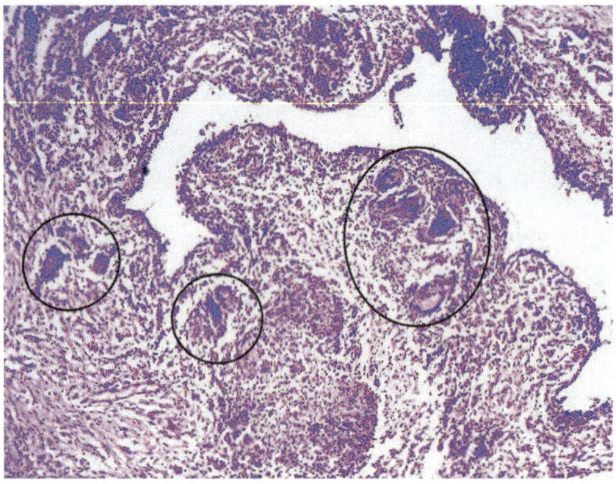

Fig. 18.6 Pulmonary tuberculosis. Tuberculosis of the bronchus (granulomas are surrounded by round frames), diffuse focal lymphoid infiltration of the bronchus wall. Stained with hematoxylin and eosin. ×200

matosis with polyangiitis, or for areas of necrosis with necrotizing sarcoid granulomatosis.

With the progression of tuberculosis, an exudative reaction in the form of a serous fibrinous or fibrinous–purulent exudate (reminiscent of a microscopic picture of bacterial pneumonia) is formed perifocal in the lung. Around the active

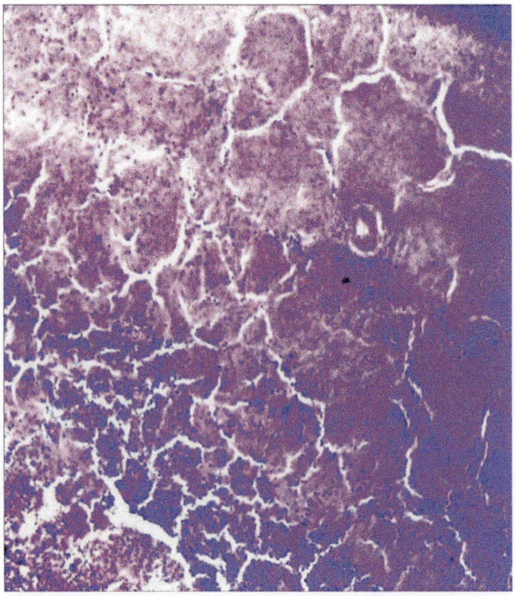

Fig. 18.7 Pulmonary tuberculosis. In caseous–necrotic masses, the outlines of the alveoli are determined. Stained with hematoxylin and eosin. ×100

foci of caseous necrosis, exudative granulomatous tissue reaction can also be formed.

With tuberculous inflammation in the lung, fibrosis of the pleura and interlobular septa is observed, and in the affected lymph node—fibrosis and thickening of the capsule. This is due to the lymphotropic properties of mycobacteria and their circulation through the described structures, rich in lymphatic capillaries and blood vessels. Granulomas can be located along the interlobular partitions.

With histological bacterioscopy according to Z-N and IHC studies, pathogens of tuberculosis are detected in caseous-necrotic masses on the surface and cytoplasm of macrophages, neutrophilic leukocytes. A histobacterioscopic examination with a Z-N stain indicates the presence of acid- and alcohol-resistant bacteria (Fig. 18.8). An IHC study with tuberculosis antibodies establishes that acid-resistant bacteria belong to the genus Mycobacteria (Fig. 18.9). Species identification is carried out by PCR with the detection of

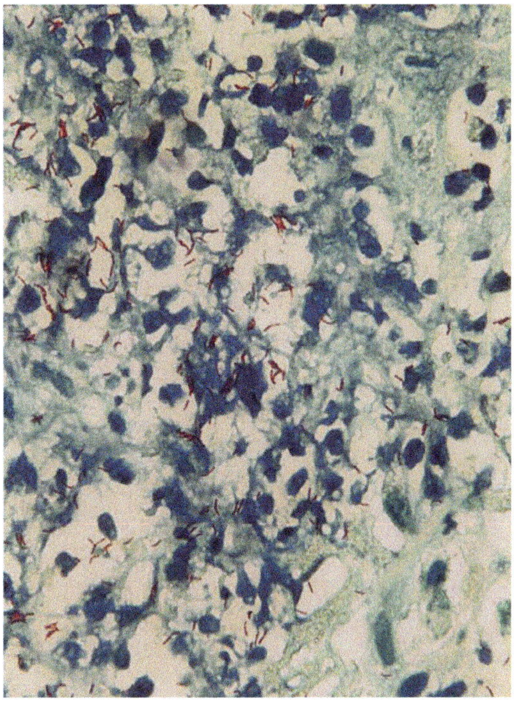

Fig. 18.8 Acid-resistant bacteria in the focus of tuberculosis inflammation (colored red). Z-N staining ×1000

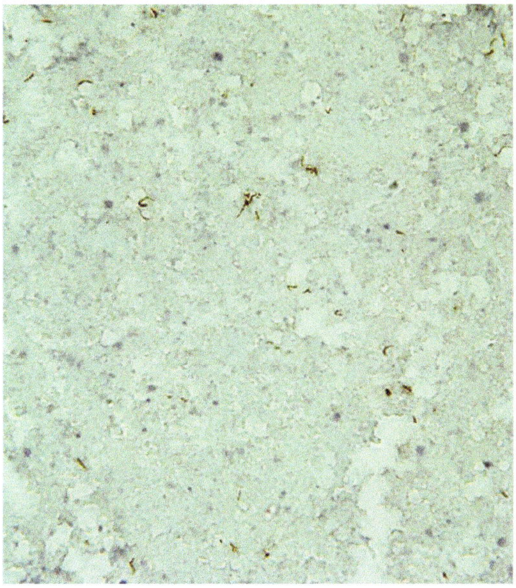

Fig. 18.9 Mycobacteria in the focus of tuberculosis inflammation (colored brown). IHC reaction with Myc. tuberculosis mouse monoclonal antibody. ×1000

Myc. tuberculosis DNA both from native and paraffin-embedded material. The type of mycobacteria can also be determined using bacteriological culture on special media.

18.2.2 Peculiarities of Tuberculosis Associated with HIV Infection

With HIV-associated tuberculosis (stage 3 of HIV infection), due to the cytopathic effect of the human immune deficiency virus (HIV) on CD4 + lymphocytes and macrophages, which are the main component of cellular immunity characteristic of tuberculosis, there is a loss of signs of granulomatous inflammation. There is a lack of features of the so-called specificity of the inflammatory process or their minimal manifestation in the form of fuzzy clusters and strands of epithelioid cells that do not form granulomas with single giant multinucleated cells (Fig. 18.10). Alterative–exudative tissue reactions predominate with the formation of purulent necrotic tuberculous lesions, which have the appearance of microabscesses or pyemic lesions, with a pronounced perifocal exudative reaction (Fig. 18.11). The zone of perifocal exudative reaction can many times exceed the volume of the tuberculous lesion itself. Against the background of pronounced exudation and a sharp plethora of lung tissue, the miliary and submiliary foci of tuberculous inflammation are microscopically difficult to distinguish.

There are no phenomena of a wave-like course of the process, which is confirmed by the monomorphism of purulent–necrotic foci and reflects the rapid development and spread of tuberculosis (the so-called acute progression) (Figs. 18.12 and 18.13). Signs of delimitation and organization of foci of tuberculous inflammation are not determined (Fig. 18.14). When stained according to Z-N, acid-resistant bacteria are usually found in large numbers, diffusely or in the form of small clusters, located mainly in necrotic masses (Fig. 18.15).

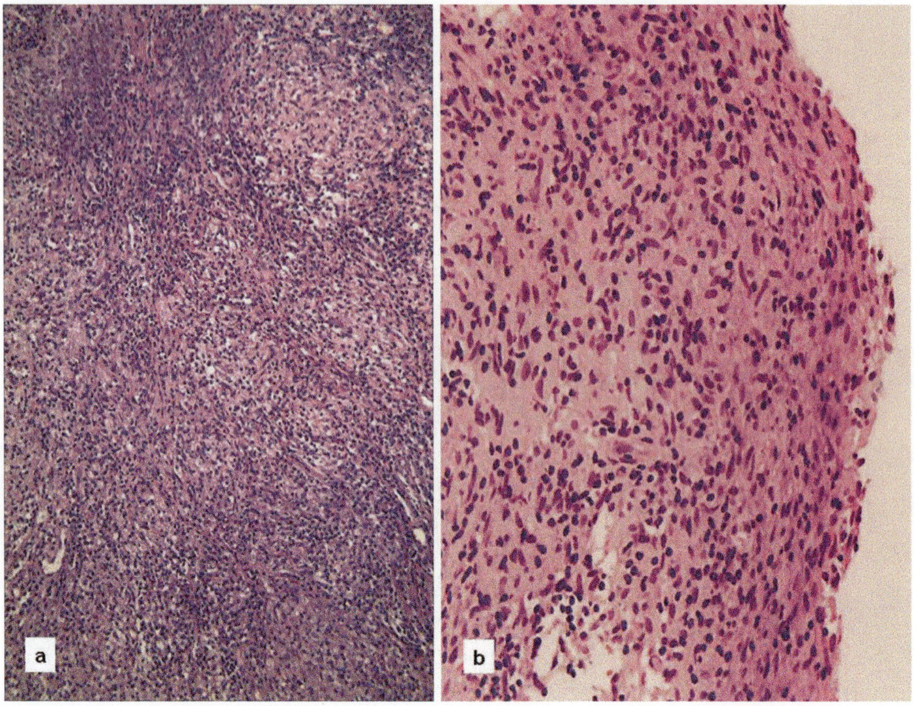

Fig. 18.10 HIV-associated tuberculosis. (**a**) Strands of epithelial cells that form very fuzzy small granuloma-like structures and (**b**) in the bronchial mucosa, fuzzy strands of epithelial cells without the formation of granulomas. Stained with hematoxylin and eosin. (**a**) ×100 and (**b**) ×200

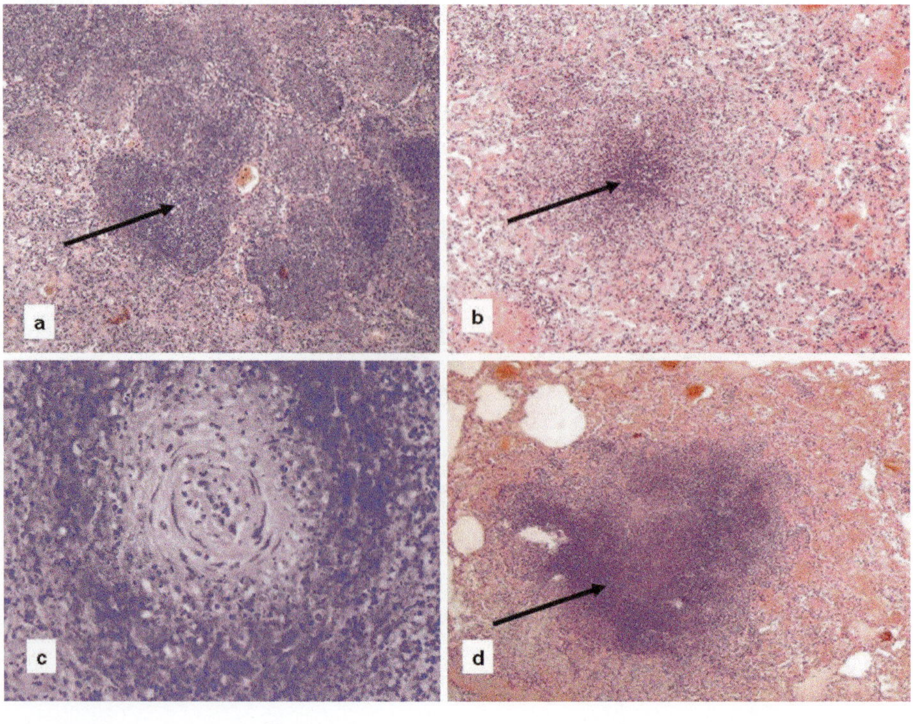

Fig. 18.11 HIV-associated tuberculosis. (**a–d**) Purulent–necrotic foci of tuberculosis inflammation (indicated by arrows), perifocal expressed exudative reaction. Stained with hematoxylin and eosin. (**a**) ×40; (**b, d**) ×100; (**c**) ×400

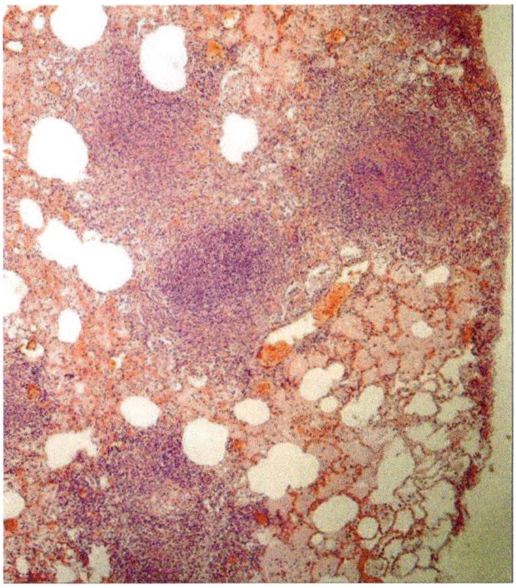

Fig. 18.12 Monomorphic purulent–necrotic foci in the lung in HIV-associated tuberculosis (for comparison, Fig. 18.13). Stained with hematoxylin and eosin. ×100

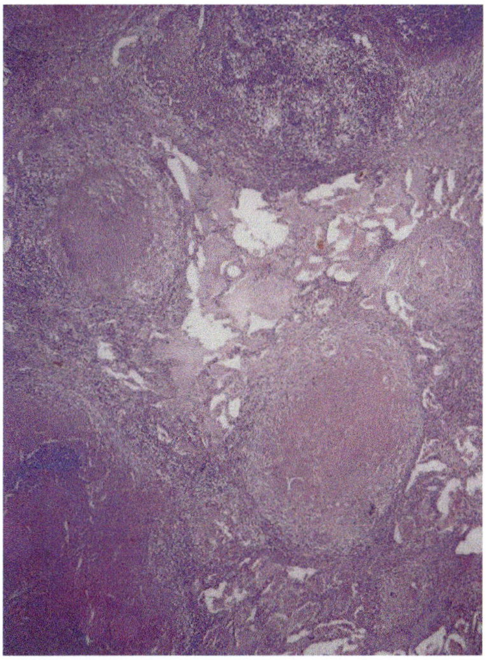

Fig. 18.13 Tuberculosis dissemination in the lung in tuberculosis without HIV infection, there are signs of a wave-like flow of the process, foci of tuberculosis dissemination of various stages. Stained with hematoxylin and eosin. ×100

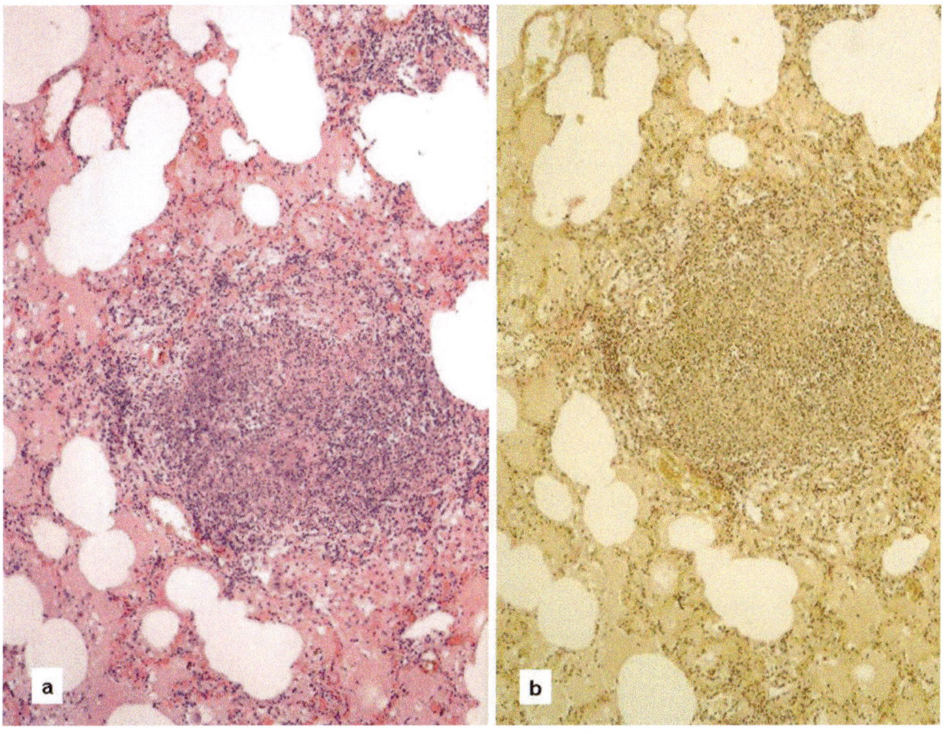

Fig. 18.14 HIV-associated tuberculosis. Absence of signs of organization of a tuberculous focus of inflammation. (**a**) Hematoxylin and eosin staining and (**b**) van Gieson staining. ×100

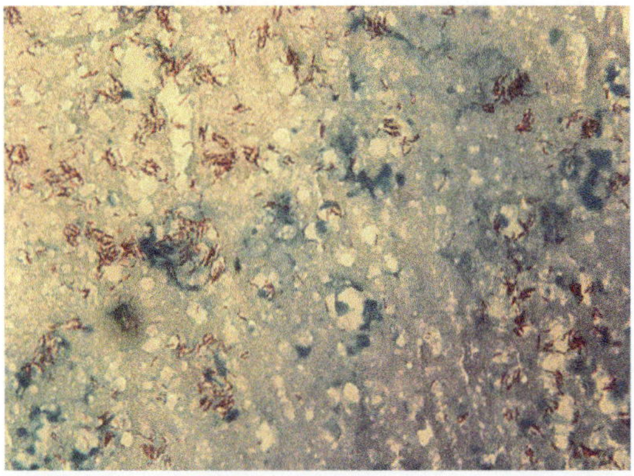

Fig. 18.15 HIV-associated tuberculosis. A large number of acid-resistant bacteria in the focus of tuberculosis inflammation. Stained by Ziehl–Nielsen. ×1000

Mycobacteria can also be detected by IHC studies with tuberculosis antibodies, however, in the later stages of HIV infection, the effectiveness of IHC studies and histological bacterioscopy according to Z-N is almost identical and reaches 80% and higher.

Morphological differential diagnosis is recommended to be carried out with pyemic foci in sepsis caused by pyogenic microbial flora, with bacterial pneumonia with areas of microabscesses, with mycotic lesion. Miliary necrotic lesions without granulomatous reaction are similar to lesions in pneumocystosis. In this situation, the pneumocystis etiology of the process can be confirmed using the PAS reaction, Grokkott staining, or an IHC reaction with antibodies to pneumocystis (Fig. 18.16).

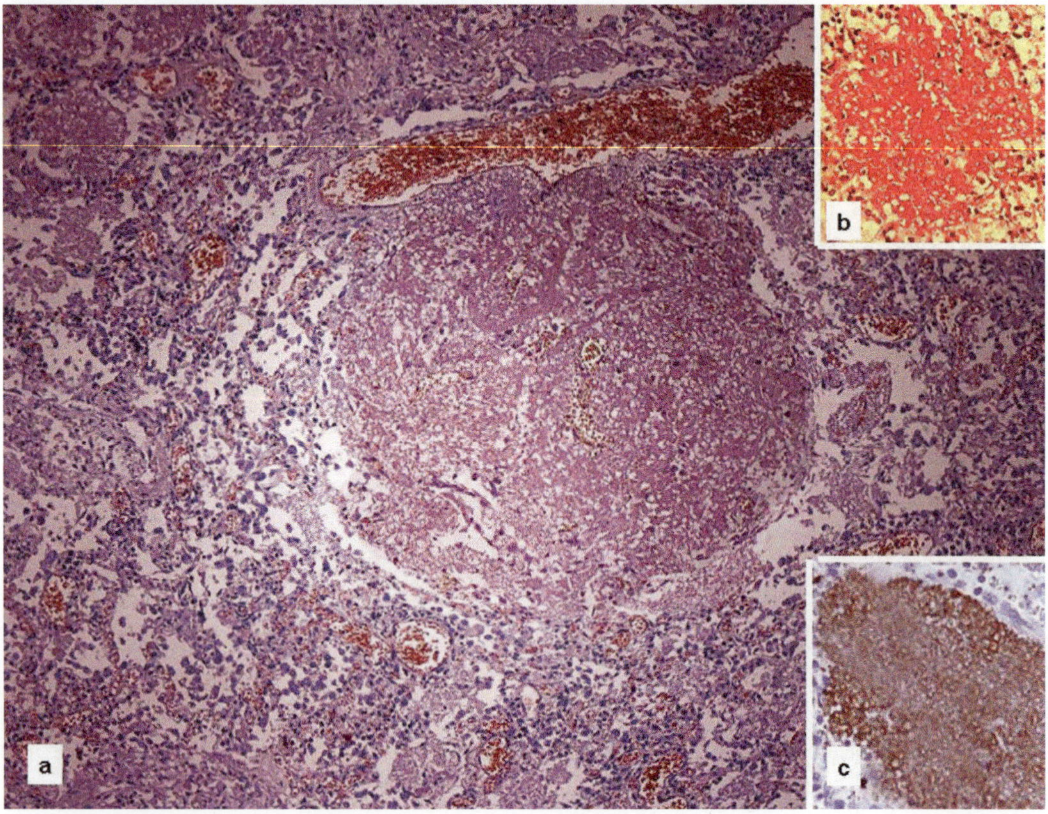

Fig. 18.16 Perivascular miliary lesion of pneumocystosis in the lung in HIV infection, similar to necrotic miliary lesion in tuberculosis. (**a**) Staining with hematoxylin and eosin; (**b**) PAS reaction; (**c**) IHC reaction with monoclonal anti-*Pneumocystis jiroveci* antibodies. (**a**) ×4; (**b**, **c**) ×400

18.3 Mycobacteriosis Caused by Nontuberculous Mycobacteria

The microscopic picture is similar to that of tuberculosis. Microscopically, the prevalence of the macrophage component of granulomatous inflammation is noted, including along the edge of the focus of necrosis and in the walls of the decay cavities, as well as the formation of macrophage–giant cell granulomas and granulomatous reactions according to the type of foreign bodies (Fig. 18.17).

The detection of acid-resistant bacteria with histological bacterioscopy according to Z-N or mycobacteria during IHC studies is provided as in tuberculosis.

Negative PCR test for Myc. tuberculosis DNA in the morphological picture of granulomatous necrotic inflammation and positive histobacterioscopy according to Z-N can be considered an indirect diagnostic sign of nontuberculous mycobacteriosis.

18.4 HIV-Associated Nontuberculous Mycobacteriosis *M. avium*, *M. avium* Intracellulare (*M. avium* Complex, MAC)

In the study of this form, granuloma-like clusters from monomorphic histiocyte-like cells with a light, fine-grained cytoplasm, with areas

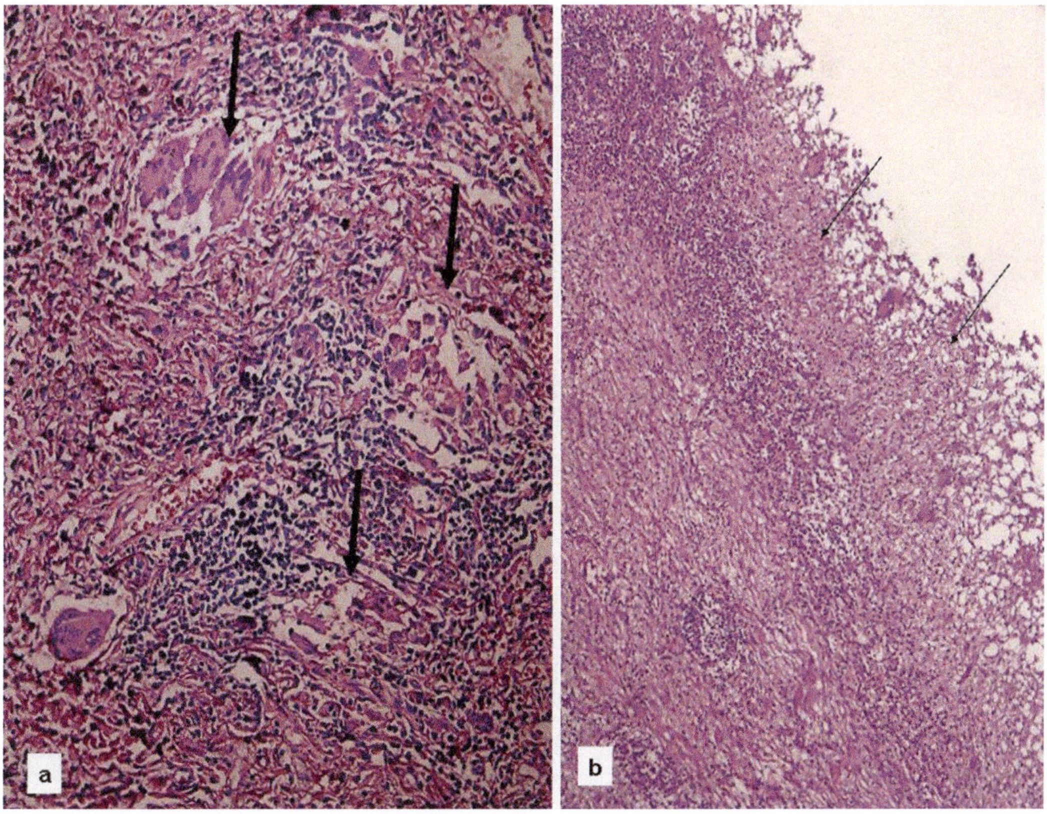

Fig. 18.17 Mycobacteriosis caused by non-tuberculosis mycobacteria. (**a**) The area of inflammation in tubercular pneumonia caused by *M. xenopii*; macrophage and giant cell granuloma (arrows); (**b**) chronic wall of the cavity of the lung in nontuberculous mycobacteriosis caused by *M. kansasii*; the inner layer of the cavity decay predominantly by macrophages (arrows), isolated giant cells type Langhans. Stained with hematoxylin and eosin. (**a**) ×200 and (**b**) ×100

of caseous necrosis erased by epithelioid or granulomatous reaction with small fuzzy macrophage–epithelioid granulomas were revealed (Fig. 18.18). There are macrophage granulomas without an epithelioid cell reaction, which can be mistaken for a site of a tumor of histiocytic origin, clear cell cancer, or for ordinary small macrophage infiltrate.

Acid-resistant bacteria were determined by Z-N stain. The causative agent is located in the cytoplasm of macrophages in huge amounts that could not be counted (Fig. 18.19). A similar pattern is observed with an IHC reaction with tuberculosis antibodies (Fig. 18.20). Species identification was carried out by PCR using Myc. avium DNA.

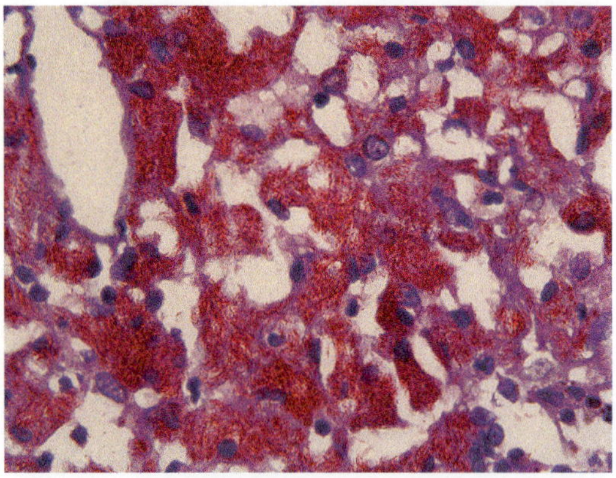

Fig. 18.19 HIV-associated mycobacteriosis caused by non-tuberculosis mycobacteria MAC. A large number of acid-resistant bacteria (incalculable) in the cytoplasm of macrophages. Stained by Ziejl–Nielsen. ×1000 (see also Fig. 13.86)

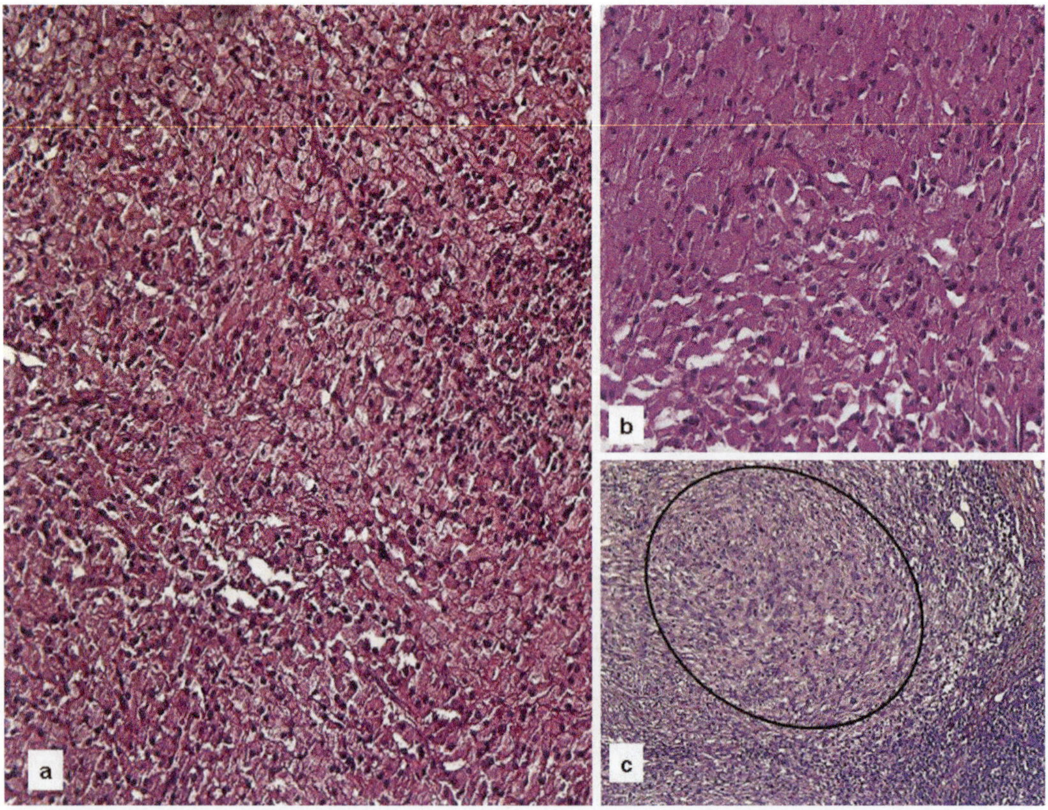

Fig. 18.18 HIV-associated mycobacteriosis caused by non-tuberculosis mycobacteria MAC. (**a**) The focus of inflammation is represented by monomorphic rounded or polygonal macrophages with a light fine-grained cytoplasm; (**b**) a fragment of the previous figure; (**c**) an indistinct macrophage–epithelial granuloma (indicated by a round frame). Stained with hematoxylin and eosin. (**a**, **c**) ×100; (**b**) ×200 (see also Fig. 13.85)

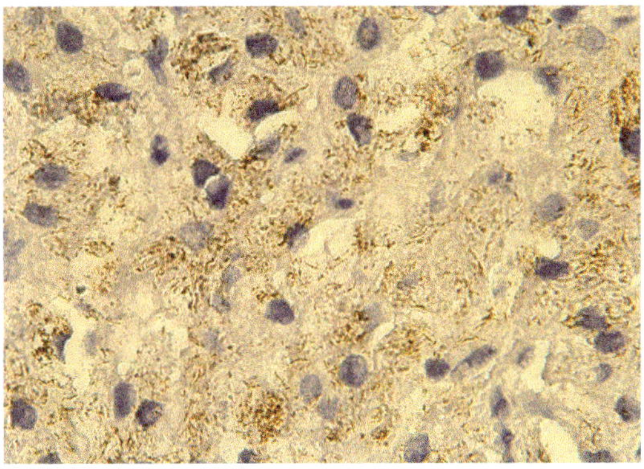

Fig. 18.20 HIV-associated mycobacteriosis caused by non-tuberculosis mycobacteria MAC. A large number of acid-resistant bacteria (incalculable) in the cytoplasm of macrophages. IHC reaction with *M. tuberculosis* mouse monoclonal antibody. ×1000 (see also Fig. 13.88)

18.5 Sarcoidosis—A Chronic Multisystem Disease Belonging to the Group of Granulomatous Diseases of an Unknown Nature

For sarcoidosis, monomorphic non-fusing (including closely spaced, but not fusing) "stamped" granulomas with annular fibrosis are typical (Fig. 18.21). Fibrosis along the edge of granulomas is well defined by any staining on the connective tissue elements (according to van Gieson, Masson, and Mallory) (Figs. 18.22 and 18.23). Granulomas are macrophage–epithelioid, macrophage–epithelioid–giant cells, without leukocytes and necrosis in the center of granulomas.

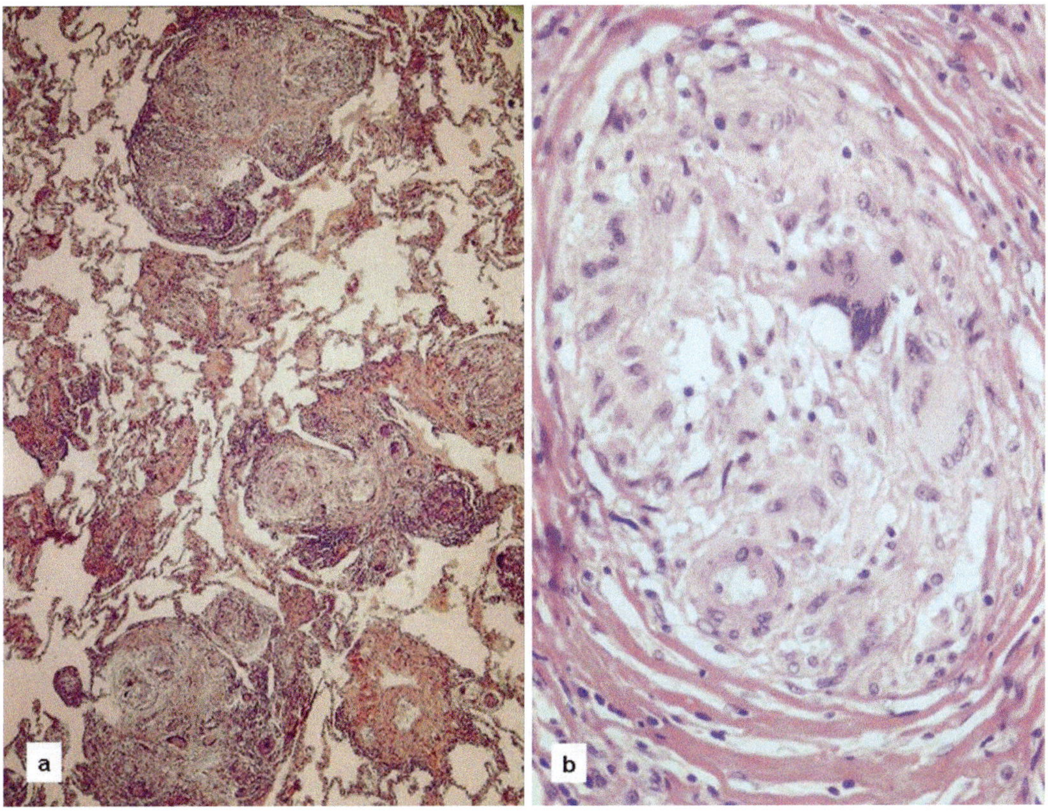

Fig. 18.21 Sarcoidosis. (**a**) Monomorphic, clearly defined, non-merging granulomas without necrosis and without white blood cells in the center and (**b**) granuloma with annular fibrosis ("stamped" granuloma). Stained with hematoxylin and eosin. (**a**) ×40 and (**b**) ×400

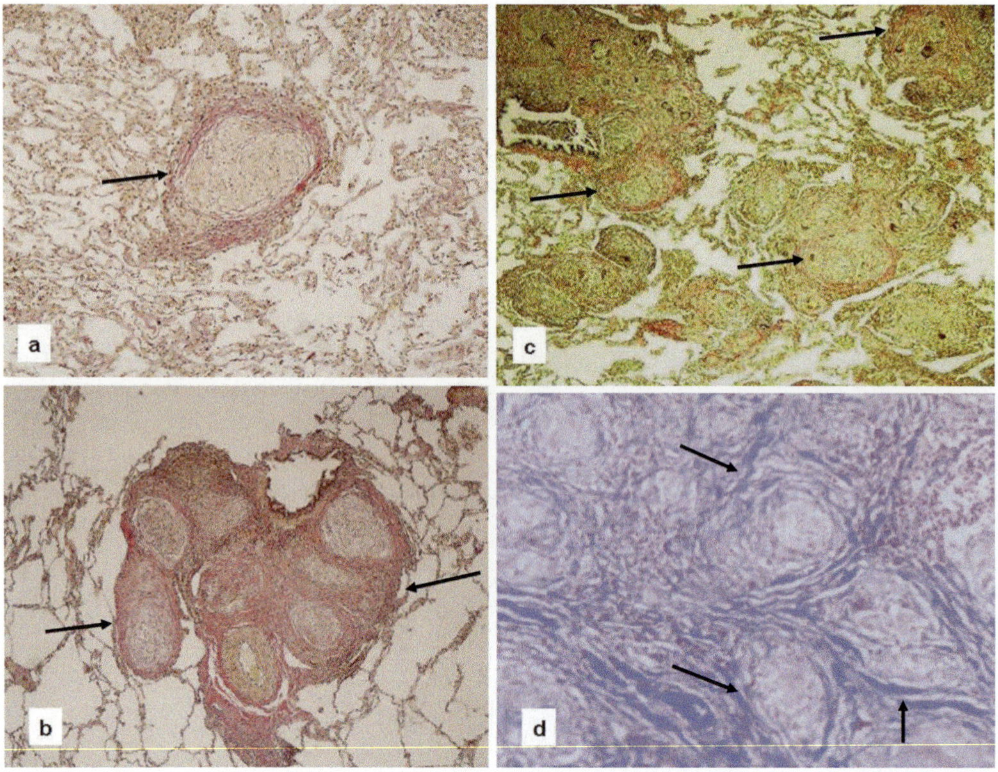

Fig. 18.22 Sarcoidosis of the lung. Monomorphic granulomas with annular fibrosis ("stamped" granulomas, indicated by arrows). (**a–c**) van Gieson stain; (**d**) Mallory stain. (**a**, **c**) ×40; (**b**) ×100; (**d**) ×200

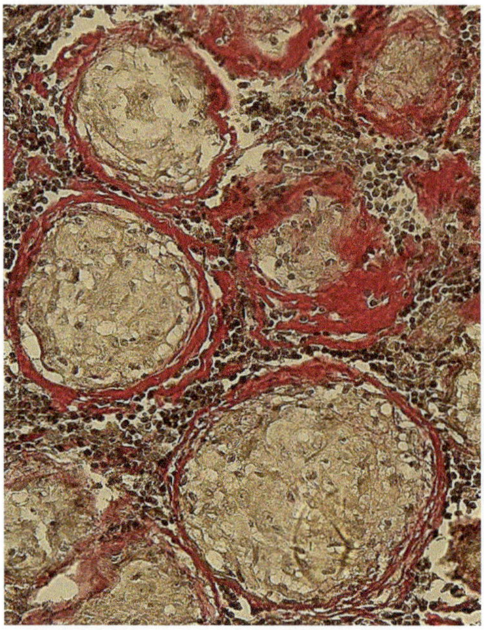

Fig. 18.23 Sarcoidosis of intrathoracic lymph nodes. "Stamped" granulomas with annular fibrosis. Color by van Gieson. ×200

Occasionally, with an acute onset of the disease, granulomas with a microfocus of fibrinoid necrosis in the center occur, which may be mistaken for tuberculous inflammation (Fig. 18.24). In single granulomas with sarcoidosis, small clusters of lymphoid cells can be found (Fig. 18.25), while with tuberculosis, neutrophilic leukocytes are usually detected in the center of the granulomas. These details need to be examined in detail at high magnification of the microscope. In giant multinucleated cells, in some cases, one can find small basophilic or weakly basophilic, often calcified, fuzzily layered structures—conchoidal bodies (Schaumann bodies or Schaumann inclusions) (Fig. 18.26). Lymphoid shaft along the periphery of the granuloma with sarcoidosis, in contrast to tuberculosis, is not expressed, the lymphoid reaction with sarcoidosis in areas of granulomatous inflammation may be minimal or absent.

The lung tissue in the perifocal areas is airy (Fig. 18.27), the alveolar septa are thin, without inflammatory infiltration, intact. Unlike tubercu-

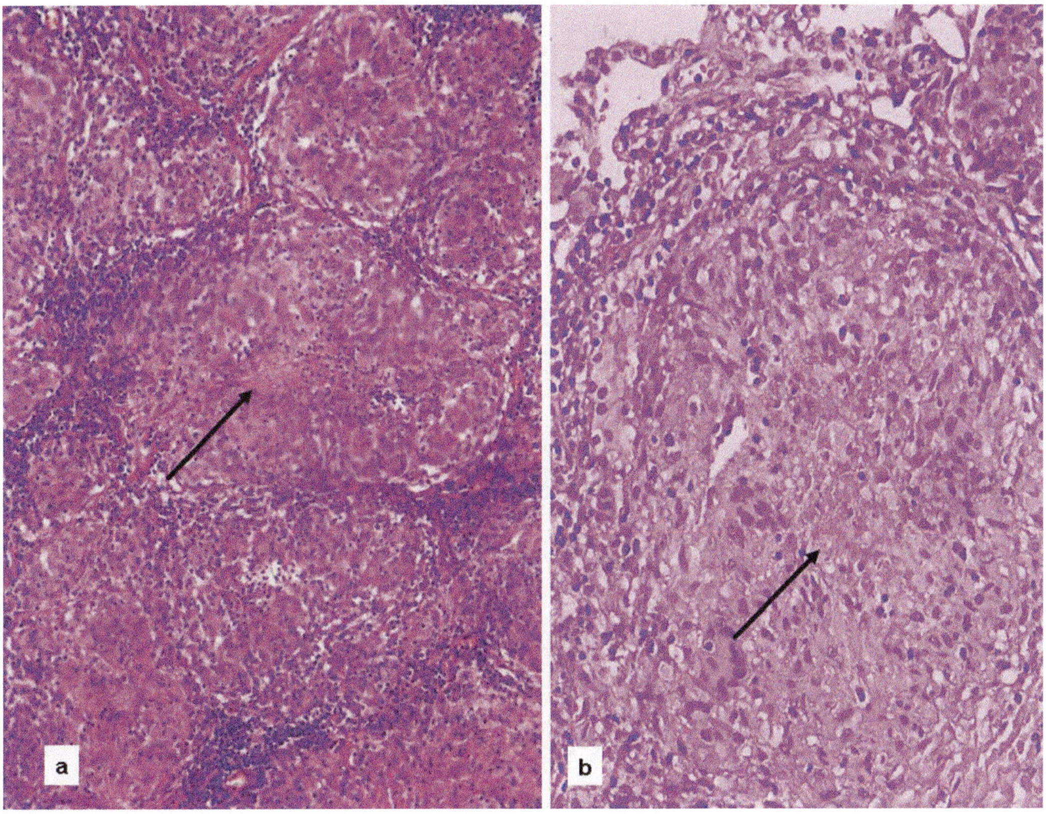

Fig. 18.24 Fibrinoid micronecrosis in the center of the granuloma in sarcoidosis (indicated by arrows). (**a**) Sarcoidosis of the lung; (**b**) sarcoidosis of the intrathoracic lymph node. Stained with hematoxylin and eosin. (**a**) ×200 and (**b**) ×100

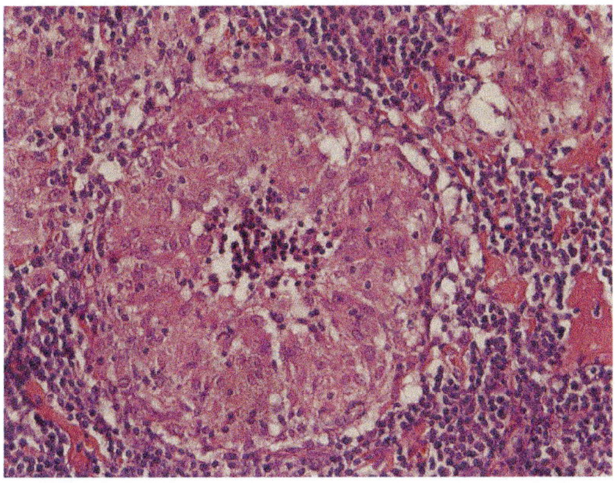

Fig. 18.25 Sarcoidosis. Lymphocytes in the center of the granuloma. Stained with hematoxylin and eosin. ×400

losis, the interlobular septa of the lung with sarcoidosis are thin, without fibrosis and inflammatory infiltration. In the foci of granulomatous inflammation, there are no reactive changes in the vessels or minimal, the endothelium is usually not changed. The narrowing of the lumen and obliteration of the vessel is not determined. When granulomas are located in the mucous membrane of the bronchi, the respiratory epithelium is intact (Fig. 18.28). When studying the lymph node affected by sarcoidosis, the fact that the capsule of the lymph node is thin, intact (Fig. 18.29) is noteworthy. This is one of the signs that can allow morphologically differentiating sarcoidosis and tuberculous lymphadenitis.

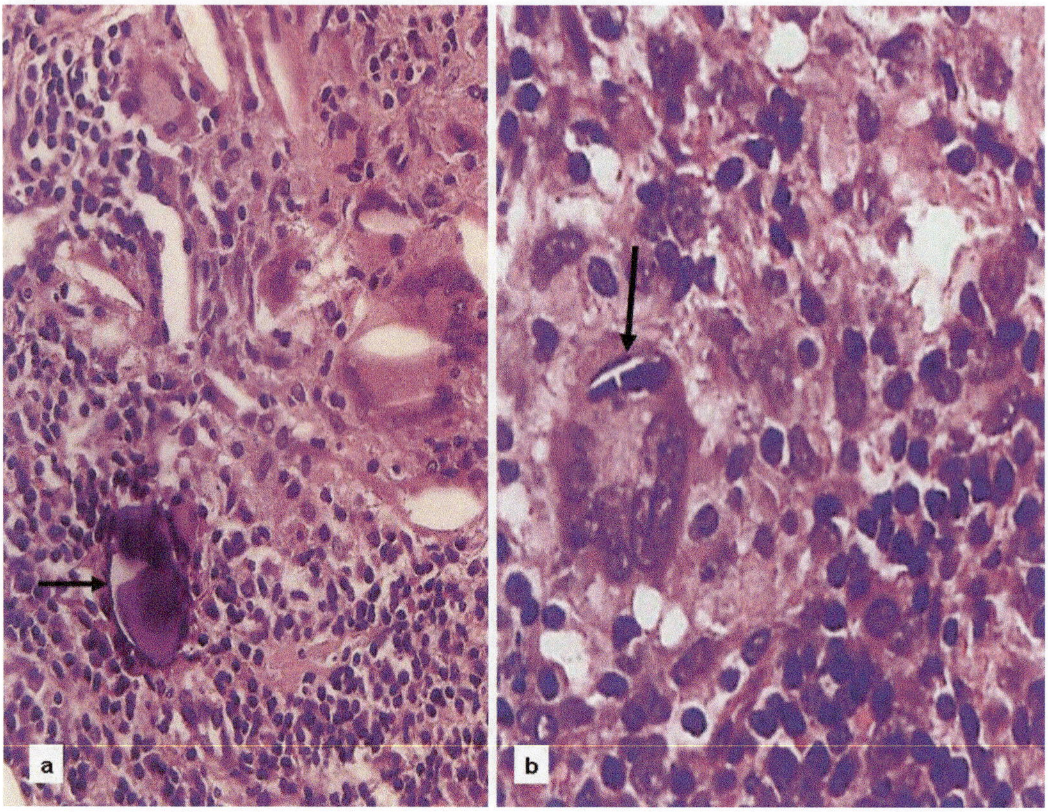

Fig. 18.26 Conchoidal corpuscles (Schaumann's corpuscles) in the granuloma (indicated by arrows). Stained with hematoxylin and eosin. ×400

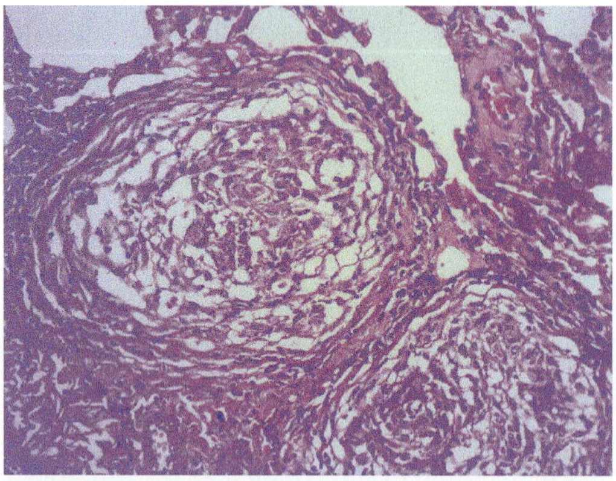

Fig. 18.27 Sarcoid granuloma, missing perifocal lymphoid shaft. Stained with hematoxylin and eosin. ×200

With tuberculosis, the capsule of the affected lymph node is thickened due to fibrosis.

With histological bacterioscopy according to Z-N, acid-resistant bacteria are absent (Fig. 18.30). The PAS reaction does not reveal fungal structures.

18.6 Necrotizing Sarcoid Granulomatosis (NSH)

This is a productive vasculitis of small arteries and veins with the formation of massive clusters of sarcoid-like granulomas, accompanied by ischemic necrosis of varying severity and prescription, the nature of which remains unclear.

In cases of necrotizing sarcoid granulomatosis in the lungs, the foci of hyalinized or organized fibrinoid necrosis with the outlines of collapsed and obliterated vessels, as well as the shadows of the "immured" monomorphic granules of the "stamped" type (Figs. 18.31 and 18.32) are determined. These changes are well defined with his-

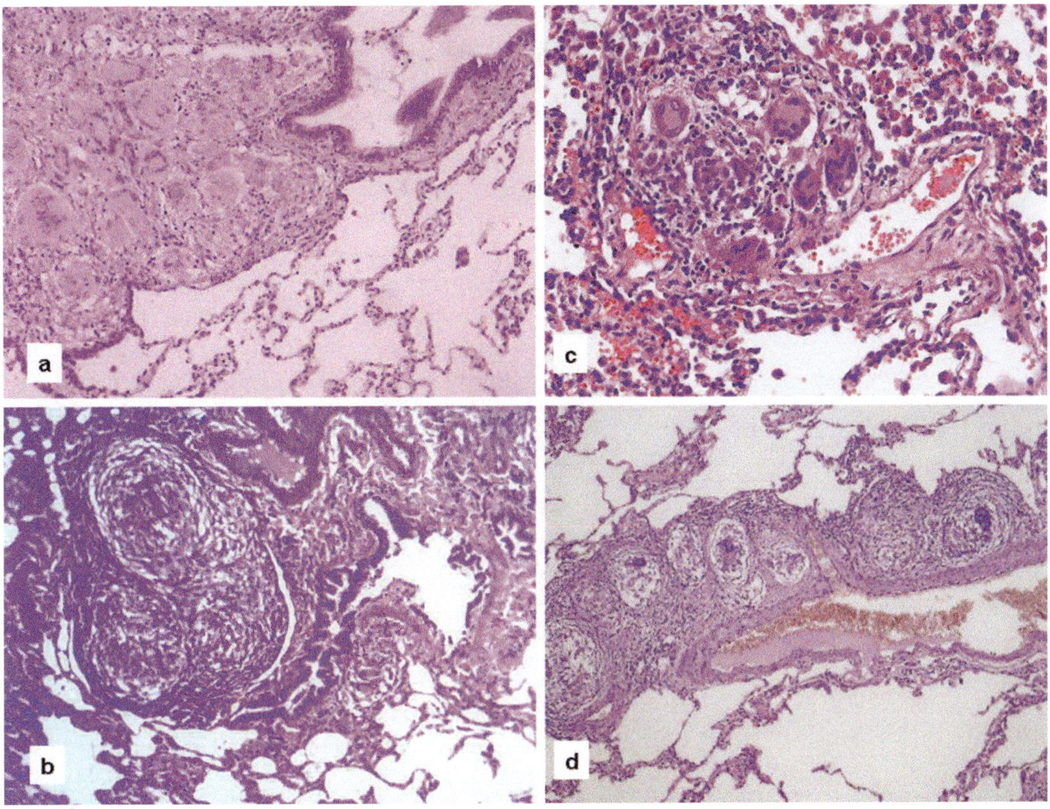

Fig. 18.28 Sarcoidosis of the lung. (**a**, **b**) Peribronchial granuloma, no lymphoid reaction around the granulomas and in the bronchial mucosa, intact respiratory epithelium; (**c**, **d**) perivascular granulomas, no lymphoid reaction in the vascular wall, endothelium intact. Stained with hematoxylin and eosin. (**a**, **c**) ×200; (**b**, **d**) ×100

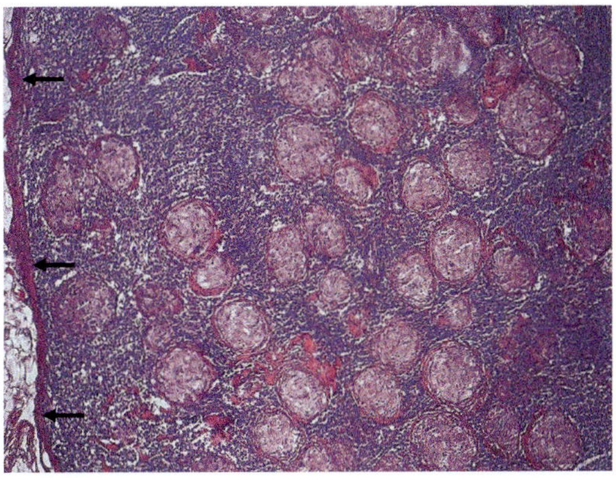

Fig. 18.29 Sarcoidosis of the lymph node. "Stamped" granulomas with annular fibrosis, a thin intact capsule of the lymph node (indicated by arrows). Stained with hematoxylin and eosin. ×100

tochemical stains on elastic and connective tissue. The contours of foci of hyalinosis are uneven due to the presence of multiple granulomas along the edge; there is no capsule of foci of hyalinosis (Fig. 18.33). Decay cavities may form in necrotic masses.

Along the periphery of hyalinosis there is a zone of granulomatous inflammation, represented by granulomas of a sarcoid type—small, monomorphic, mainly closely spaced, but not merging. Granulomas are macrophage–giant cells and epithelioid–macrophage–giant cells, without leukocytes and, for the most part, without necrosis in the center. In individual granulomas, the formation of a microsection of fibrinoid necrosis can be noted, and the reaction from

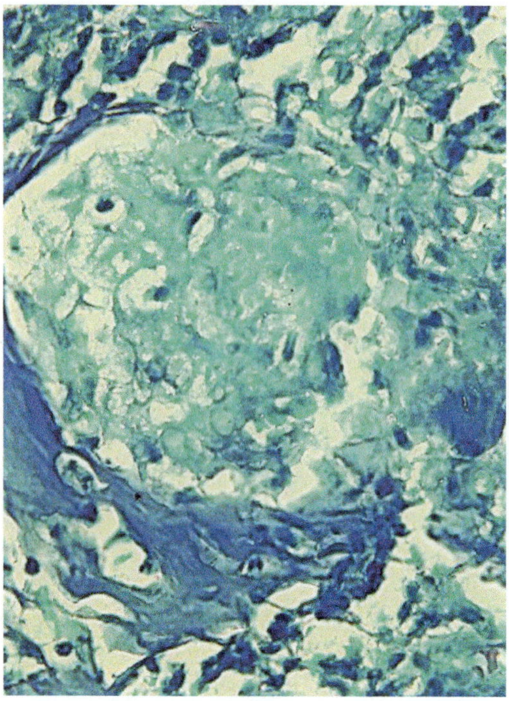

Fig. 18.30 Granuloma in sarcoidosis. Negative result of Ziehl–Nielsen histobacterioscopy, no acid-resistant bacteria. ×1000

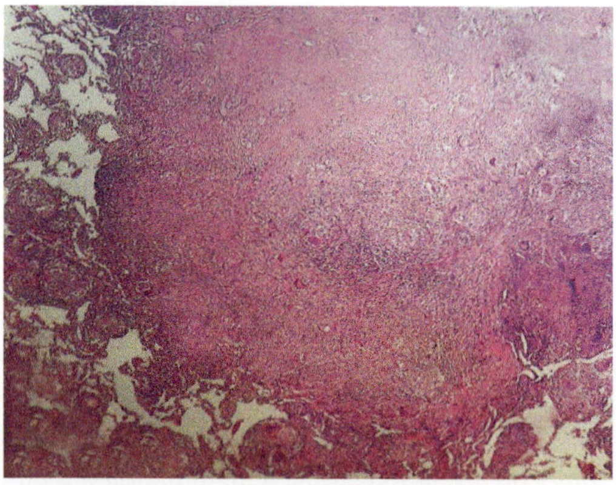

Fig. 18.31 Necrotizing sarcoid granulomatosis. Hyalinizing focus of necrosis in the lung, without signs of encapsulation, with granulomas on the periphery. Stained with hematoxylin and eosin. ×100

eosinophilic leukocytes is occasionally determined. Most granulomas are "stamped" in appearance due to annular fibrosis of varying severity (Figs. 18.34 and 18.35).

Near the areas of hyalinized necrosis, blood vessels with signs of granulomatous inflammation are detected. The most typical lesion of the small branches of the pulmonary artery is less likely to affect the veins (Fig. 18.36). Granulomas are usually localized in the middle layer of the vascular wall, deform ("stretch") the elastic framework or adventitia. In this case, narrowing of the lumen of the vessel or its partial or complete obliteration is observed (Fig. 18.37). Changes in the elastic framework are well defined by histochemical studies of elasticity (e.g., orcein) (Fig. 18.38). The elastic structures are well visualized when impregnated with silver according to Grokkott, although this technique is usually used to detect mycotic structures.

When in histobacterioscopy according to Z-N, acid-resistant bacteria are not detected, IHC studies of mycobacteria are also not determined. Perifocal lung tissue is airy, with thin intact interalveolar septa (Fig. 18.39). In a number of cases, changes in the microvasculature are revealed with alveolar–hemorrhagic phenomena in the form of plethora, diapedesis of erythrocytes, and hemorrhages.

Most often, necrotizing sarcoid granulomatosis must be differentiated from tuberculosis, sarcoidosis, and granulomatosis with polyangiitis (formerly Wegener's granulomatosis).

18.7 Hypersensitive Pneumonitis (Exogenous Allergic Alveolitis)

This is included in the group of diffuse parenchymal lung diseases with a known etiology and belongs to granulomatous diseases (noninfectious granulomas).

In hypersensitive pneumonitis, predominantly macrophage–giant cell granulomas merge with the predominance of multinucleated foreign body cells, as well as epithelioid–macrophage granulomas (Fig. 18.40). In the cytoplasm of giant multinucleated cells, conchoidal bodies are determined (small basophilic or weakly basophilic, often calcified, fuzzily layered structures—Schaumann

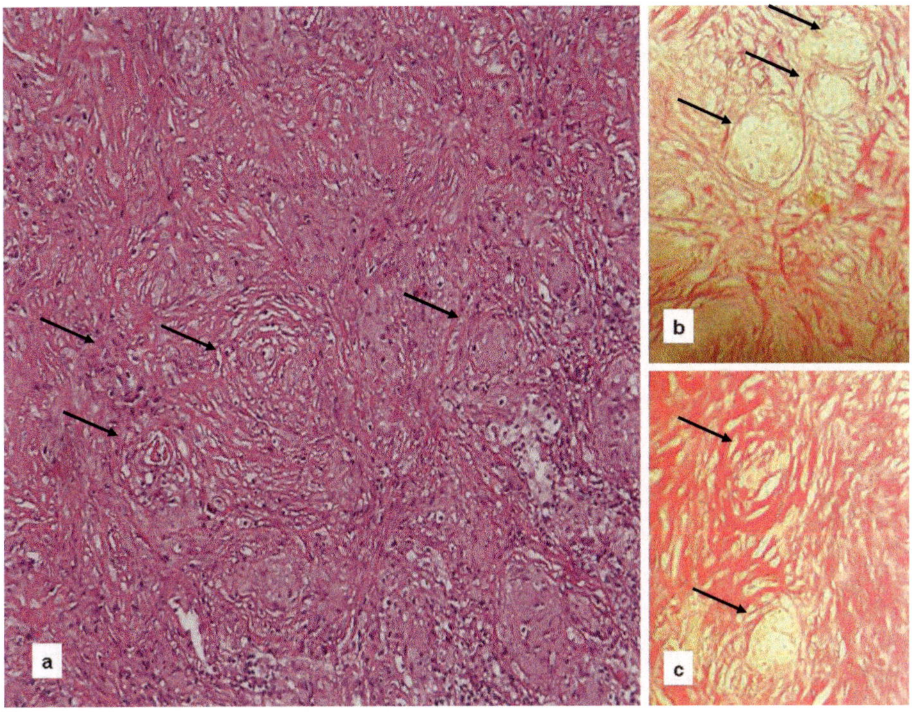

Fig. 18.32 Necrotizing sarcoid granulomatosis. Hyalinizing focus of necrosis in the lung, with the outlines (shadows) of granulomas (indicated by arrows). (**a**) Hematoxylin and eosin staining; (**b**, **c**) Van Gieson staining. ×200

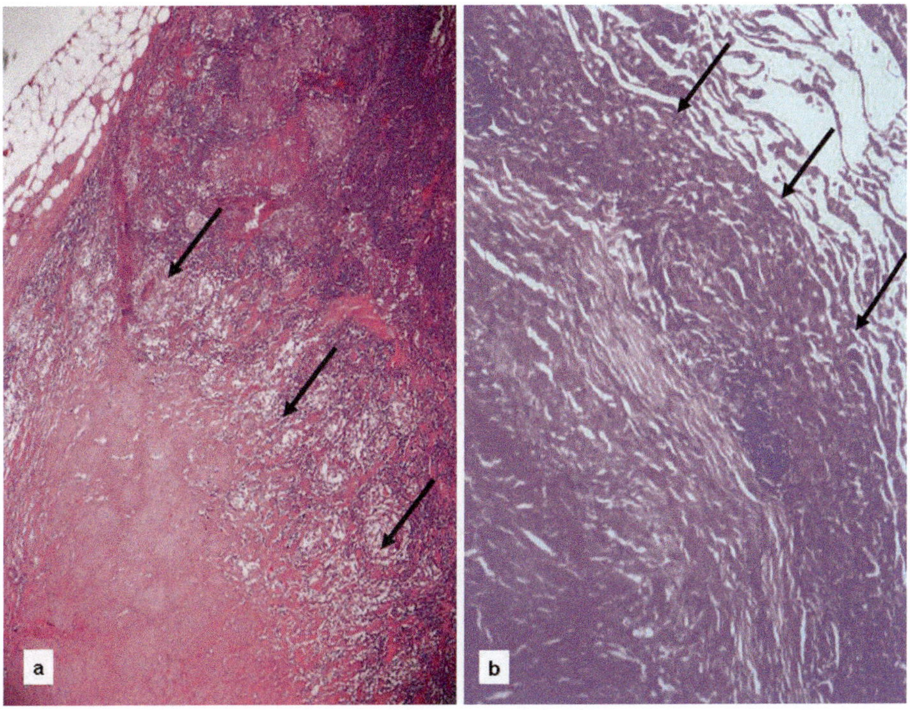

Fig. 18.33 (**a**) Necrotizing sarcoid granulomatosis. Absence of the focus capsule, along the edge of the hyalinizing necrosis focus granulomatous inflammation (indicated by arrows); (**b**) Focal tuberculosis (for comparison)—encapsulated focus of caseous necrosis (capsule indicated by arrows). Stained with hematoxylin and eosin. ×100

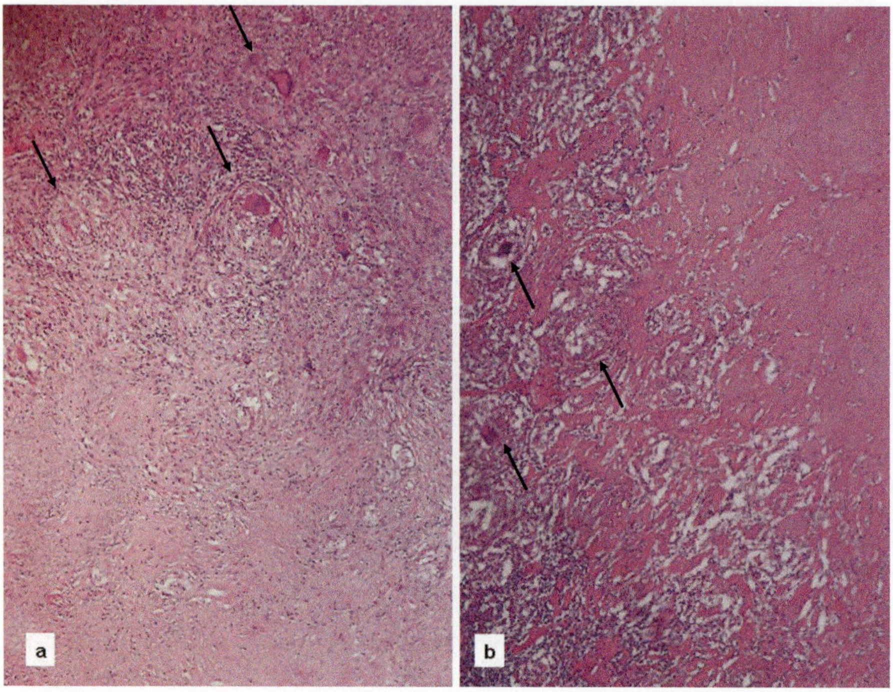

Fig. 18.34 Necrotizing sarcoid granulomatosis. Absence of a capsule of the focus, along the edge of the hyalinizing focus of necrosis granulomatous inflammation (individual granulomas are indicated by arrows). Staining with hematoxylin and eosin; (**a**) ×100 and (**b**) ×200

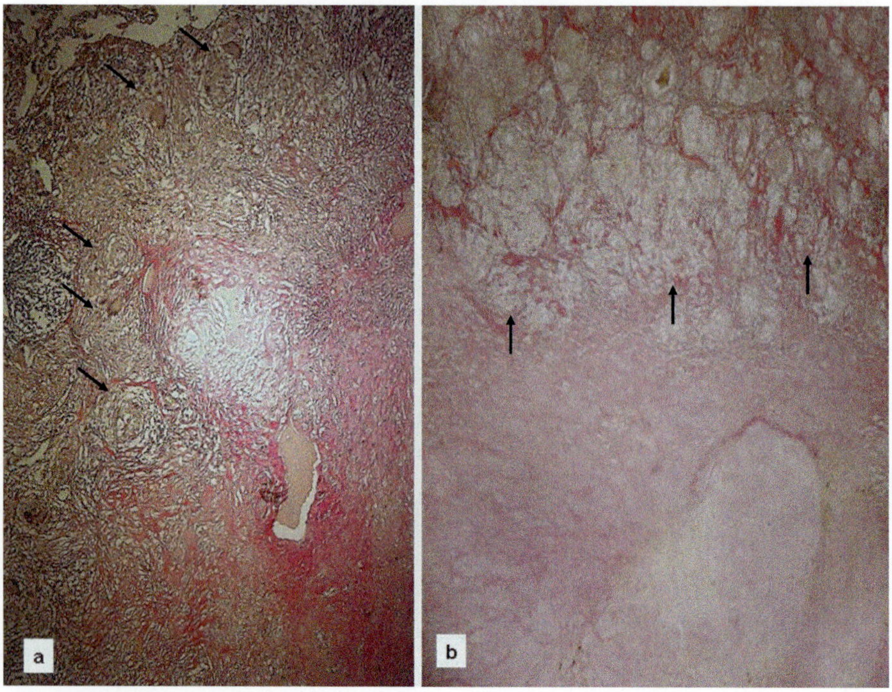

Fig. 18.35 Necrotizing sarcoid granulomatosis. Absence of a capsule of the focus, along the edge of the hyalinizing focus of necrosis granulomatous inflammation (individual granulomas are indicated by arrows). Staining by Van Gieson. ×100

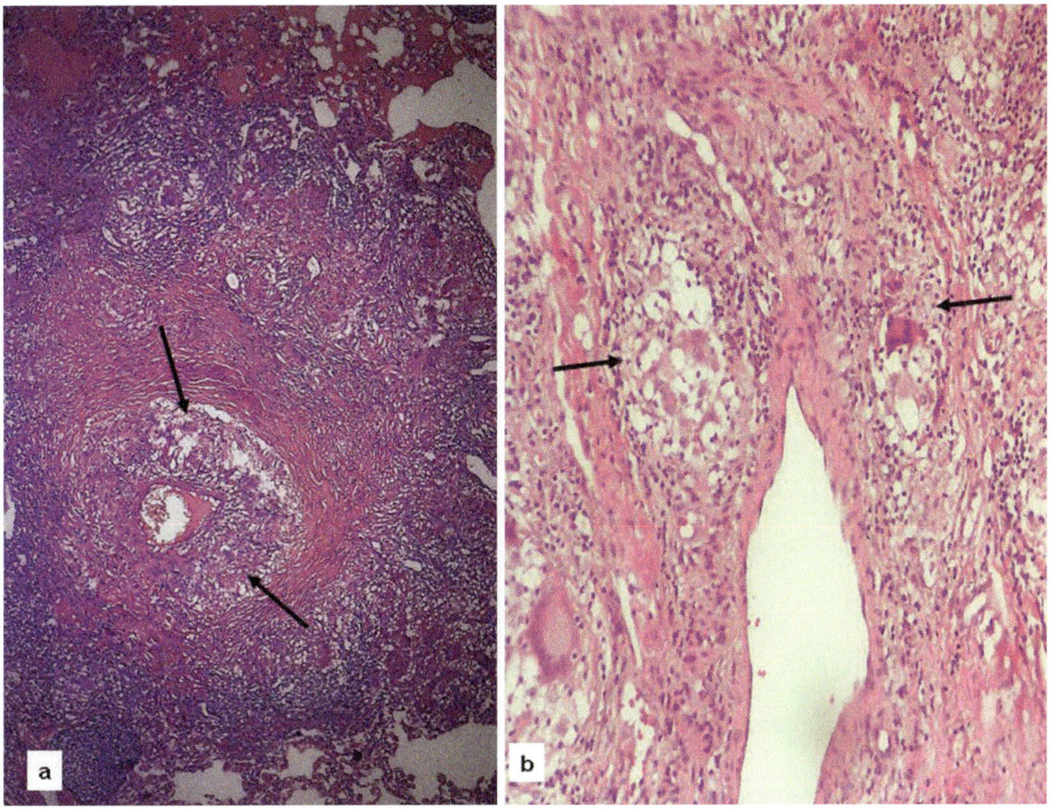

Fig. 18.36 Necrotizing sarcoid granulomatosis. Granulomatous vasculitis, the vessel wall is sharply thickened (granulomas in the vessel wall are indicated by arrows). Stained with hematoxylin and eosin. (**a**) ×100 and (**b**) ×200

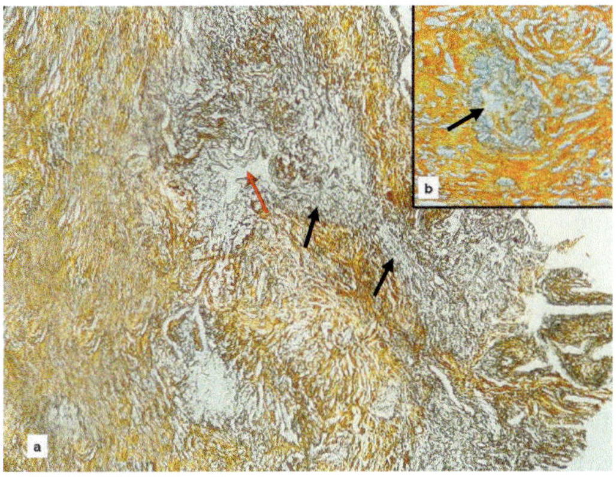

Fig. 18.37 Necrotizing sarcoid granulomatosis. Obliterated vessels in the area of hyalinizing necrosis (the preserved lumen of the vessel is indicated by a red arrow, obliterated areas are indicated by black arrows). Silver impregnation. (**a**) ×100 and (**b**) ×200

bodies or Schaumann inclusions), asteroid bodies, cholesterol crystals (Figs. 18.41 and 18.42). Exudative changes with edema and plasma impregnation of the vascular walls develop perifocal; there are clusters of siderophages in the lumen of the alveoli, serous exudate with an abundance of eosinophilic leukocytes, eosinophilic leukocytes in the lumen of blood vessels (Fig. 18.43). The alveolar septa are thickened due to significant edema, plethora of capillaries, polymorphic cell infiltration with a large number of eosinophilic leukocytes (Fig. 18.44). The result of hypersensitive pneumonitis may be the formation of a "netlike" lung, while granulomas are not always microscopically determined (Fig. 18.45).

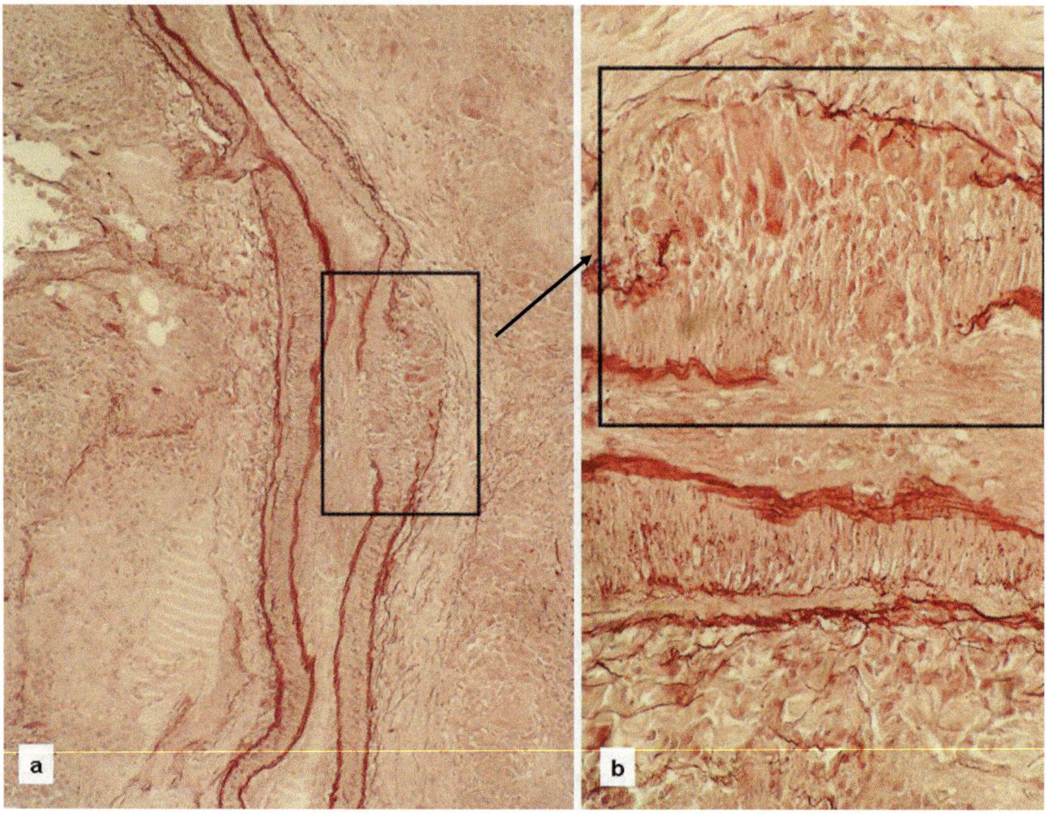

Fig. 18.38 Necrotizing sarcoid granulomatosis. Granulomatous vasculitis. Violation of the integrity of elastic fibers of the vascular wall in the area of granulomatous vasculitis (the area is framed). Stained by orsein. (**a**) ×100 and (**b**) ×400 (fragment of Fig. "**a**")

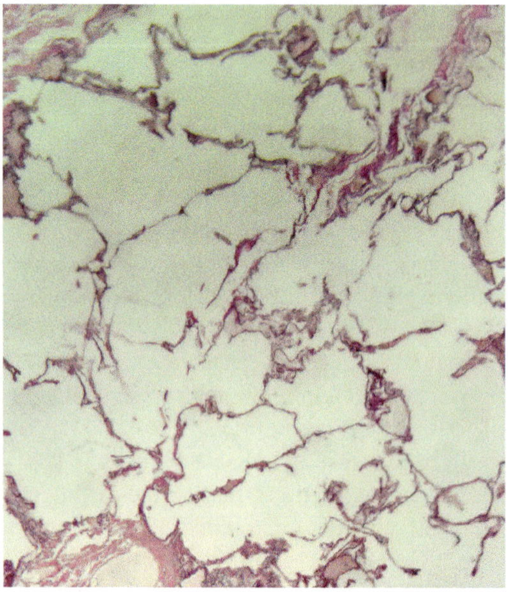

Fig. 18.39 Necrotizing sarcoid granulomatosis. Air intact lung tissue with thin interalveolar partitions outside the lesions. Stained by Van Gieson–Weigert. ×100

18.8 Mycotic Lesions

In many observations, clinicians and pathologists do not possess the data of mycological studies, which does not allow us to accurately determine the type of pathogen, which forces us to expound on these lesions in total. With fungal lesions, the formation of macrophage–epithelioid–giant cell granulomas with an abundance of giant cells of foreign bodies (Fig. 18.46) is noted. There are foci of necrosis with severe infiltration of necrotic masses by eosinophilic leukocytes, sometimes with the development of areas of abscess formation.

In the peripheral areas, reactive productive vasculitis develops. In addition, with an invasive mycotic process, a fungal vascular lesion develops with an invasion of the vascular wall by fungal mycelium—mycotic vasculitis, mycotic thrombovasculitis (Figs. 18.47, 18.48, and 18.49).

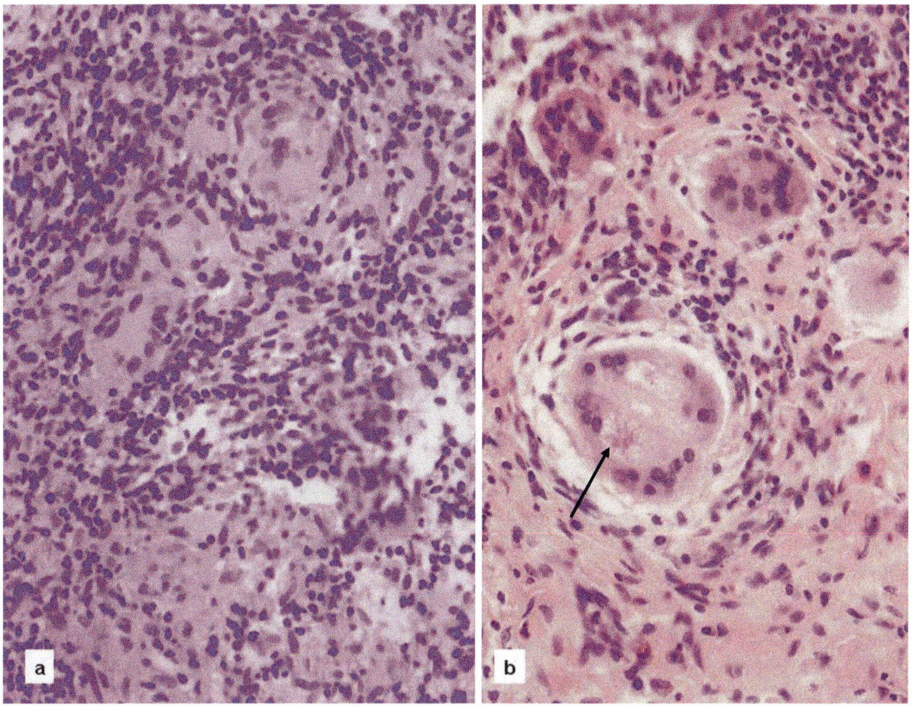

Fig. 18.40 Hypersensitive pneumonitis (exogenous allergic alveolitis). (**a**) Macrophage–epithelioid–gigantocellular granuloma; (**b**) macrophage–gigantocellular granuloma (the arrow indicates the asteroid body). Granulomas contain a large number of giant multinucleated cells. Stained with hematoxylin and eosin. ×400

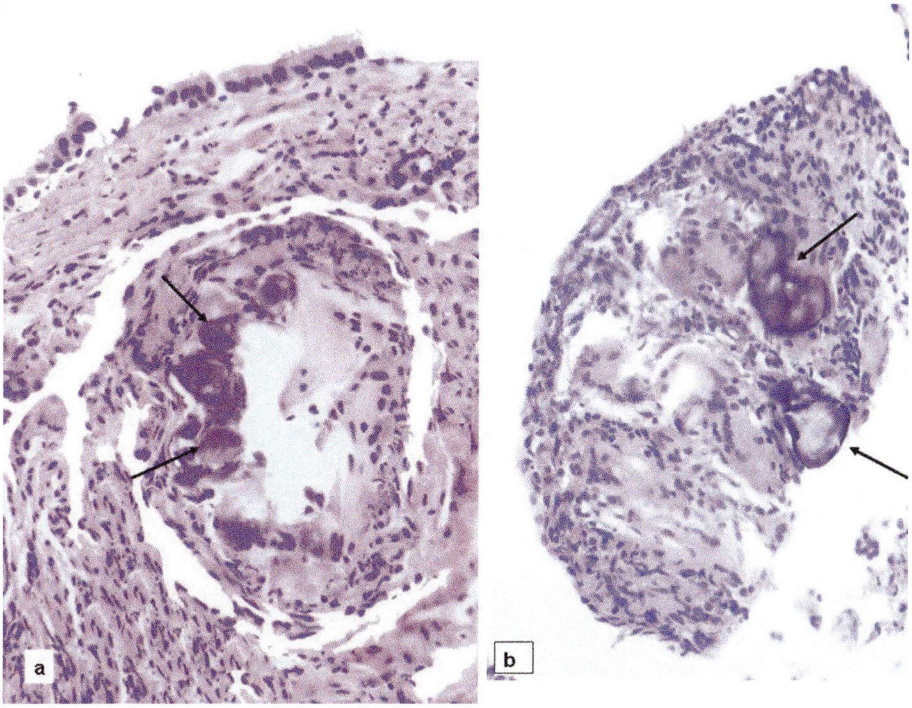

Fig. 18.41 Hypersensitive pneumonitis (exogenous allergic alveolitis). Conchoidal corpuscles (Schaumann corpuscles), indicated by arrows. Stained with hematoxylin and eosin. ×400

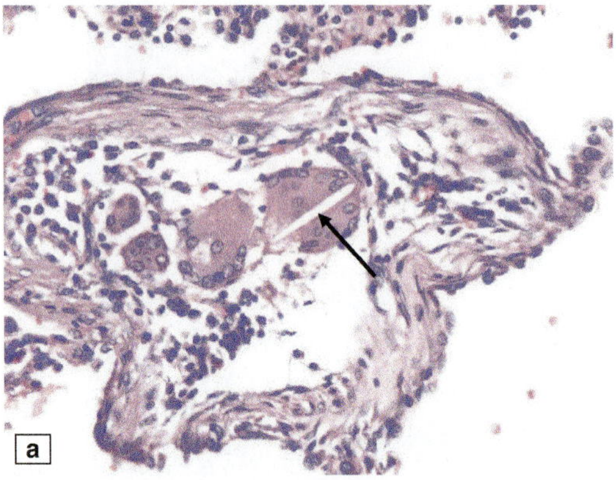

Fig. 18.42 Hypersensitive pneumonitis (exogenous allergic alveolitis). Cholesterol crystal indicated by an arrow. Stained with hematoxylin and eosin. ×400

In the adjacent lung tissue with active mycotic inflammation, an exudative perifocal reaction is noted with the presence in the exudate of disseminated multinucleated macrophages and eosinophilic leukocytes. With the development of mycotic pneumonia, the granulomatous component is not always determined. In the lumen of the alveoli, fibrinous–purulent exudate with an abundance of eosinophilic leukocytes and a pronounced hemorrhagic component in the form of hemolyzed and non-hemolyzed red blood cells is detected, scattered giant multinucleated cells, erased fuzzy granulomas, and fungal structures can be found.

The structures of the fungus can be determined by observing microscopy stained with

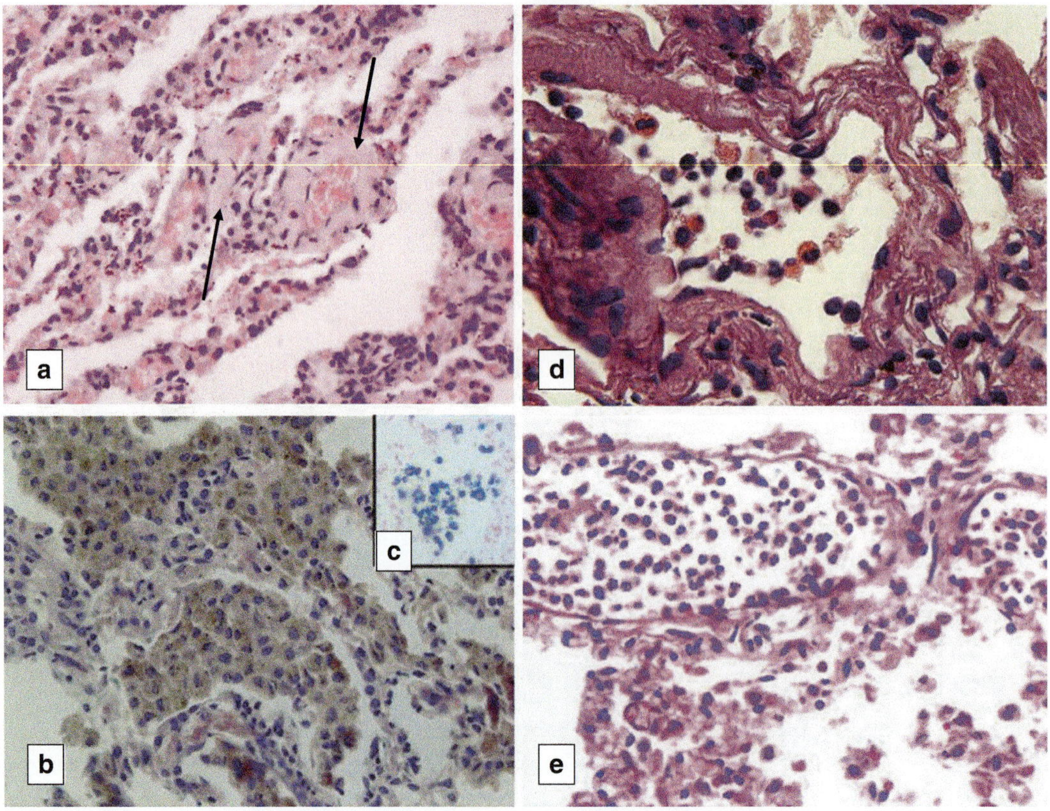

Fig. 18.43 Hypersensitive pneumonitis (exogenous allergic alveolitis). Exudative changes in the lung tissue. (**a**) Signs of increased vascular permeability, plasma impregnation of the vessel walls (indicated by arrows); (**b**, **c**) siderophages in the lumen of the alveoli; (**d**, **e**) eosinophilic leukocytes in the lumen of the vessels. (**a**, **b**, **d**, **e**) Hematoxylin and eosin staining; (**c**) Prussian blue reaction. (**a**, **b**) ×400; (**c**, **e**) ×200; (**d**) ×1000

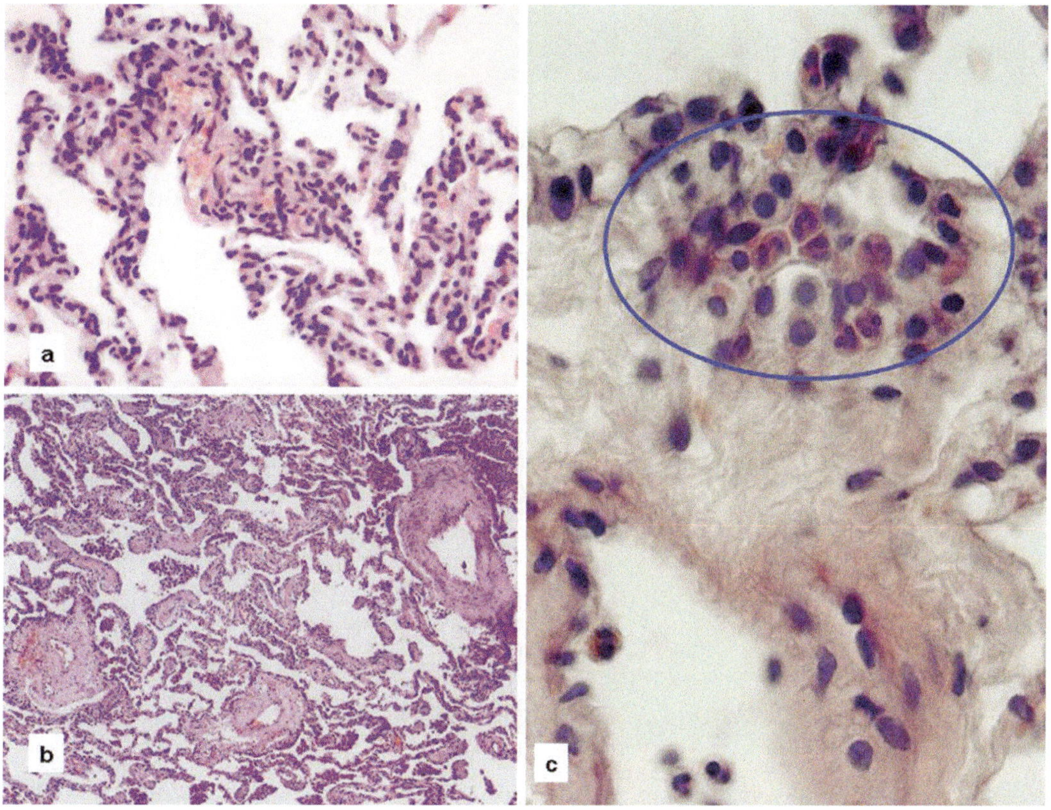

Fig. 18.44 Hypersensitive pneumonitis (exogenous allergic alveolitis). Exudative changes in the lung tissue. (**a**, **b**) Interalveolar septa are thickened due to edema and cellular infiltration; (**c**) eosinophilic infiltration of the interalveolar septa (circled with a round frame). Stained with hematoxylin and eosin. (**a**) ×200, (**b**) ×100, (c) ×1000

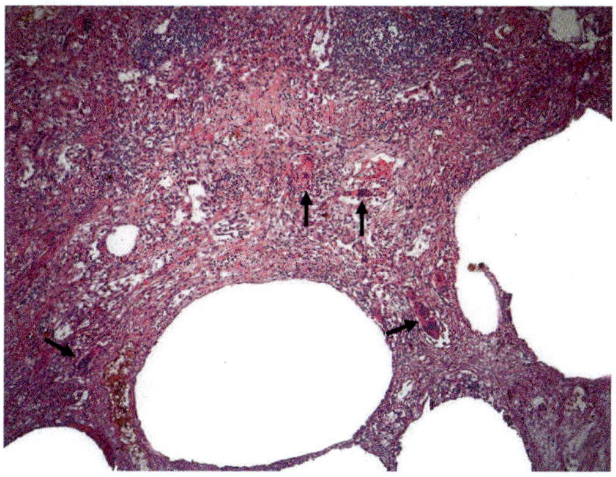

Fig. 18.45 "Cellular" light, single small fuzzy granulomas (indicated by arrows). Stained with hematoxylin and eosin. ×200

H-E, especially with chromomycosis. When histobacterioscopic (histomycoscopic) examination, the structure of the fungus is usually well visualized. These can be elements of mycelium, pseudomycelium, conidia, budding forms, and others. They are detected in necrotic masses, in the walls of blood vessels, in thrombotic masses, in the cytoplasm of giant cells of foreign bodies—Candida, Aspergillum, Mucor, Histoplasma, Blastomycetes, Cryptococci, etc.). The most commonly used is the PAS reaction, in which the glycoproteins of the shell of the fungal structures are stained reddish crimson (Fig. 18.50). However, it must be remembered that approximately 15% of the fungi are PAS-

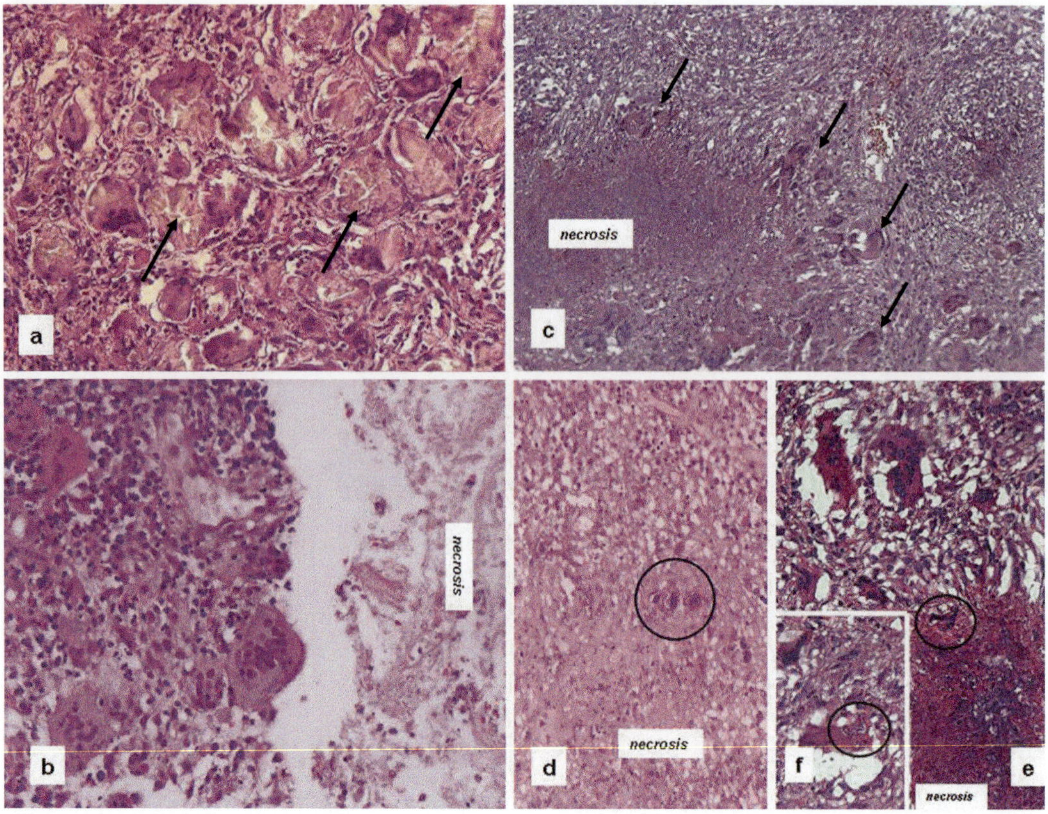

Fig. 18.46 Granulomas in mycoses. (**a**) Giant cell granuloma around structures in aspergillosis (indicated by arrows); (**b**) macrophages–giant cell granuloma at mycosis; (**c**) granulomatous–necrotic inflammation when fungal growth on the edge of severe necrosis giant cell reaction (arrows); (**d**) the site of inflammation in histoplasmosis (Histoplasma circled round frame); (**e**) granulomatous–necrotic inflammation in lesion due to Mucor, giant cell reaction at the edge of the necrotic center, necrotic masses mushroom of Mucor type (circled with a round frame); (**f**) a giant cell of the type of foreign bodies with phagocytosis of a fungus of the type of Mucor. Staining with hematoxylin and eosin. (**a**, **b**, **d**, **e**) ×400; (**c**) ×100; (**f**) ×1000. (See also Figs. 14.2–14.4)

negative. In this regard, the application of silver staining according to Grokkott (Gomori–Grokkott), in which the structure of the fungus is painted black (Fig. 18.51), is relevant. A combination of PAS stain with alcian blue is also used, which allows better identification of Cryptococci (Fig. 18.52). One can also use Gram stain or its modified versions—according to Gram-Weigert, according to Brown–Hopps, in which it is possible to verify gram-positive and gram-negative structures of the fungus that change their properties over time (Fig. 18.53). Z-N staining allows in most of the cases to define fungi, stained dark blue, and quite clearly visible against a pale blue background (Fig. 18.54).

Most often it is necessary to conduct a morphological differential diagnosis between the mycotic and mycobacterial (tuberculosis, nontuberculous mycobacteriosis) process.

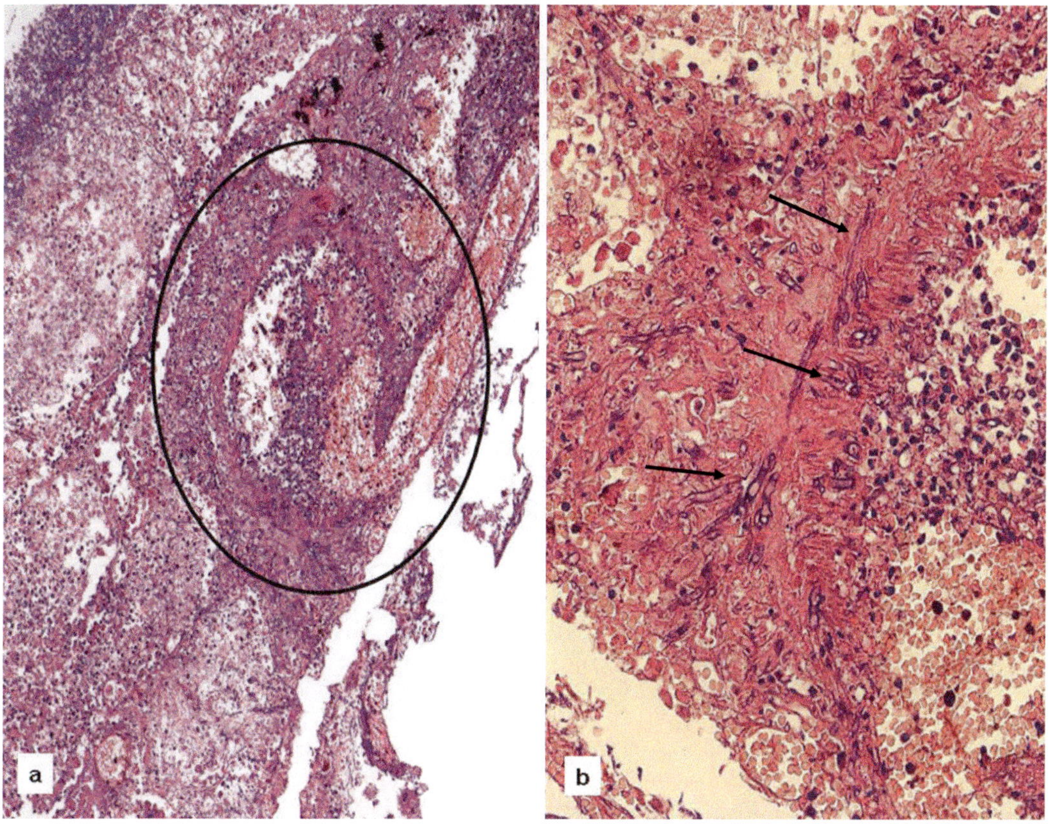

Fig. 18.47 Thrombovascular mycotic lung. (**a**) Blood vessel with signs of thrombovascular (circled in a round frame) in the focus of mycotic lesions; (**b**) the mycotic thrombovascular, mycotic invasion of the vascular wall (separate structures of the fungus in the vascular wall is indicated by the arrows). Stained with hematoxylin and eosin. (**a**) ×200 and (**b**) ×1000

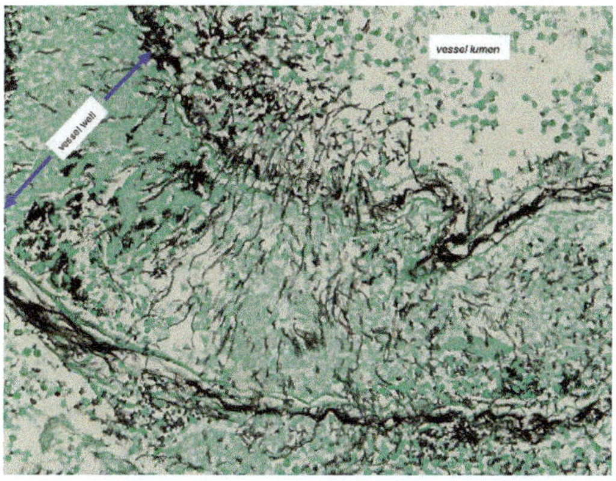

Fig. 18.48 Mycotic vasculitis, invasion of the fungus into the vessel wall (mycelium of the fungus is black). Grocott coloring. ×1000

18.9 Actinomycosis

Actinomycetes are an extensive taxonomic group of gram-positive microorganisms capable of forming branching filaments resembling mushroom mycelium at certain stages of development, which allowed them to be assigned to the mushroom kingdom earlier. In modern microbiology, actinomycetes are considered as actinobacteria. Actinomycosis is characterized by the development of granulomatous inflammation (infectious granulomas).

Actinomycotic foci can have the most diverse appearance—from miliary, to larger formations and abscesses.

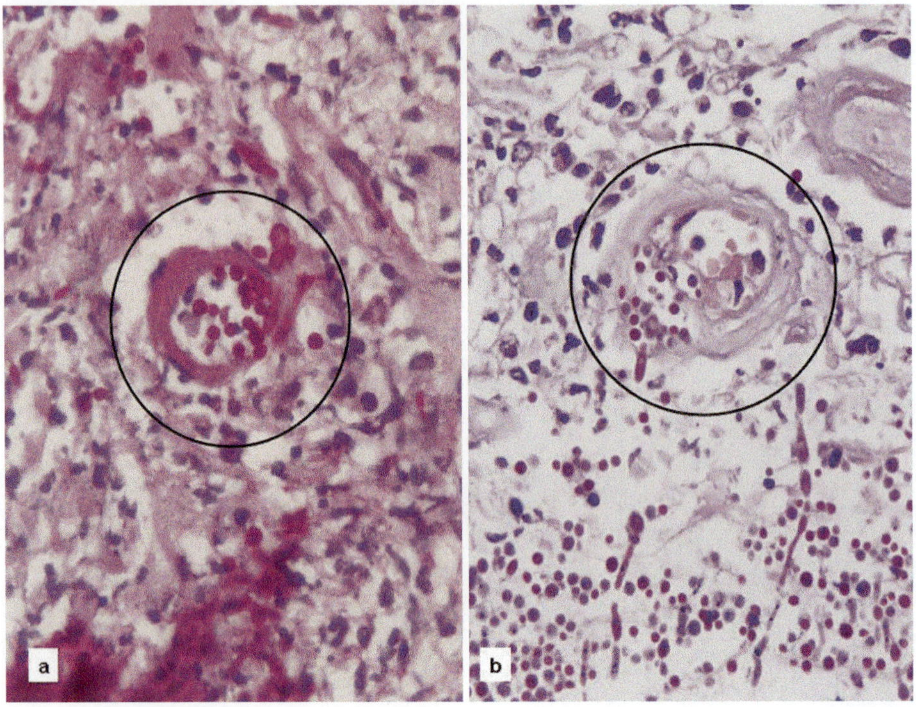

Fig. 18.49 Mycotic vasculitis, fungal invasion into the vessel wall (the vessel with infestations is surrounded by a round frame; the mycelium of the fungus is crimson red). PAS reaction ×1000

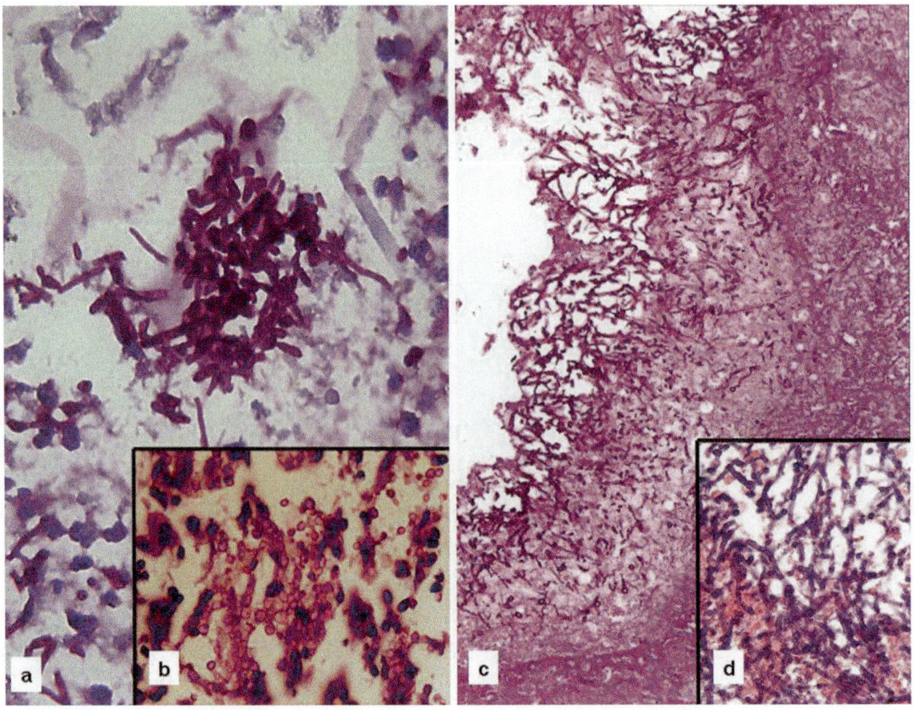

Fig. 18.50 Fungi. (**a–c**) PAS reaction, fungal structures are colored crimson red, (**b**) round-shaped cryptococci; (**d**) hematoxylin and eosin staining (for comparison). (**a**, **b**, **d**) ×1000 and (**c**) ×200

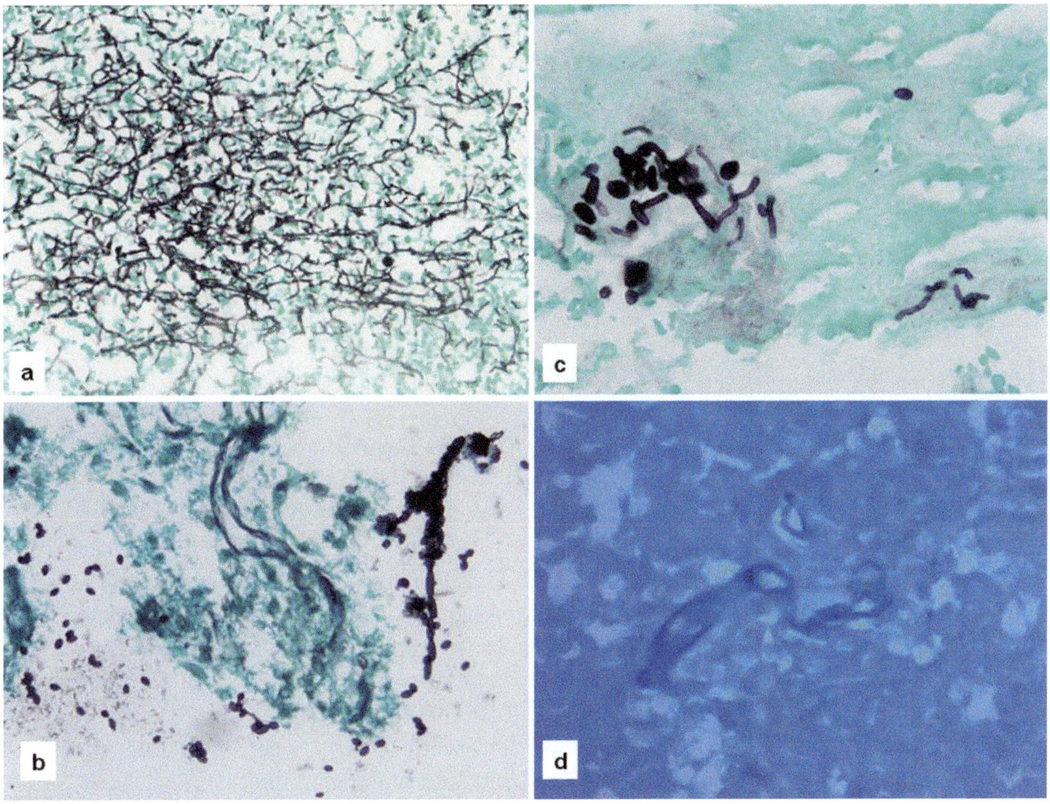

Fig. 18.51 Mushrooms. The structure of the fungi is colored black (**d**—Mucor mushroom, very weakly accepts various stains). (**a**) ×100 and (**b–d**) ×1000

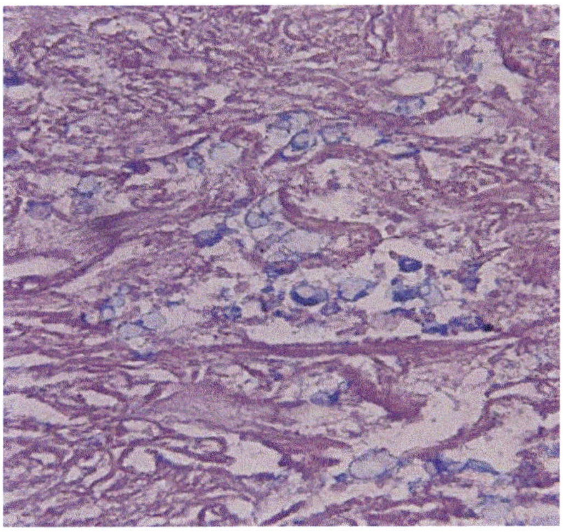

Fig. 18.52 Mushrooms. Stained by Alcyan blue, the rounded structures of the fungus (cryptococci) are stained blue. ×1000

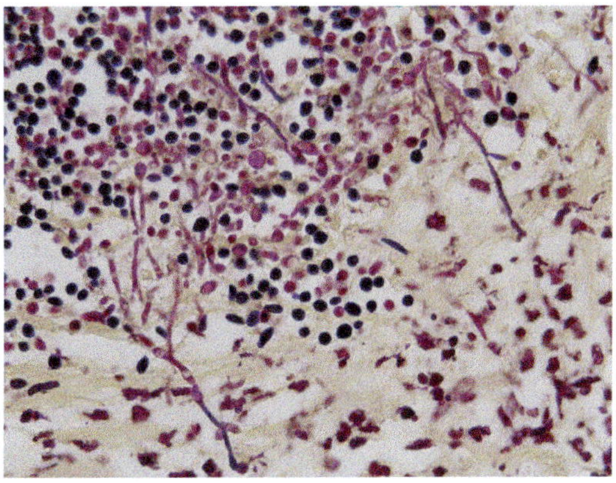

Fig. 18.53 Mushrooms. Brown–Hopps stain, the structure of the fungus is gram-positive (red) and gram-negative (dark blue) depending on the different degrees of maturity of the mycelium. ×1000

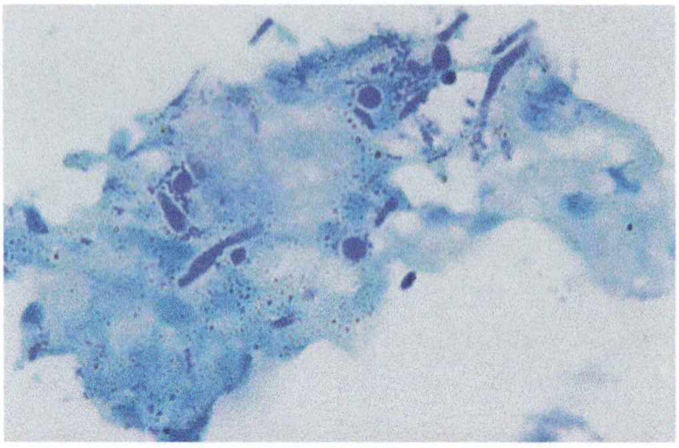

Fig. 18.54 Mushrooms. Stained by ZIehl–Nielsen, the structures of the mushroom are colored dark blue

Actinomycotic granuloma is characterized by the formation in its center of a site of necrosis and microabscesses from neutrophilic and eosinophilic leukocytes with the presence of actinomycetic structures in the form of radiant druses (See Fig. 11.10). Further to the periphery, there is a zone of granulation tissue with an abundance of capillaries and the presence of lymphoid, epithelioid, multinuclear giant cells such as Langhans's and the type of foreign bodies, plasma, xanthoma cells, fibroblasts. Sometimes one can identify hyaline balls. Coarse fibrosis and scars are formed in the outcome of actinomycotic inflammation.

In histobacterioscopy using the PAS reaction, actinomycetes have a weakly or moderately pronounced positive reaction (Fig. 18.9.3); when stained according to Z-N, they are blue (light blue) (Fig. 18.9.4). Actinomycetes are stained well according to Brown–Hopps in a dark blue color, like gram-positive structures (Fig. 18.9.5).

18.10 Tularemia

Francisella tularensis is the etiological agent of tularemia, a serious and occasionally fatal disease of humans and animals. In humans, ulceroglandular tularemia is the most common form of the disease caused by F. tularensis type A and is usually a consequence of a bite from an arthropod vector that has previously fed on an infected animal. The pneumonic form of the disease occurs rarely but is the likely form of the disease should this bacterium be used as a bioterrorism agent. Nowadays such form of the disease is diagnosed extremely rare and we had no opportunity to see any cases.

Nearby in many parts of the world, it is not a rarely diagnosed another form of the disease with much milder course due to Francisella tularensis subsp. holarctica (type B). There are data that in lungs and lymph node, necrotic granulomas could be noted. We had no opportunity to observe any proven cases.

18.11 Granulomatosis of Chlamydial and Mycoplasma Etiology

Mycoplasmas and chlamydia are taxonomically far apart, but the pathological processes they cause are both clinically and morphologically close to each other. Although there are numerous data indicating their ability to cause chronic infectious lesions against the background of immunopathological processes with the formation of granulomas, in the human pathology, they are almost not studied. The foregoing served as the basis for citing some results of our own research.

In nine observations of patients aged 15–72, the analysis of pathological changes and the detection of macrophage granulomas without necrosis with small vacuolization of macrophage cytoplasm containing small PAS-positive inclusions required an IHC study of the diagnostic material of the lymph node and the focus of lung tissue using sera against antigens of *Mycoplasma pneumoniae*, *Chlamydia trachomatis*, *Toxoplasma gondii*, CD68. In four patients, *M. pneumoniae* was detected, in four—*C. trachomatis*. Clinical peculiarities in these patients compared to those having granulomatosis of a different nature were not identified.

The general nature of the changes in the study of surgical and biopsy material was similar. Microscopic examination of lung tissue detected focal carnification, in some places thickening of the interalveolar septa, and some places, marked thickening of the walls of blood vessels with perivascular fibrosis was noted. In the lumen of the alveoli, numerous alveolar macrophages with slightly enlarged finely vacuumed cytoplasm containing PAS-positive inclusions. Acid-resistant bacteria, when stained by Z-N, are not found.

We give several observations as an example.

Patient L. Ch., From the anamnesis, it is known that at the age of 12 she suffered from polyarthritis of the hand, received treatment with prednisone for 12 months. She had complaints of frequent colds, periodic cough. She had not previously had tuberculosis and denied contact. Changes in the lungs were first detected when seeking medical help in connection with an increase in body temperature to 39 °C with the appearance of pain in the chest without irradiation. Received nonspecific antibiotic therapy, during which a slight improvement in the state of health was noted, however, radiological dynamics were not obtained.

During a clinical examination in a blood test, hemoglobin 103 g/L, red blood cells 4.17×10^{12}, white blood cells 4.8×10^{9} without formula shifts, accelerated ESR up to 40 mm/h. When assessing the function of external respiration, it was found that the vital capacity of the lungs and airway are within normal limits. Markers of viral hepatitis, HIV, and RW are negative. Cytological and immunological studies of mycobacterium tuberculosis were not detected.

When R-examination from May 5th, 2012—the root of the lung is unstructured, the local area of reduction of pneumatization in the reed segment according to the type of "frosted glass." 12.05. was detected drainage infiltration in the basal part of the upper lobe of the left triangular shape, the base in the direction of the costal pleura. The dynamic of radiologic data showed a decrease in infiltration in length and severity, with preservation only in the basal sections of S2 with the formation of pleurodiaphragmatic adhesions. On CT scan dated 28th May, in addition to interstitial infiltration, a 3.5×2.5 lymph node with point destruction at the lateral pole reveals a bifurcation angle in the upper left lobe between B2 and B3. The lumens of the bronchi are not changed. In S6 and S8 on the left, one identified lesion is 0.9 and 0.5, respectively. Pleurodiaphragmatic adhesions on both sides.

PET from June 29th on a series of tomograms of the chest in the basal part S3 of the left lung revealed a focus of pathological accumulation of radiopharmaceuticals.

In order to verify the diagnosis, a video thoracoscopic operation was prescribed: a biopsy of the mediastinal lymph node with an edge resection of the left lung.

An extensive histological study was performed, paraffin sections were stained with hematoxylin and eosin, Z-N, PAS, IHC study was also performed to detect C trachomatis, M. pneumoniae antigens.

Microscopic examination of lung tissue determines focal carnification, in places thickening of the interalveolar septa (Fig. 18.55). Marked thickening of the walls of blood vessels with perivascular fibrosis. Marked proliferation of the alveolar epithelium, an increase in the number of macrophages expressing CD68 (Fig. 18.56). In the lumen of the alveoli, numerous alveolar macrophages with a slightly enlarged finely vacuumed cytoplasm containing PAS-positive inclusions (Fig. 18.57) expressing the *M. pneumoniae* antigen. Antigens of other pathogens in the IHC study were not identified. Acid-resistant bacteria when stained according to Z-N were not found.

Macrophages are located in the tissue of the lymph nodes against the background of moderate

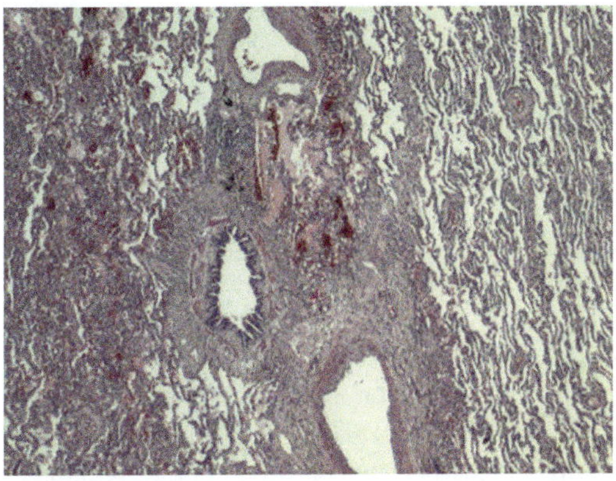

Fig. 18.55 General view of the lung in surgical specimen from patient Ch. H.-E. ×100

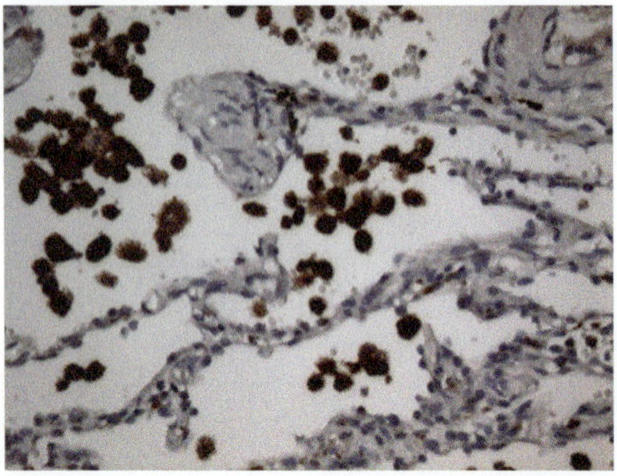

Fig. 18.56 Predominance of CD68 macrophages in the same case. IHC ×400

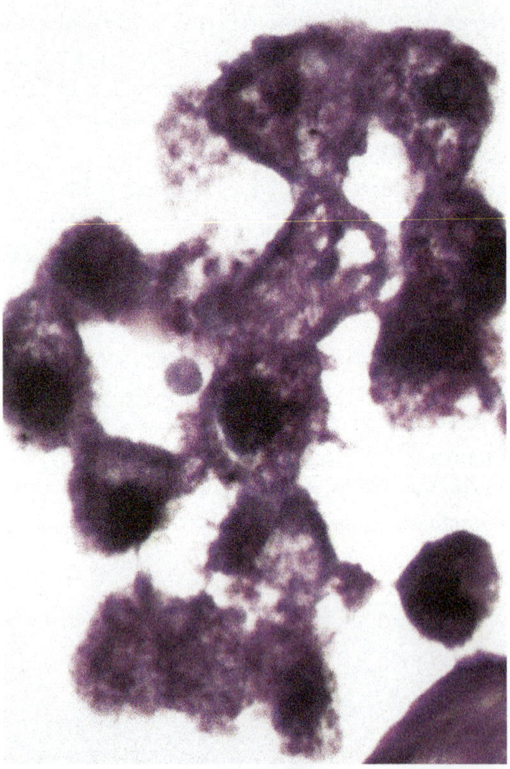

Fig. 18.57 Vacuolated macrophages with small inclusions in the same case. PAS ×1000

or significantly pronounced lymphoid emptying and diffuse focal anthracosis, including giant multinucleated CD68-positive cells, which in places form small granulomas without signs of necrosis in the center (Fig. 18.58). In the cyto-

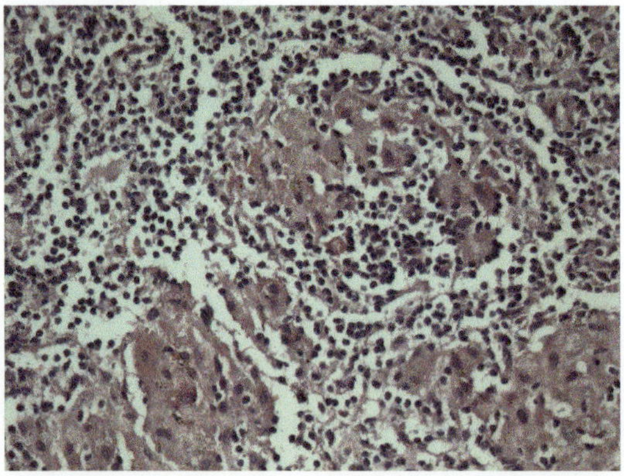

Fig. 18.58 Granuloma in lymph node of the same patient. H.-E. ×400

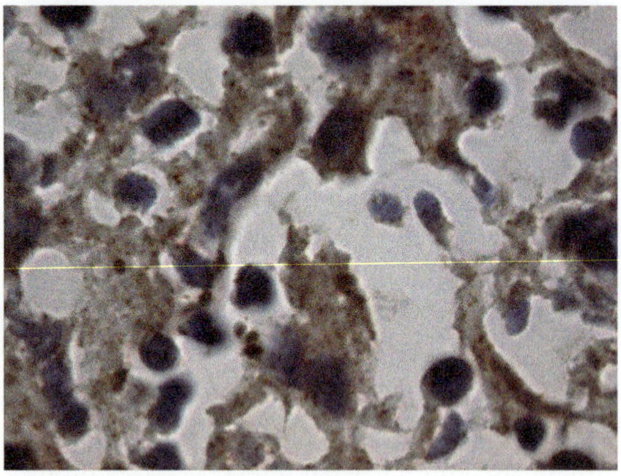

Fig. 18.59 Antigen of *Mycoplasma pneumonia* in lymph node of the same patient. IHC ×1000

plasm of multinuclear giant cells in the tissue of the lymph nodes, including their sinuses, there are small-granular PAS-positive structures expressing the M. pneumoniae antigen (Fig. 18.59). No expression of *C. trachomatis*, toxoplasma antigens was detected. Conclusion: desquamative–macrophageous pneumonia with interstitial and perivascular fibrosis. Macrophageal granulomas of the lymph nodes. The etiology of these changes is mycoplasma. There is no data for the tumor process.

After discharge from the hospital, the patient came under the supervision of a medical center, when contacted, the patient complained of weakness, fatigue, cough, chest pain, and subfebrile temperature. On examination, the skin and visible mucous membranes are clean, peripheral lymph nodes are not enlarged. A slight shortening of percussion sound in the paravertebral regions was noted above the lungs. By auscultation, against the background of hard breathing, scattered dry and single wet rales were heard, respiratory rate up to 24 per minute. In a clinical blood test, moderate anemia (hemoglobin is reduced to 96 g/L), leukocytopenia (to 4.3 × 109), in the formula, a left shift to nine nuclear bacilli, and accelerated ESR up to 40 mm/h. For 3 weeks, the patient underwent a course of antibacterial therapy intravenously in combination with plasmapheresis, symptomatic therapy. As a result of the treatment, the patient's condition and well-being completely normalized, by the third week the chest pain, cough, low-grade fever completely disappeared. Control clinical, laboratory and radiological data testified to the almost complete recovery of the patient. Later on, contact with the patient for several years is maintained by telephone. The patient considers herself practically healthy for lung pathology.

Slices related to a transbronchial biopsy of the son of a patient examined for suspected sarcoidosis were also consulted. Small non-necrotic epithelioid–macrophage granulomas with giant cells of foreign bodies, partially consisting of vacuolated cells, were revealed, which made the morphological picture similar to that observed in the lymph nodes in the mother (Fig. 18.60). Additional studies revealed intracellular PAS-positive inclusions and mycoplasma antigen both perivascular

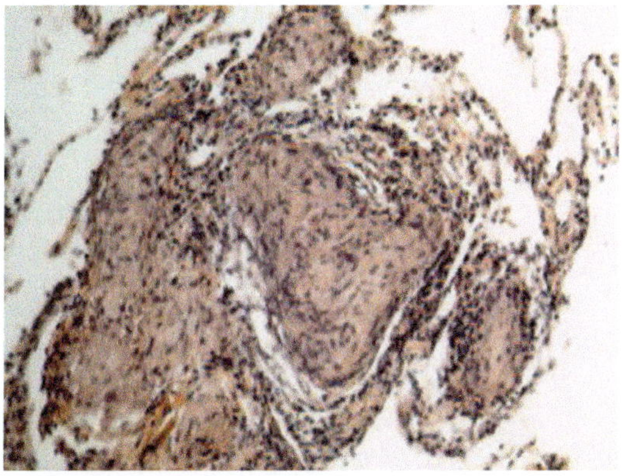

Fig. 18.60 Granuloma in transbronchial biopsies of the son of the patient. H.E. ×200

and, to a lesser extent, in granuloma cells. C. trachomatis antigen not detected. After the treatment, the condition improved, the diagnosis of sarcoidosis by clinicians was withdrawn.

Mycoplasma etiology of chronic lesions of the lungs and regional lymph nodes in this observation can be considered proven. Not only the results of IHC studies but also quite characteristic histological changes testify to her favor. In addition, the clinical history, manifestations, and effectiveness of targeted therapy do not contradict this diagnosis. The conducted studies allow the exclusion of other etiological factors discussed in the literature. Although there is no indication in the available literature on the ability of mycoplasmas to lead to the formation of granulomas, their occurrence fits well with the recently refined characterization of the properties of this pathogen associated with various immunopathological reactions. In particular, their ability to act as a trigger for autoimmune reactions with the appearance of autoantibodies to many internal organs in the blood, the initiation of the formation of circulating immune complexes, the activation of excessive T-cell reactions, the stimulation of lymphocytes to blast transformation is known. The relationship of mycoplasmas with chronic lung diseases accompanied by fibrosis has been proven for a long time. The activity of the inflammatory process in this observation was also evidenced by the results of PET, which could not exclude the tumor process. Of interest is the development of similar lesions in the patient's son, which suggests the presence of a family focus. It cannot be ruled out that joint injuries that the patient had in her teens and are currently worrying about have mycoplasma etiology as well.

Patient K.P. (37 years). Complaints of general weakness, fatigue, discomfort in the chest when breathing. A routine R-examination in October revealed changes in the lungs. Consulted by phtysiatrist without signs of tuberculosis. CT scan of the chest cavity was recommended. The results of microbiological, serological, and PCR diagnostics for tuberculosis were negative. With MSCT of the organs of the chest cavity, numerous foci from 0.1 to 0.8 cm are determined in the lung tissue. Infiltrative changes in the lung tissue were not determined. Along the right upper lobar bronchus, the formation of lymph nodes with uneven walls with a thickness of up to 0.7 cm and a length of up to 1.7 cm was determined. The course and patency of the trachea, main, lobar bronchi were preserved. Enlarged lymph nodes of almost all groups are visualized: upper paratracheal—0.7 × 0.6 cm, lower—1.3 × 0.9 cm, 1.7 × 1.3 cm, bifurcation—up to 1.8 × 1.7 cm, right bifurcation—up to 1.6 × 1.7 cm, left—up to 1.5 × 1.6 cm. The fluid in the pleural cavities was not determined. Bone-destructive changes in the scan area were not determined. Conclusion: CT picture of disseminated lung lesions, adenopathy of the intrathoracic lymph nodes.

Transbronchial lung biopsy from S3, S4, S5, S8, S9, S10, right lung, (seven biopsy specimens). Histological examination in a biopsy of sections of lung tissue with several small epithelial unicellular (macrophage) granulomas without giant cells, to which dense lymphocytic infiltrates are attached in places. Macrophageous granuloma in the lung, pronounced small vacuolization of both macrophages and ciliated epithelial cells (Fig. 18.61). There is no necrosis. Acid-resistant microbiota is not detected. Small intracellular PAS-positive inclusions were revealed (Fig. 18.62) Conclusion: granulomatosis of unspecified nature. There is no evidence of tuberculosis. It is necessary to exclude mycoplasmosis and chlamydia. IHC study of lung and lymph node tissue: in the study of the expression of antigens of Mycobacterium tuberculosis complex, Mycoplasma pneumoniae, Toxoplasma gondii was not detected. Numerous CD 68+ cells were revealed (macrophages). The expression of C. trachomatis antigens in the tissue of the lung and lymph node was revealed (Fig. 18.63).

Diagnosis: chronic granulomatous inflammation caused by Chlamydia.

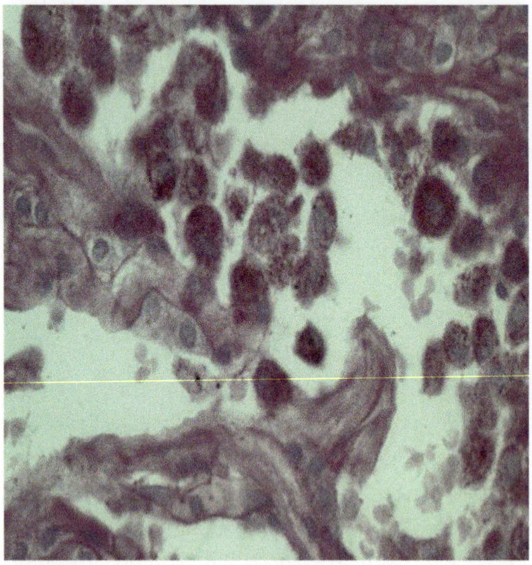

Fig. 18.62 Numerous PAS-positive inclusions in macrophage's cytoplasm PAS ×1000

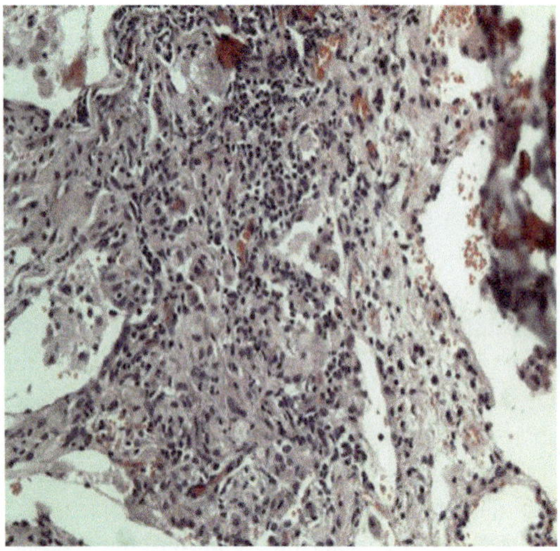

Fig. 18.61 Macrophageous granuloma in surgical specimen of patient K. H.E. ×200

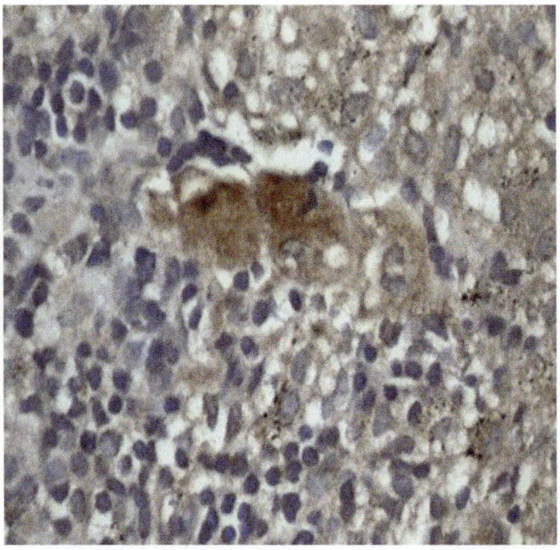

Fig. 18.63 Antigen of *C. trachomatis* in lymph node of the same patient. IHC ×400

18.12 Bronchocentric Granulomatosis

Bronchocentric granulomatosis is a rare disease characterized by necrotizing granulomatous inflammation of the wall of the bronchi and bronchioles, with chronic inflammatory changes in the adjacent lung parenchyma. The etiology of the disease is unknown, it occurs in patients with bronchial asthma, in people with a congenital immune defect. In addition, the disease is often associated with the presence of pulmonary aspergillosis, and this type of granulomatosis is considered an allergic reaction to fungi. However, it is possible that other structures penetrating the respiratory tract can also act as allergens. It is believed that bronchocentric granulomatosis is not always an independent process but maybe a manifestation of various pulmonary or systemic diseases.

During histological examination, it is noteworthy that the process is mainly associated with the bronchi. In the lung, ectazed bronchi are detected, mainly cartilage-free, with dense lymphoid or mononuclear wall infiltration, with signs of granulomatous inflammation, with areas of destruction of the mucous membrane or completely of the bronchial wall with the destruction of all its layers. Fibrinoid-like areas of necrosis of the bronchial wall may form. Respiratory epithelium is usually with dystrophic changes, but squamous metaplasia is not characteristic. Granulomas in the bronchial wall are usually small, fuzzy, with a predominance of macrophages—macrophage, macrophage–epithelioid, with an admixture of giant multinucleated cells. Clearly formed granulomas may not be observed, there are fuzzy small clusters of epithelioid cells, scattered multinuclear giant cells (Fig. 18.64). In the lumen of the affected and nearby

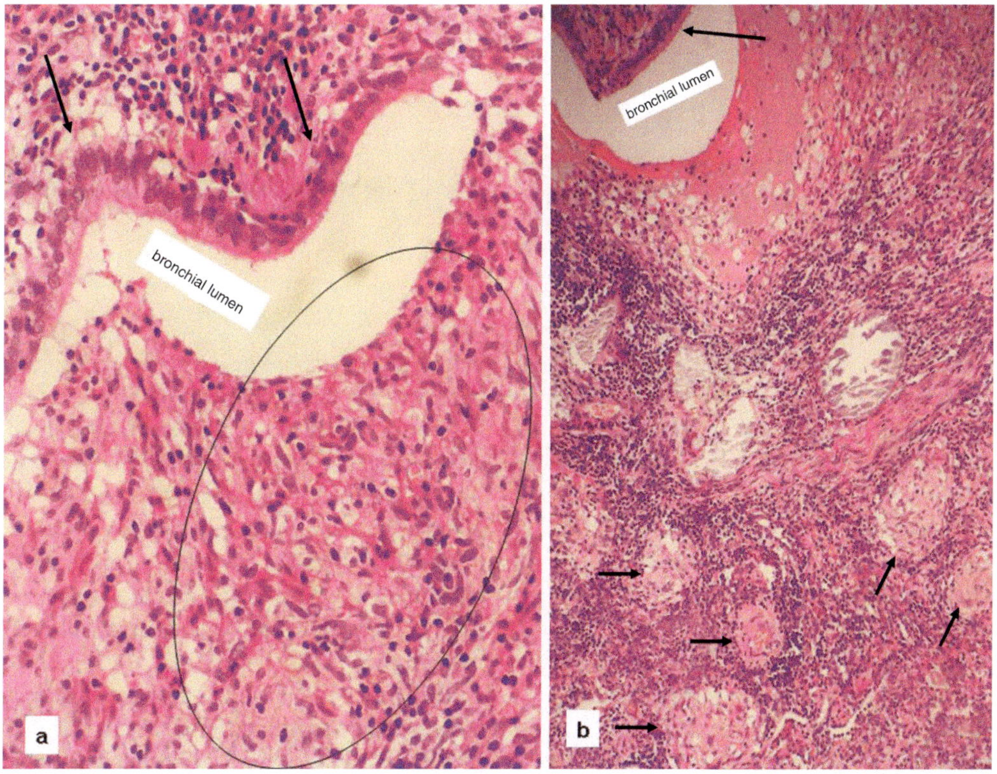

Fig. 18.64 Bronchocentric granulomatosis. Bronchus with a section of destruction with epithelial cell reaction (**a**) and granulomatous reaction (**b**). Preserved bronchial mucosa covered with respiratory epithelium is indicated by long arrows (**a**, **b**); the section of destruction of the bronchial mucosa with epithelial cell reaction is circled by an oval frame (**a**); granulomas in the section of destruction of the bronchus are indicated by short arrows (**b**). Staining with hematoxylin and eosin. (**a**) ×400; (**b**) ×200

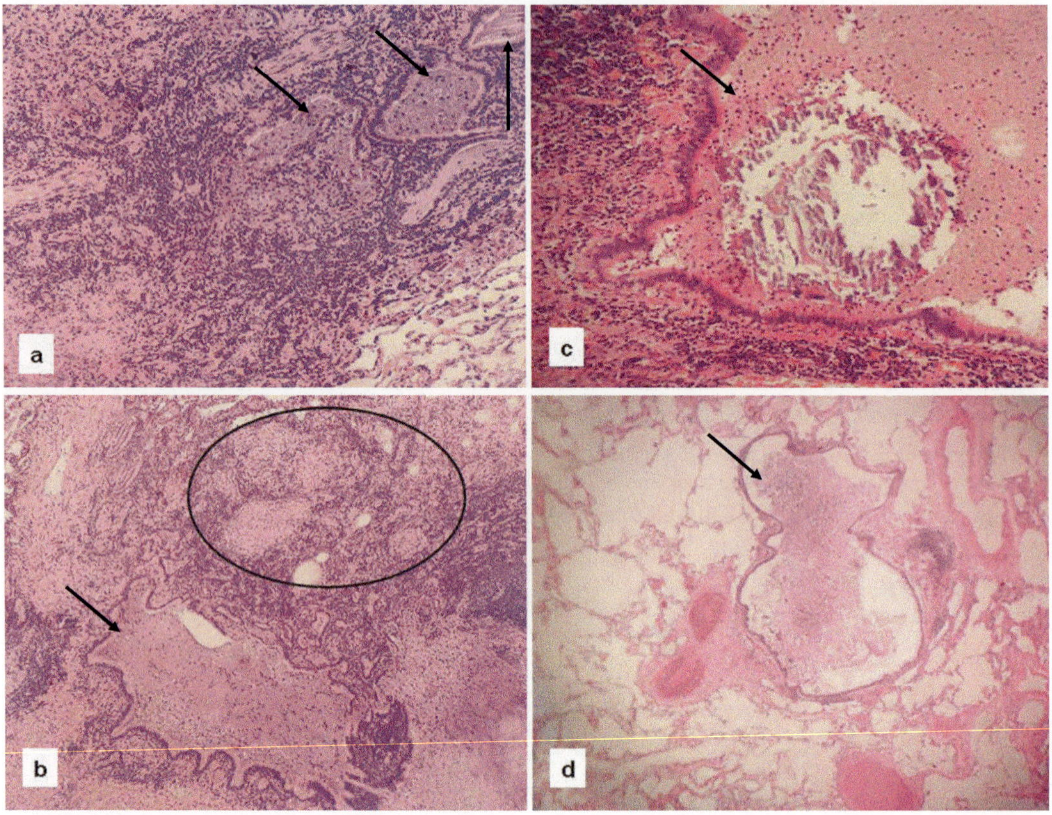

Fig. 18.65 Bronchocentric granulomatosis. Ectasia of small cartilaginous bronchus filled with eosinophilic protein exudate (indicated by arrows). (**a–c**) Perifocally expressed lymphoid reaction and areas of granulomatous inflammation (outlined in Fig. "**b**"); (**d**) PAS-negative content in the lumen of the bronchus with ectasia, perifocally air lung tissue with thin intact interalveolar partitions. (**a–c**)—hematoxylin and eosin staining; (**d**)—PAS reaction. (**a**) ×100; (**b**, **d**) ×40; (**c**) ×200

bronchi, a weakly eosinophilic fine-grained protein exudate is determined, PAS-negative, although in some cases mucus is found in the lumen of the bronchi (respectively, the PAS reaction in these areas is positive). There is a "mosaic" arrangement of protein exudate and mucus both in individual bronchi and in the lumen of one bronchus. In the lumen of the affected bronchi, one can detect detritus, small areas of granulation tissue with granulomas, which are probably particles of the destroyed bronchial wall, as well as neutrophilic and eosinophilic leukocytes, and in large quantities. Alveoli adjacent to the described bronchi are ectazed and contain the above-described protein PAS-negative content in the lumen (Fig. 18.65). In the peripheral areas of the lung, a mostly dense lymphoid infiltrate or polymorphic cell infiltration is formed with the presence of mononuclear cells (macrophages, plasma cells, lymphocytes, with the predominance of the latter in the composition of the infiltrate) and leukocytes. The number of leukocytes, neutrophilic and eosinophilic, can be different, up to microabscesses sites. In many cases, eosinophilic white blood cells predominate, especially in cases due to the presence of aspergillus in the lungs. In the lymphoid infiltrate, granulomas are located both in the form of rather extensive sections of granulomatous inflammation, and scattered, in a small amount. Granulomas are both single and with a tendency to merge, mainly macrophage–giant cell and macrophage–epithelioid, as well as giant cell granulomas with a predominance of giant cells such as foreign bodies (Fig. 18.66).

Outside the affected areas, the lung tissue is airy, with thin intact interalveolar septa. With histological bacterioscopy according to Z-N, acid-

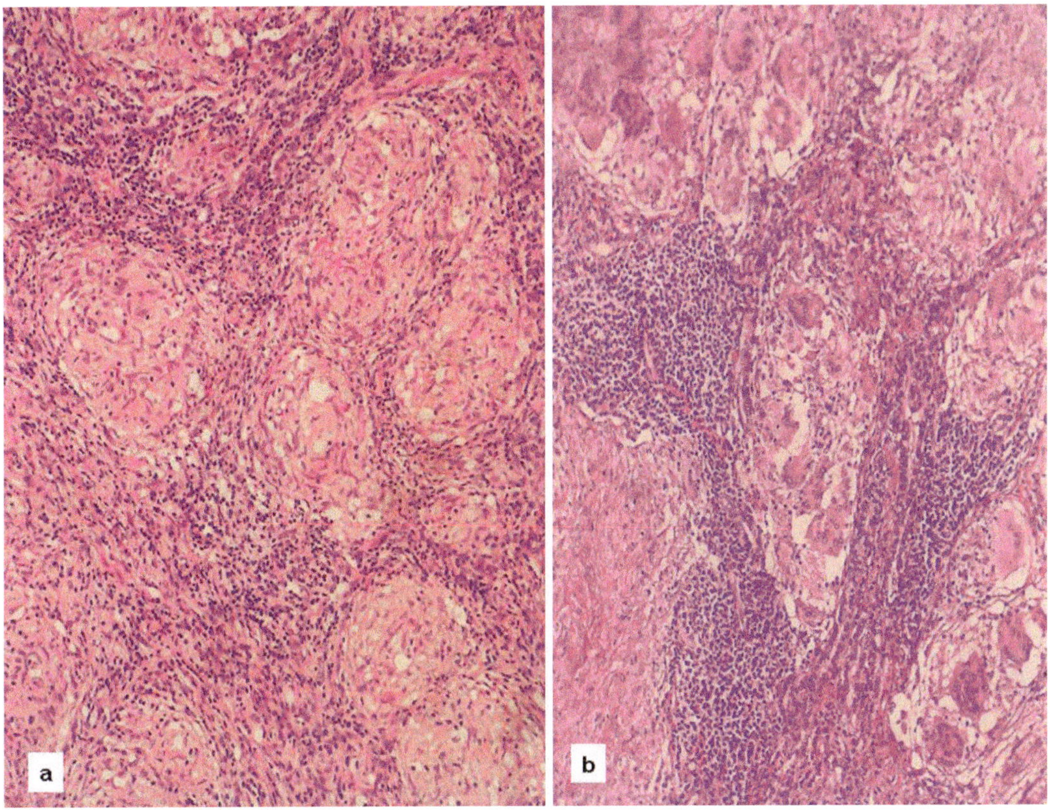

Fig. 18.66 Bronchocentric granulomatosis. Granulomas in the lung—macrophage–epithelioid–giant cellular (**a**), macrophage–giant cellular with a predominance of giant multinucleated cells (**b**). Staining with hematoxylin and eosin. ×200.1000

resistant bacteria are not detected either in areas of granulomatous inflammation, or in areas of destruction of the bronchi, or the contents of the lumen of the bronchi. When staining for mushrooms, according to the literature, in some cases mycotic structures are detected, however, in our studies, fungi were not found.

Differential diagnosis should be carried out primarily with tuberculosis, various mycoses, exogenous allergic alveolitis (in which productive bronchiolitis may develop), interstitial lung diseases.

18.13 Granulomatosis with Polyangiitis

Granulomatosis with polyangiitis (formerly Wegener's granulomatosis)—granulomatous systemic vasculitis with damage to small and medium blood vessels (capillaries, venules, arterioles, and arteries), with the predominant involvement of the respiratory system and kidneys, an autoimmune process. It is a systemic necrotizing vasculitis. Refers to granulomatous inflammation of an unknown nature.

For granulomatosis with polyangiitis, a triad of morphological signs is characteristic: foci of necrosis of a "geographical form", granulomatous–necrotic thrombovasculitis, polymorphic cell granulomas.

Foci of fibrinoid necrosis have an irregular shape with irregular contours (the so-called geographical necrosis) (Fig. 18.67), in necrotic masses there can be eosinophilic infiltration, both focal and massive diffuse. Necrotic masses, due to a large number of destroyed and collapsing leukocytes and the abundance of nuclear detritus,

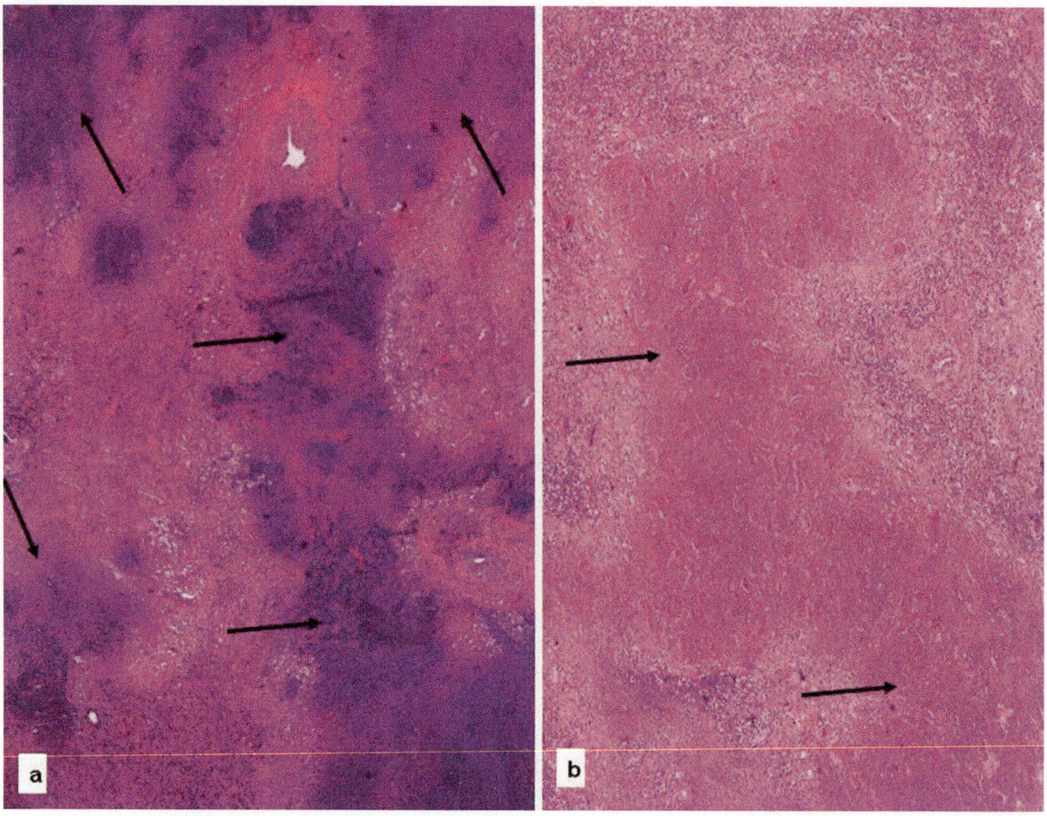

Fig. 18.67 Granulomatosis with polyangiitis (formerly Wegener's granulomatosis). Foci of fibrinoid necrosis of irregular "geographical" shape (indicated by arrows), in Fig. "**a**"—with a pronounced basophilic tinge. Stained with hematoxylin and eosin. ×100

acquire a basophilic shade (the so-called dirty necrosis). In the foci of necrosis, decay cavities can form.

In blood vessels of small and medium caliber, destructive necrotic granulomatous vasculitis and thrombovasculitis are detected. The walls of the vessels are sharply thickened, edematous, with areas of fibrinoid necrosis of various sizes, polymorphic cell infiltration, including eosinophilic leukocytes, plasma cells, giant multinucleated and epithelioid cells, fuzzy granulomas (Fig. 18.68). In the surrounding infiltrate, the contours of the walls of blood vessels with inflammatory changes can be difficult to find. Thrombotic masses (granulomatous–necrotic thrombovasculitis) can be found in the lumen of blood vessels (Fig. 18.69). With the lesion of small-caliber vessels, capillaries, their walls are swollen, with signs of increased permeability of the vascular wall, infiltration by cellular elements—neutrophilic and eosinophilic leukocytes, plasma cells, lymphocytes. The severity of inflammation is different.

Polymorphic cell granulomas, fuzzy, more like extensive infiltrates. Granulomas are represented by eosinophilic and neutrophilic leukocytes, lymphocytes, plasma cells, macrophages, giant multinucleated cells. Multinucleated cells with signs of cell and nuclear polymorphism (Fig. 18.70).

The histobacterioscopic examination does not reveal acid-resistant bacteria and fungal structures.

Differential morphological diagnosis must first be carried out with tuberculosis, the mycotic process, as well as with rheumatoid lesions of the lung and other types of systemic vasculitis.

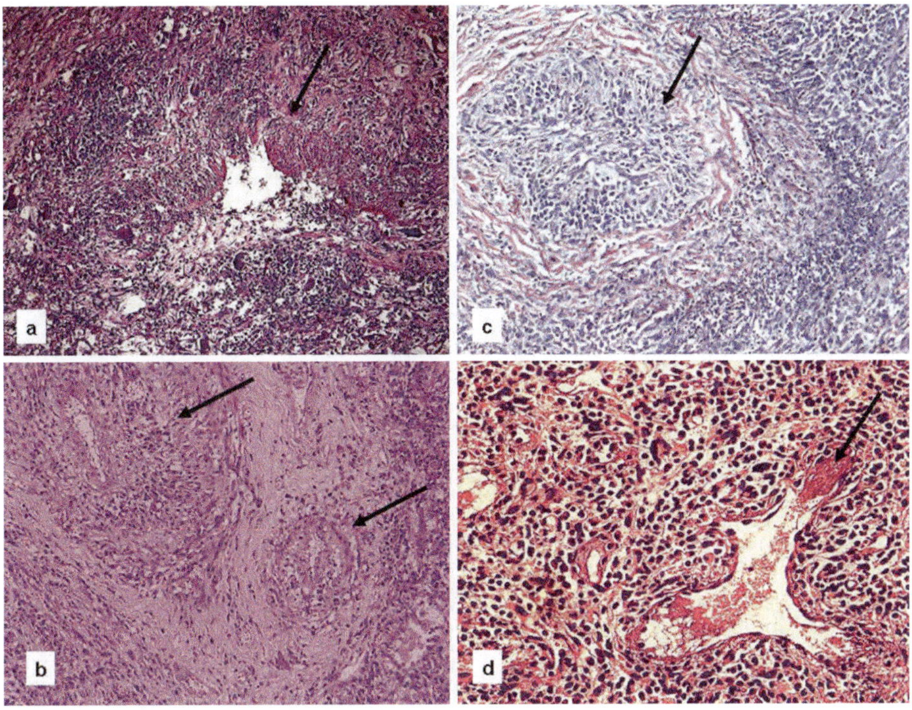

Fig. 18.68 Granulomatosis with polyangiitis (former Wegener's granulomatosis). Granulomatous destructive vasculitis (affected vessels are indicated by arrows). Stained with hematoxylin and eosin. ×200

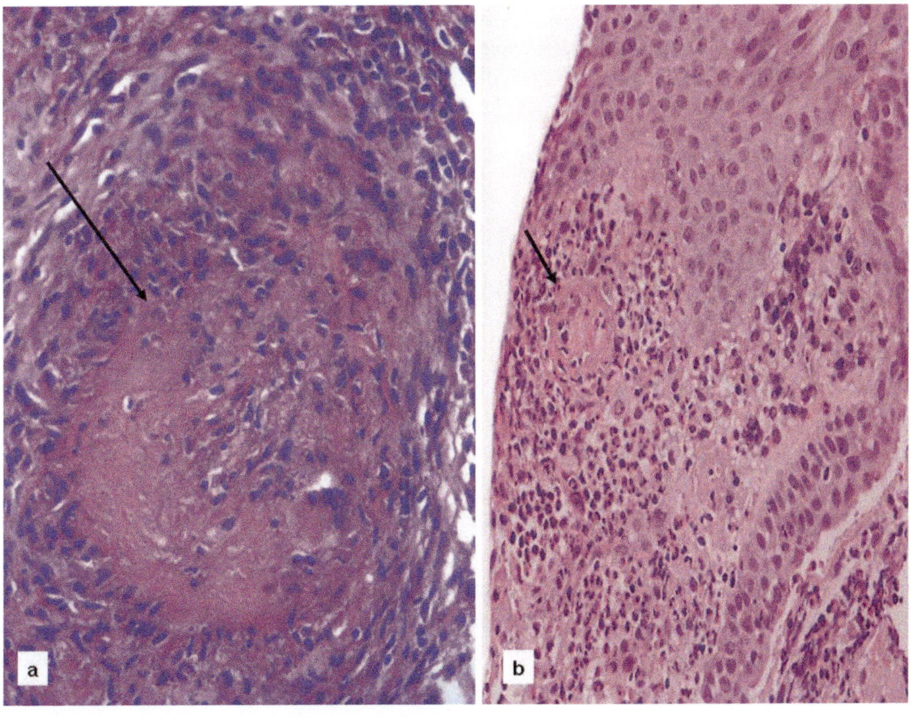

Fig. 18.69 Granulomatosis with polyangiitis (former Wegener's granulomatosis). Thrombovascular: (**a**) lung; (**b**) the mucous membrane of the bronchus (vessels indicated by arrows). Stained with hematoxylin and eosin. ×200. (**a**) ×400 and (**b**) ×100

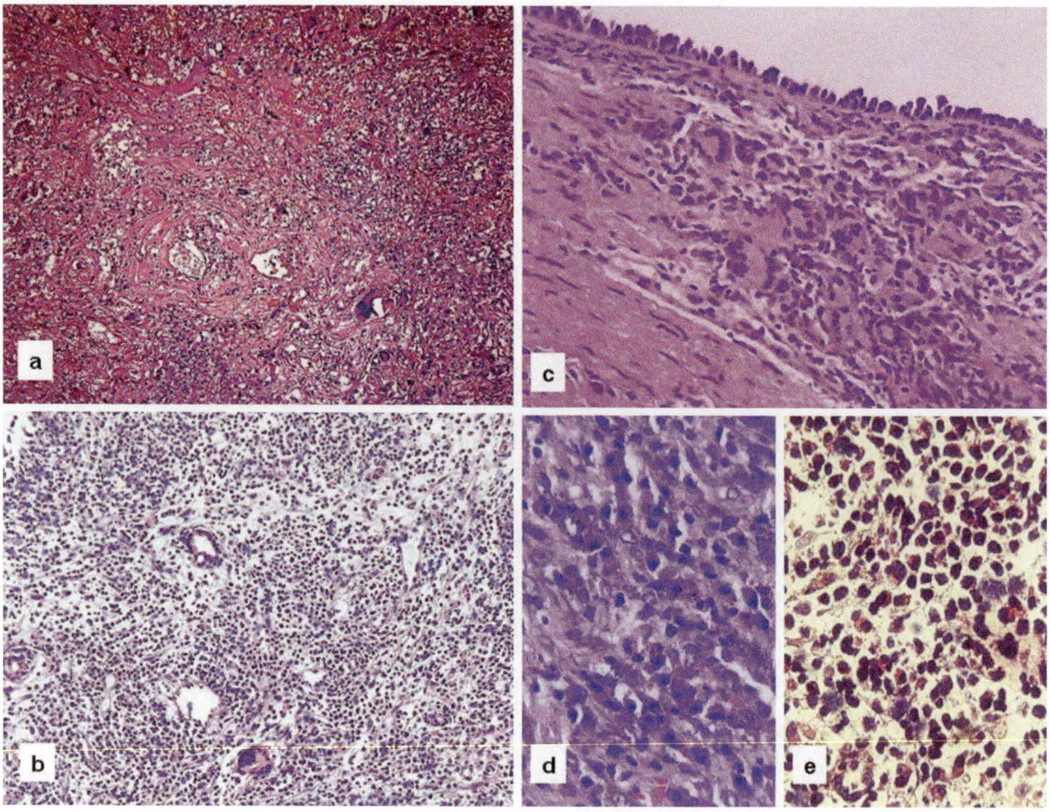

Fig. 18.70 Granulomatosis with polyangiitis (former Wegener's granulomatosis). Polymorphocellular granulomas. (**a**, **b**) In the lung; (**c**) in the bronchial mucosa; (**d**) expressed plasmocytic reaction; (**e**) expressed eosinophilic reaction. Stained with hematoxylin and eosin. (**a**) ×100; (**b**, **c**) ×200; (**d**, **e**) ×1000

18.14 Histiocytosis X

Histiocytosis X (histiocytosis from Langerhans cells, eosinophilic granuloma, pulmonary granulomatosis X, pulmonary Langerhans cell granulomatosis)—belongs to the group of diseases characterized by the development of eosinophilic granulomas. The etiology of the process has not been established; it is assumed that histiocytosis X is based on an immunopathological process that promotes the proliferation of histiocytes and eosinophilic leukocytes.

Langerhans cells are a subtype of dendritic cells that develop with the participation of transforming growth factor-β (TGF-β) and are mainly localized in the epithelial tissues—the epidermis and mucous membrane of the tracheobronchial tree, are antigen-presenting cells, regulatory cells of the macrophage system. Langerhans cells are large, 15–25 nm in size, with fuzzy borders, an eosinophilic cytoplasm, a bean-shaped nucleus with a convoluted nuclear membrane, and the absence of nucleoli. With histiocytosis X, Langerhans cell proliferation is noted, changes in the antigen-presenting function of macrophages lead to the accumulation of immune complexes, their deposition in the walls of blood vessels and bronchioles, and activation of the macrophage system.

Histological examination in the early stages of histiocytosis X shows marked local bronchocentric tissue destruction, signs of destructive bronchiolitis with the formation of bronchocentric and peribronchiolar granulomas with the accumulation of pigmented alveolar macrophages are observed. Later, a tabular (star-shaped) type of granuloma is formed, spreading along the alveolar septa (Fig. 18.71). Granulomas are formed from Langerhans cells; granulomas also include smaller histiocytic cells, eosinophilic leukocytes, fibroblasts, and plasma cells, lymphocytes (Fig. 18.72). According to the literature, granulomas have a significant number of CD4 + T cells in contact with Langerhans cells that express costimulatory molecules. In granulomas, clusters of pigmented macrophages are often detected (Fig. 18.73). The composition of the granulomas is unstable and can vary significantly even within the same slice. With the progression of the process, characteristic stellate fibrous scars are formed, surrounded by cystic cavities, which are formed due to the traction expansion of peripheral alveoli.

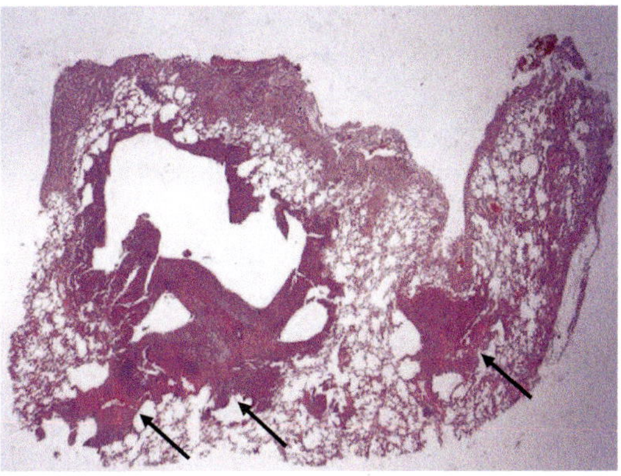

Fig. 18.71 Histiocytosis X. Stellate granulomas in the lung (indicated by arrows). Stained with hematoxylin and eosin. ×4

Perifocal changes in the lung are in the form of desquamate interstitial pneumonia. An IHC study with histiocytosis X reveals positive staining of Langerhans cells when using antibodies to CD1a, to S-100 protein (Fig. 18.74). An ultrastructural study using transmission electron microscopy reveals Birbeck granules (X-bodies)

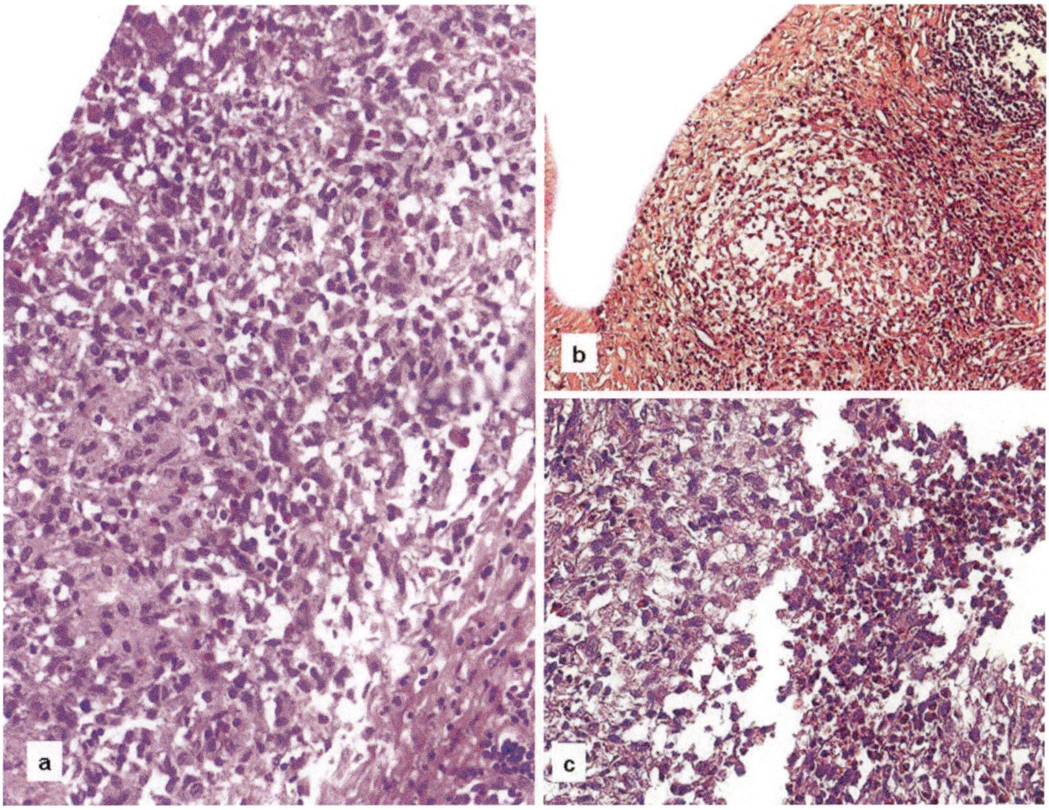

Fig. 18.72 Histiocytosis X. Macrophage granulomas with an admixture of eosinophilic leukocytes. Stained with hematoxylin and eosin. (**a**, **c**) ×400 and (**b**) ×100

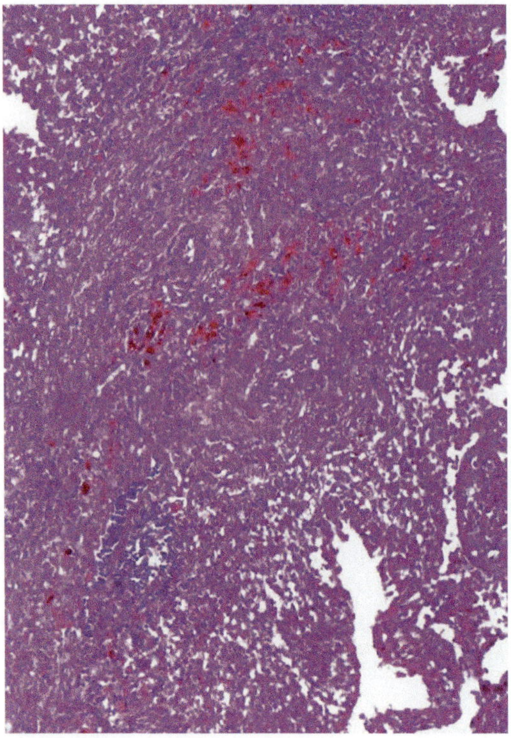

Fig. 18.73 Histiocytosis X. Pigmented macrophages in granulomas. Stained with hematoxylin and eosin. (**a**) ×400

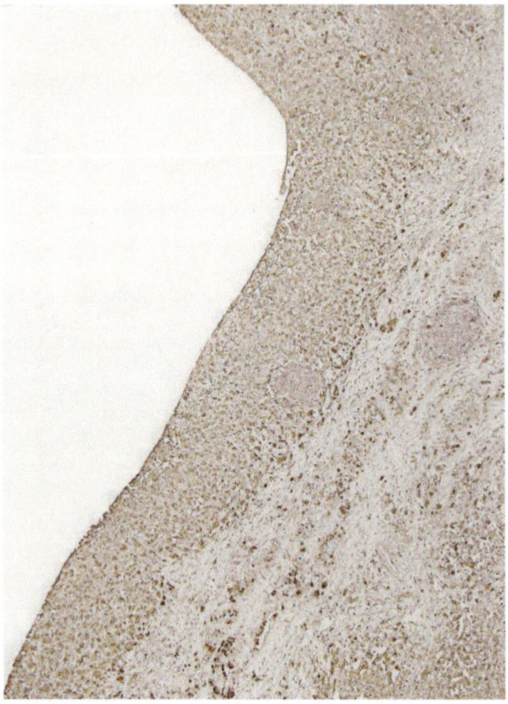

Fig. 18.74 Histiocytosis X. Positive immunohistochemical reaction for S 100

in Langerhans cells. Birbek granules are cytoplasmic inclusions in the form of a tennis racket.

18.15 Rheumatoid Damage

Rheumatoid damage to the lungs is one of the most common systemic, extra-articular manifestations of rheumatoid arthritis, and rheumatoid nodules are one of the most common variants of damage to the lung parenchyma.

Macroscopically rheumatoid nodules are whitish–yellowish encapsulated foci similar to foci of caseous necrosis in tuberculosis. In some cases, a slightly yellowish or brownish tint of necrotic masses is noted. There are nodules with the decay of necrotic masses and the formation of a cavity, which macroscopically is also easy to take for a tuberculous cavity.

Histological examination determines that rheumatoid lesion of the lung with the formation of rheumatoid nodules is accompanied by the development of foci of fibrinoid necrosis, mainly of irregular shape, there may be rounded lesions. Necrotic foci, unlike tuberculous foci, without the preserved outline of the interalveolar septa, but with "shadows" of the thrombosed vessels, which are well defined when stained according to van Gieson, as well as when stained with elastic, when stained with silver according to Grokkott (Fig. 18.75). In necrotic masses, focal or diffuse focal infiltration from eosinophilic leukocytes, in places with areas of microabscesses, is detected. Due to the abundance of nuclear detritus of destroyed leukocytes, necrotic masses take on a pronounced basophilic hue, the so-called dirty necrosis (Fig. 18.76).

Along the edge of necrosis, subcapsularly, a picket of fibroblast-like cells is formed, which can be either implicit or clearly formed around the entire necrotic focus. In addition to fibroblast-like cells, macrophages, scattered giant multinucleated cells that usually do not form granulomas, are detected along the edge of necrosis, although in some cases small, macrophage–giant cell granulomas can be noted along the edge of necrosis (Fig. 18.77).

The capsule of foci of fibrinoid necrosis can be wide or uneven, consists of coarse fibrous tissue with randomly arranged fibers (Fig. 18.78).

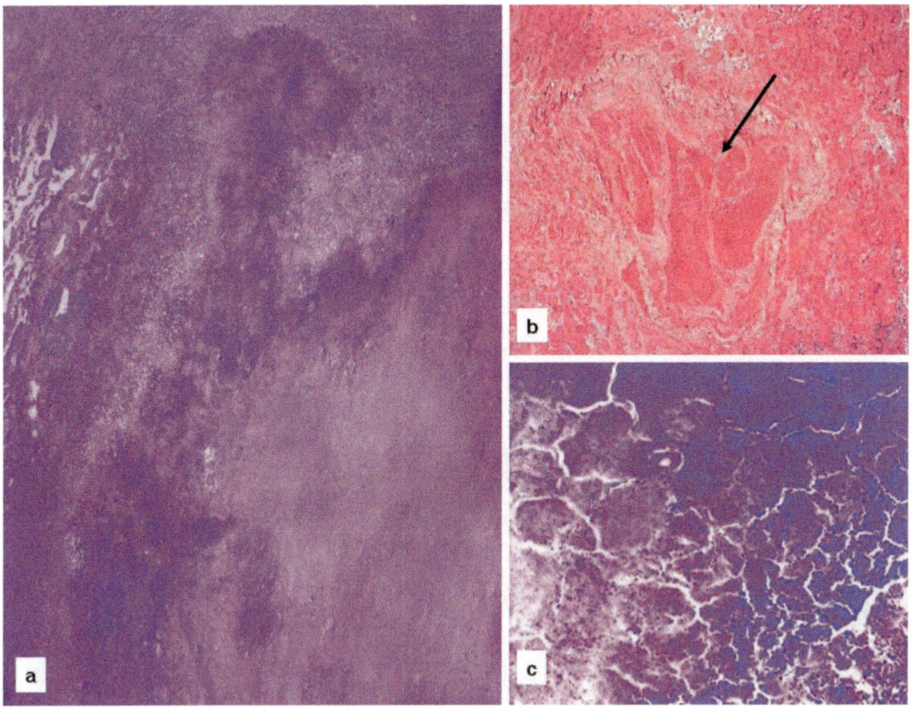

Fig. 18.75 Rheumatoid lesions of the lung. (**a**) Fibrinoid necrosis of irregular shape; (**b**) a thrombosed vessel in the focus of fibrinoid necrosis; (**c**) for comparison—a focus of caseous necrosis in tuberculosis with preserved outlines of interalveolar partitions. Stained with hematoxylin and eosin. (**a**, **c**) ×100 and (**b**) ×200

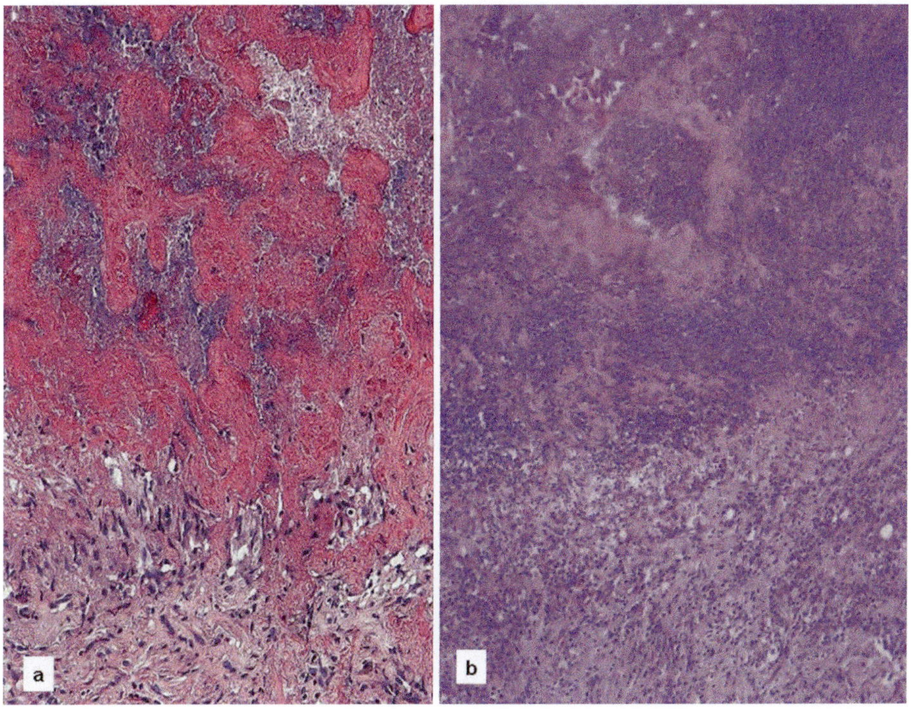

Fig. 18.76 Rheumatoid lung damage. "Dirty necrosis," necrotic masses take a pronounced basophilic hue of nuclear detritus of destroyed white blood cells. Stained with hematoxylin and eosin. (**a**) ×200 and (**b**) ×100

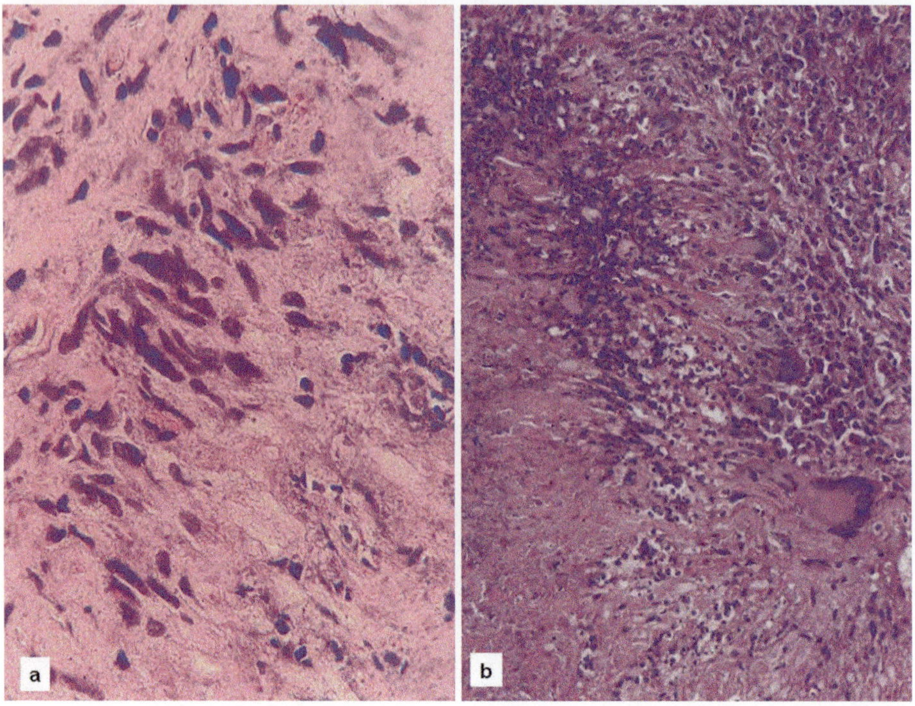

Fig. 18.77 Rheumatoid lung damage. (**a**) Along the edge of necrosis, a palisade of fibroblast-like cells; (**b**) along the edge of necrosis, fibroblast-like cells, and giant multinucleated cells. Stained with hematoxylin and eosin. (**a**) ×400 and (**b**) ×200

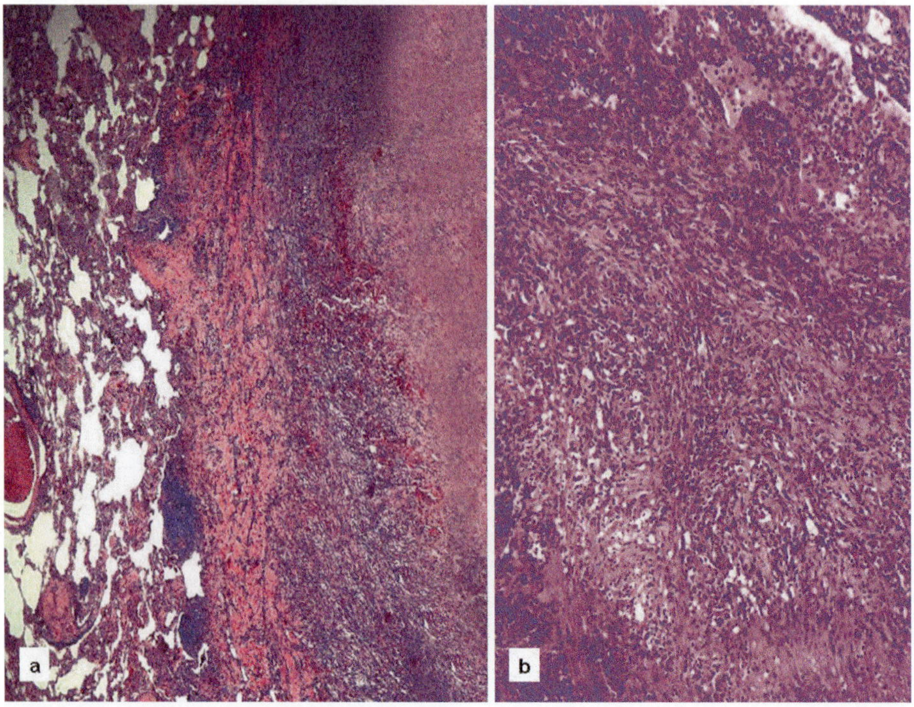

Fig. 18.78 Rheumatoid lung damage. (**a**) Fibrous capsule of the necrotic focus; (**b**) randomly located collagen fibers of the necrotic focus capsule. Stained with hematoxylin and eosin. (**a**) ×100 and (**b**) ×200

Perifocal, near the foci of necrosis, are vessels with signs of subacute, productive obliterating thrombovasculitis. The intensity of the lymphoid reaction can be different, weak, moderate, or pronounced. There are vessels with partial as well as a complete obliteration of the lumen of the vessels, obliterated vessels with the phenomena of sewerage and revascularization (Fig. 18.79). With the location of a rather large affected vessel along the edge of necrosis, part of the vessel with signs of productive obliterating vasculitis can be located outside the focus, and part in the necrotic masses, in which only its shape will be determined. In the lumen of the adjacent alveoli, clusters of siderophages are located, which are colored in a characteristic blue–green when stained according to Prussian bluc reaction (Figs. 18.80 and 18.81).

In the lung tissue outside the rheumatoid nodules, the interalveolar septa are thin, the lung tissue is usually airy, the interlobular septa are not fibrosed, but clusters of siderophages are noted in the lumen of the alveoli. In addition, there are vessels with signs of productive obliterating vasculitis, the severity of inflammatory changes in which they are usually less pronounced than in the peripheral areas. Vessels with a wall thickened due to fibrosis without inflammatory infiltration or vessels with perivascular fibrosis can be determined. There are small lymphoid or lymphoid–macrophage infiltrates with scattered giant multinucleated cells or small clusters of macrophages, without the formation of clear granulomas.

Morphological differential diagnosis is usually required primarily with foci of tuberculous dis-

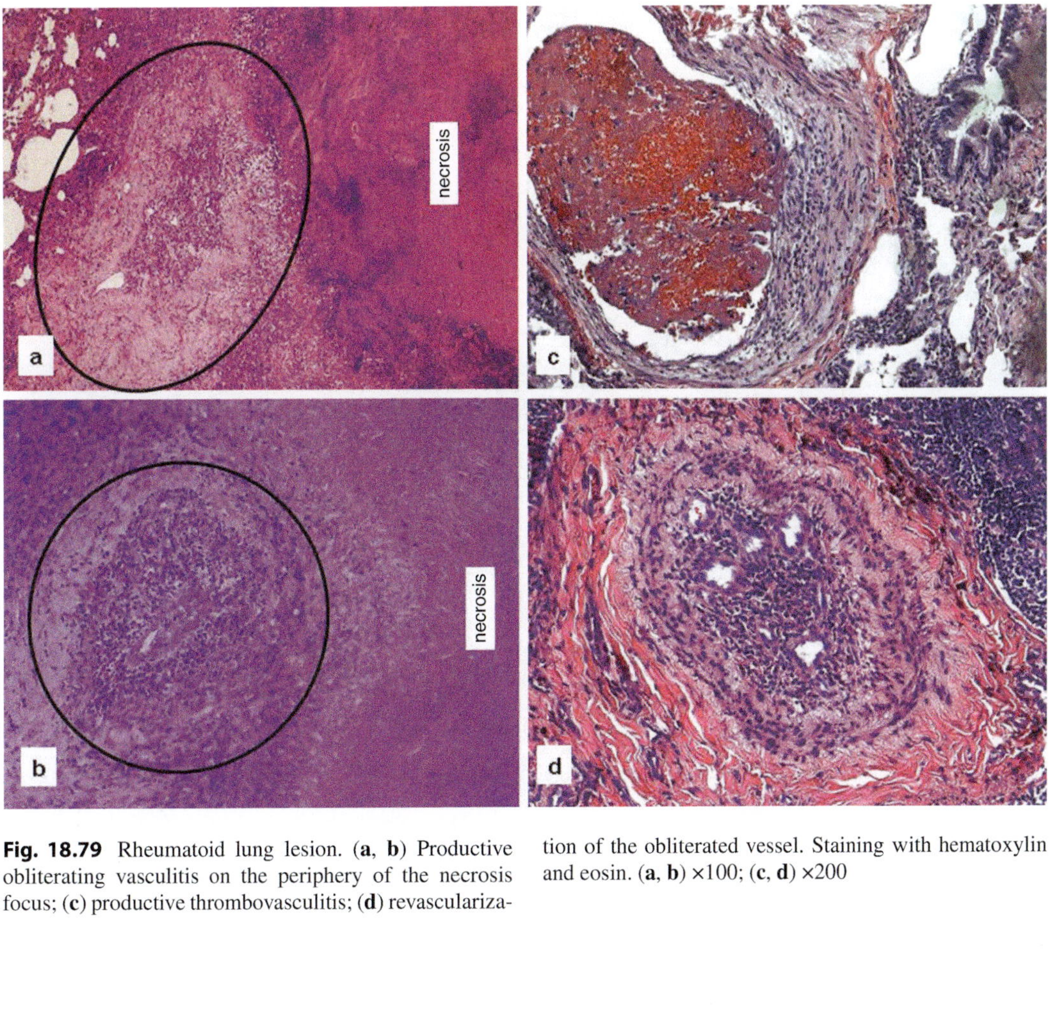

Fig. 18.79 Rheumatoid lung lesion. (**a**, **b**) Productive obliterating vasculitis on the periphery of the necrosis focus; (**c**) productive thrombovasculitis; (**d**) revascularization of the obliterated vessel. Staining with hematoxylin and eosin. (**a**, **b**) ×100; (**c**, **d**) ×200

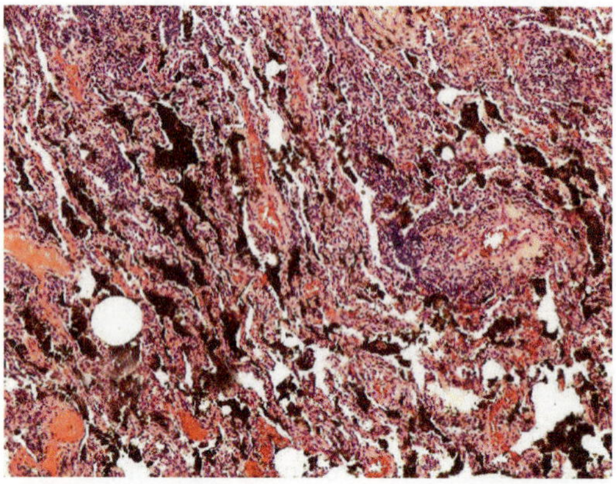

Fig. 18.80 Rheumatoid lung damage. Siderophages in the lumen of the alveoli. Stained with hematoxylin and eosin. ×100

semination, mycotic lesion, lung damage with another systemic vasculitis (primarily with granulomatosis with polyangiitis—former Wegener granulomatosis). It must be remembered that patients with rheumatoid arthritis receive immunosuppressive therapy for a long time, against the background of which pulmonary tuberculosis can develop, and therefore it is necessary to carefully conduct morphological verification of necrotic foci, determining their belonging to tuberculosis or rheumatoid lung damage. The most difficult cases are those with combined lung damage with the simultaneous development of tuberculous dissemination and rheumatoid nodules. The use of complex morphological studies with histochemical and

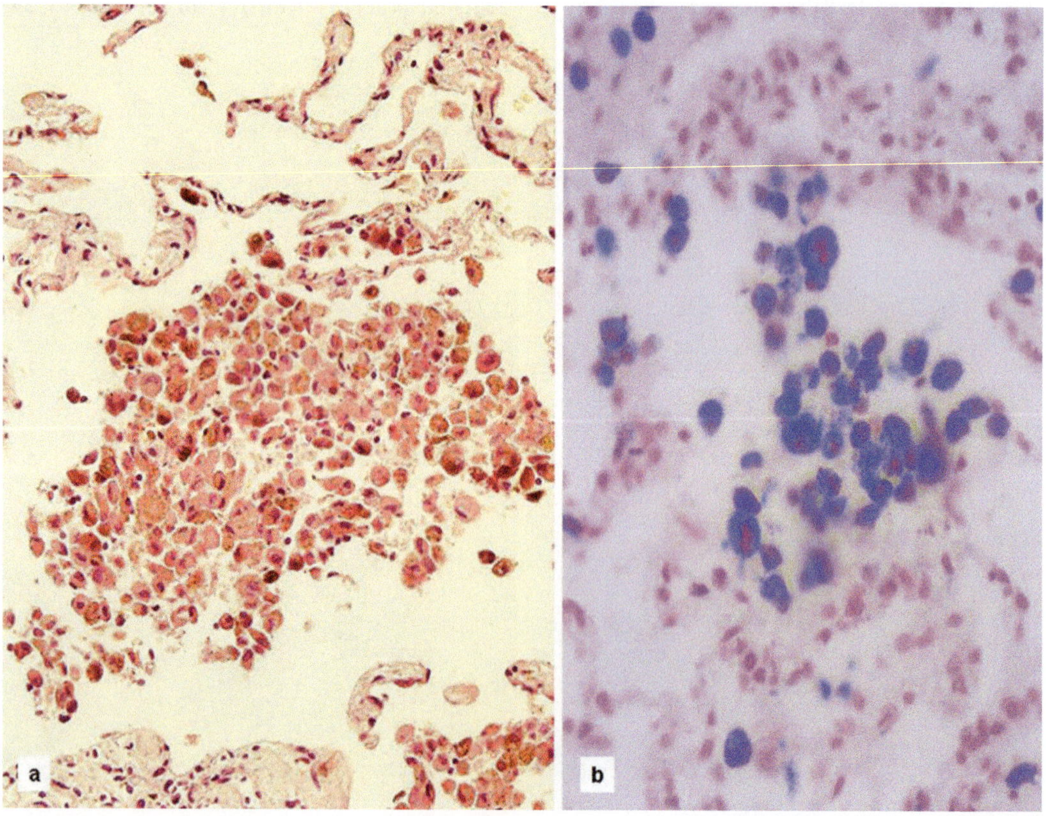

Fig. 18.81 Rheumatoid lung lesion. Siderophages in the lumen of the alveoli. (**a**) Hematoxylin and eosin staining and (**b**) Prussian blue reaction. ×200

histobacterioscopic methods, molecular biological research of the material allows us to interpret correctly the morphological picture.

18.16 Helminthiasis

In cases of pulmonary helminthiasis (the most common are echinococcosis, alveococcosis, ascariasis), granulomatous–necrotic inflammation was observed with a predominance of giant cells of foreign bodies, macrophages, eosinophilic leukocytes. Elements of helminth and eggs were found in necrosis and perifocal polymorphic cell infiltrate.

In echinococcosis, the chitinous membrane of echinococcal cysts, which has a characteristic multilayer structure and PAS-positive reaction (Figs. 18.82, 18.83, and 18.84), is histologically

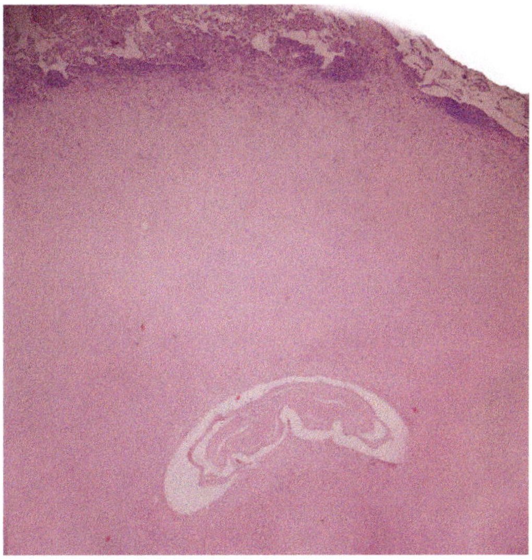

Fig. 18.82 The shell hydatid cysts in the necrotic masses. Stained with hematoxylin and eosin. ×100

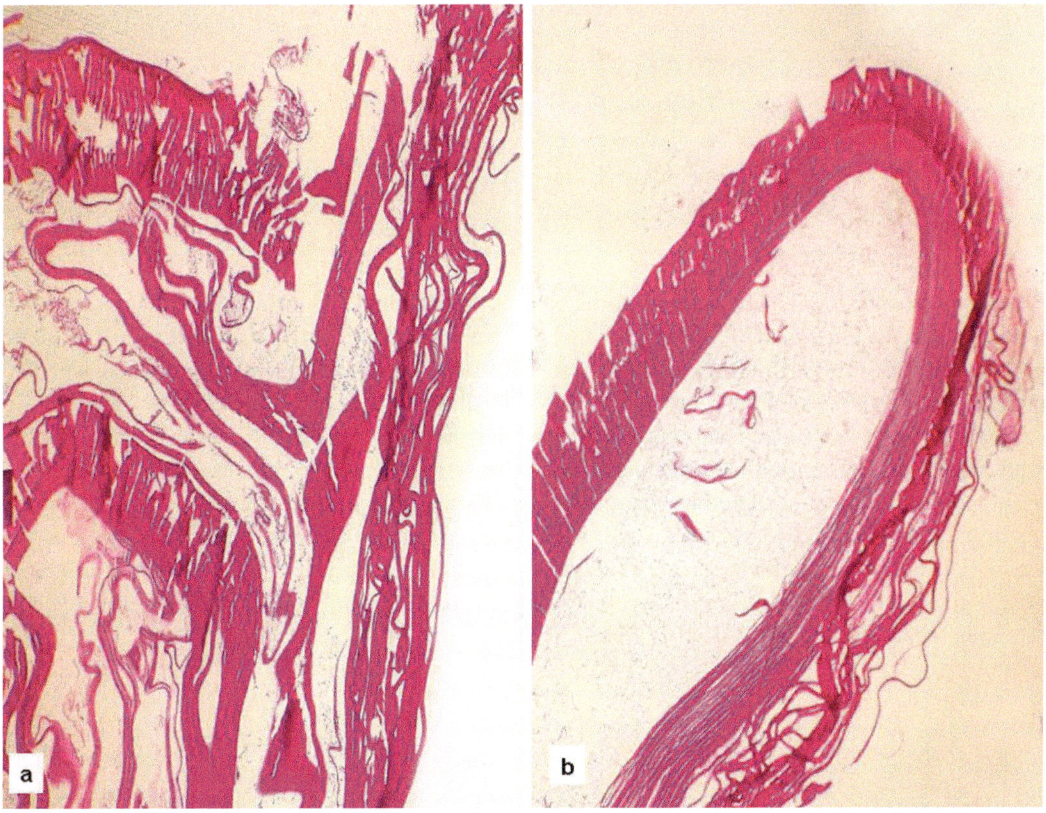

Fig. 18.83 Chitinous shell of Echinococcus. PAS × 200

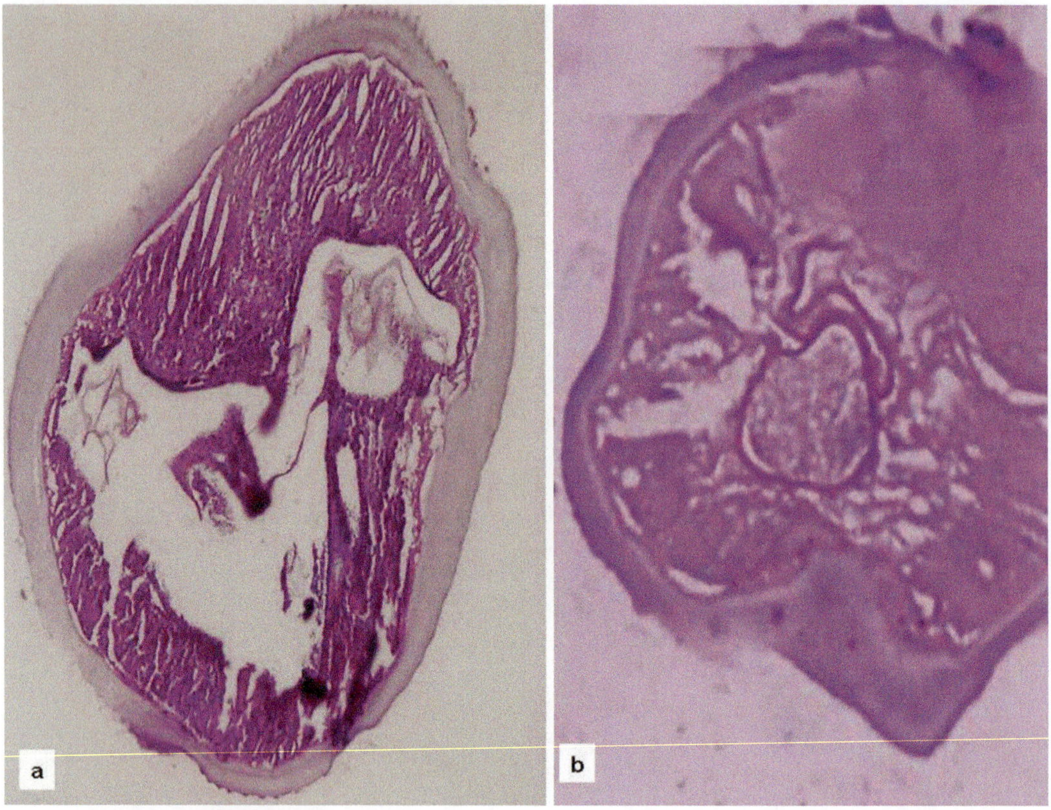

Fig. 18.84 Structure of the helminth. PAS. ×1000

found in necrotic masses. In the wall of the maternal echinococcal cyst, a shaft of epithelioid cells is subcapsularly formed, and infiltration with eosinophilic leukocytes is noted in the necrotic masses.

Perifocal exudative tissue reaction of the lung with plasma cells infiltration and an abundance of eosinophilic leukocytes scattered by giant multinucleated cells with a predominance of cells such as foreign bodies, granulomas, mainly macrophage–giant cell, although macrophage–epithelioid granulomas are also found (Fig. 18.85).

Morphological differential diagnosis must first be carried out with tuberculosis, mycotic lesions. Serial cutting of the material with the identification of the structures of helminths in necrotic foci can help in correctly determining the etiology of the process. Due to the pronounced eosinophilic reaction, it may be necessary to differentiate helminthiasis and various types of systemic vasculitis, which are also characterized by the development of necrosis and eosinophilic tissue reaction.

18.17 Granulomatous Inflammation of Foreign Bodies

Granulomatous inflammation of foreign bodies is characteristic of many processes. At the same time, a granulomatous reaction is formed around particles of foreign origin from giant multinucleated cells type foreign bodies and macrophages. Phagocytized particles are detected in the cytoplasm of multinucleated macrophages. The source of the formation of granulomatous inflammation of foreign bodies can be many factors. Below, as examples, we give only a few of them.

So, with aspiration pneumonia, food particles, plant or animal origin (e.g., muscle fibers from food) are usually located in granulomas (Fig. 18.86).

Foreign body granulomas form around the suture material, which has the characteristic appearance of weakly basophilic fibers (longitudinal or transverse) of the ligature. In the cytoplasm of multinucleated macrophages, phagocytosed particles of suture material are clearly visible. Also, after surgery, in addition to suture material, particles of talcum powder (e.g., from the gloves of a surgeon, etc.) can become a source of granulomatous inflammation (Fig. 18.87).

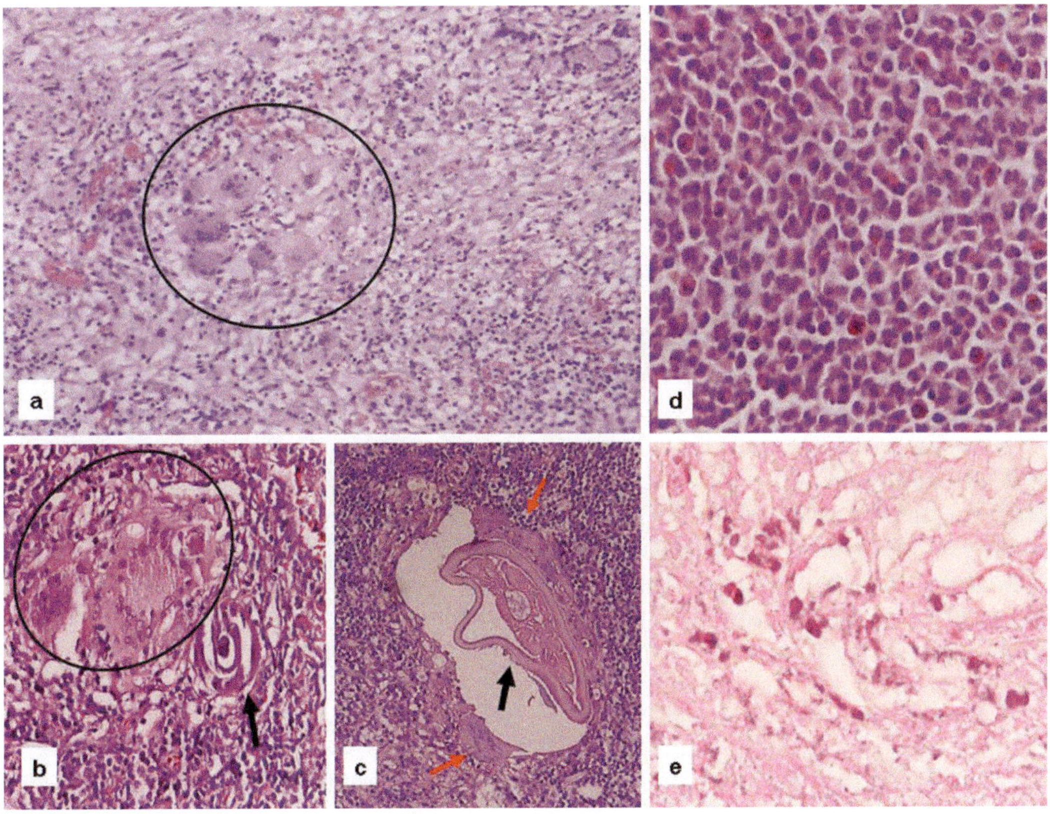

Fig. 18.85 Helminthiasis. (**a**) Giant cell granuloma in the area of inflammation in helminthiasis (circled by a round frame); (**b**) giant cell granuloma near the helminth structure (helminth indicated by an arrow, granuloma circled by a round frame); (**c**) giant cell reaction around the helminth structure (helminth indicated by a black arrow, multicellular giant cells of the type of foreign bodies indicated by red arrows); (**d**) eosinophilic reaction in the inflammatory infiltrate; (**e**) eosinophilic reaction in necrotic masses in the area of inflammation in helminthiasis. Stained with hematoxylin and eosin. (**a**, **d**, **e**) ×200; (**b**, **c**) ×400. (See also Figs. 15.3–15.7)

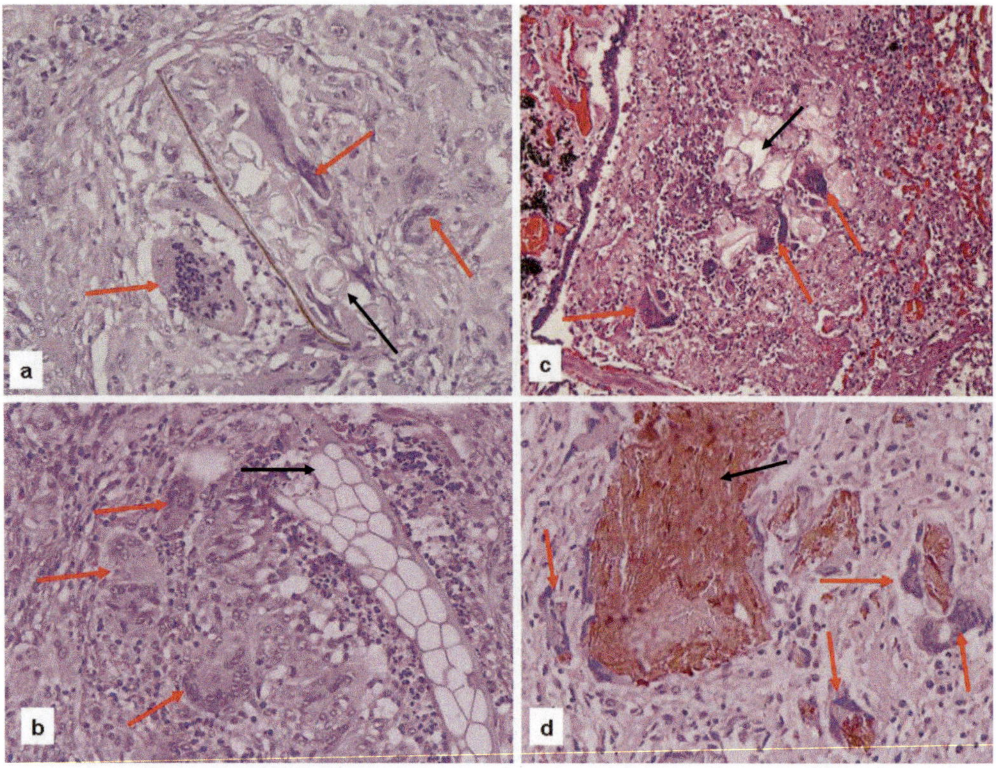

Fig. 18.86 Granulomatous inflammation of foreign bodies. Aspiration pneumonia. (**a**, **b**) Aspiration of particles of vegetable origin; (**c**) aspiration of particles of animal origin (in the lumen of the bronchus, a particle of adipose tissue); (**d**) aspiration of gastric contents with acid hematin. Foreign-aspirated particles are indicated by black arrows, giant cell reaction by red arrows. Stained with hematoxylin and eosin. ×400

Individuals taking narcotic drugs, both inhalation and intravenous, form small macrophage–giant cell granulomas in their lungs that contain foreign, weakly basophilic crystalloid structures, which give a characteristic glow during the chromatographic method of investigation. These granulomas are located in the interalveolar septa and perivascular (Figs. 18.88 and 18.89).

Oleogranulomas develop around patches of oil-based drugs or any other chemicals of a similar nature that have somehow entered the lung tissue. Macrophages in the granulomas of foreign bodies in such cases can be represented by a large number of "xanthoma" cells, i.e., macrophages with many lipid microvacuoles in the cytoplasm. In the cytoplasm of multinucleated cells of foreign bodies, one can find rather large fat vacuoles or phagocytized xanthoma cells.

Oleogranulomas develop around patches of oil-based drugs or any other chemicals of a similar nature that have somehow entered the lung tissue. Macrophages in the granulomas of foreign bodies in such cases can be represented by a large number of "xanthoma" cells, i.e., macrophages with many lipid microvacuoles in the cytoplasm. In the cytoplasm of multinucleated cells of foreign bodies, one can find rather large fat vacuoles or phagocytized xanthoma cells (Fig. 18.90).

In the case of amyloid lesion of the lung around the amyloid deposits, a giant cell reaction of the type of foreign bodies is observed in the form of scattered multinuclear giant macrophages and with the formation of granules of foreign bodies (Fig. 18.91). Histochemical stains according to Van Gieson and Congo red help differentiate amyloid masses from necrotic masses, including foci of fibrosis and hyalinosis (Fig. 18.92). IHC studies also confirm the presence of amyloid.

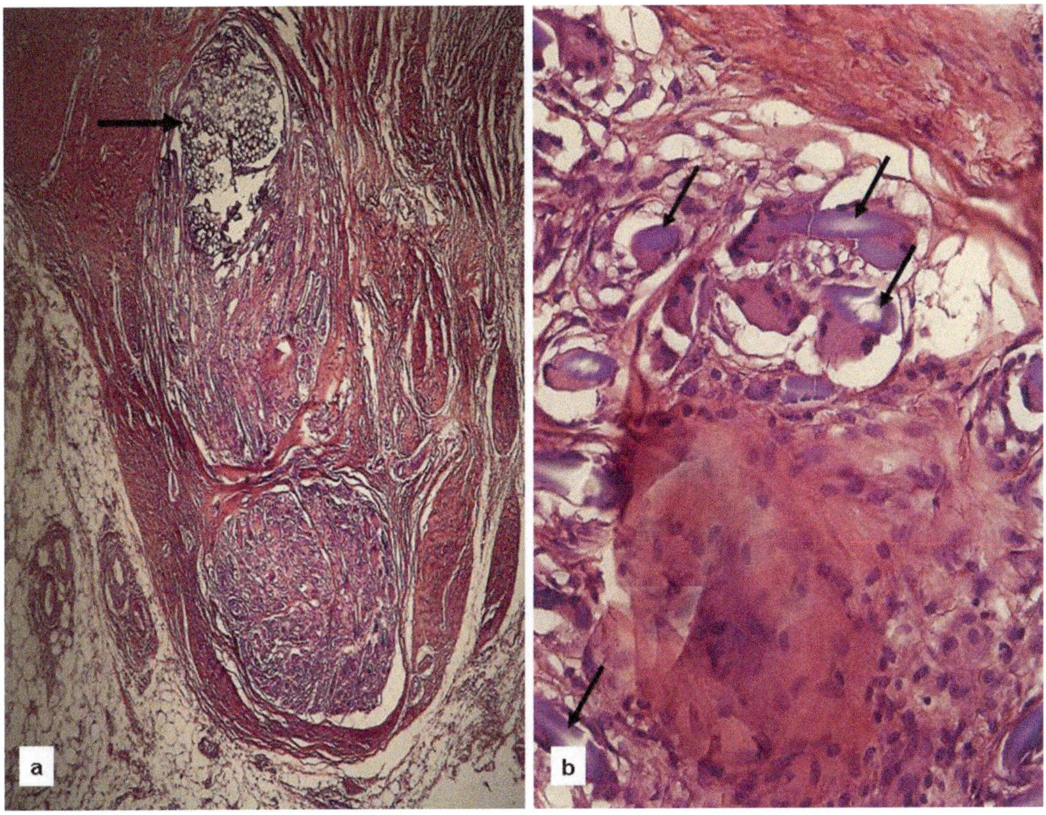

Fig. 18.87 Granulomatous inflammation of foreign bodies. Granulomas around the suture material in the soft tissues of the chest wall. (**a**) Ligature in the granuloma is indicated by an arrow; (**b**) the granuloma of foreign bodies with signs of phagocytosis of suture material particles by giant cells of the type of foreign bodies (ligature particles are indicated by arrows). Stained with hematoxylin and eosin. (**a**) ×100 and (**b**) ×1000

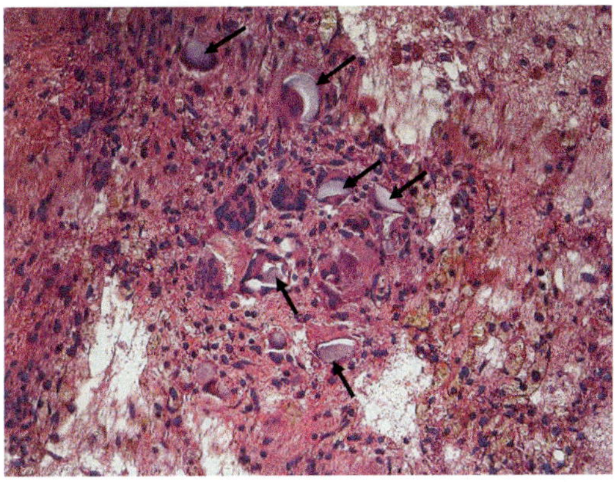

Fig. 18.88 Granulomatous inflammation of foreign bodies. Granuloma of foreign bodies in the lungs of an addict. Phagocytosis by granuloma cells of weakly basophilic crystalloid particles (the particles are indicated by arrows). Stained with hematoxylin and eosin. ×400

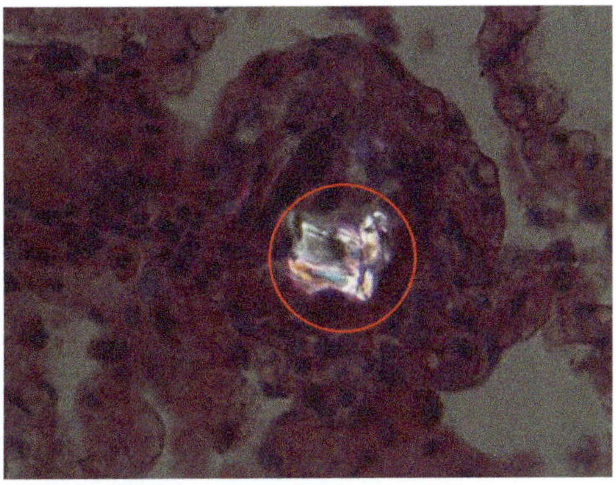

Fig. 18.89 Granulomatous inflammation of foreign bodies. Granuloma of foreign bodies in the lungs of an addict. Crystalloid structures with characteristic lighting. Polarizing microscopy. ×1000 (slice provided by Freund G. G)

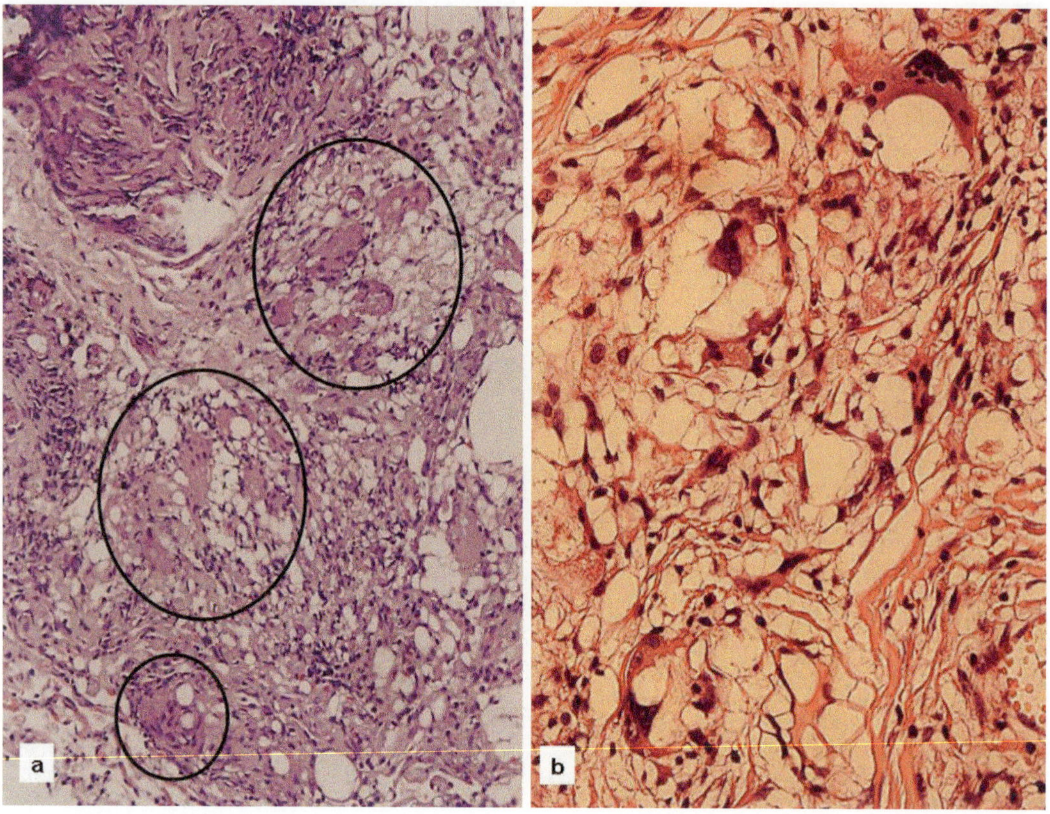

Fig. 18.90 Granulomatous inflammation of foreign bodies. Oleogranulomas in the soft tissues of the chest wall. (**a**) Granulomas of foreign bodies with signs of phagocytosis of lipocytes; (**b**) in the cytoplasm of giant multicore cells of the foreign body type, fat vacuoles, xanthoma cells. Stained with hematoxylin and eosin. (**a**) ×100 and (**b**) ×400

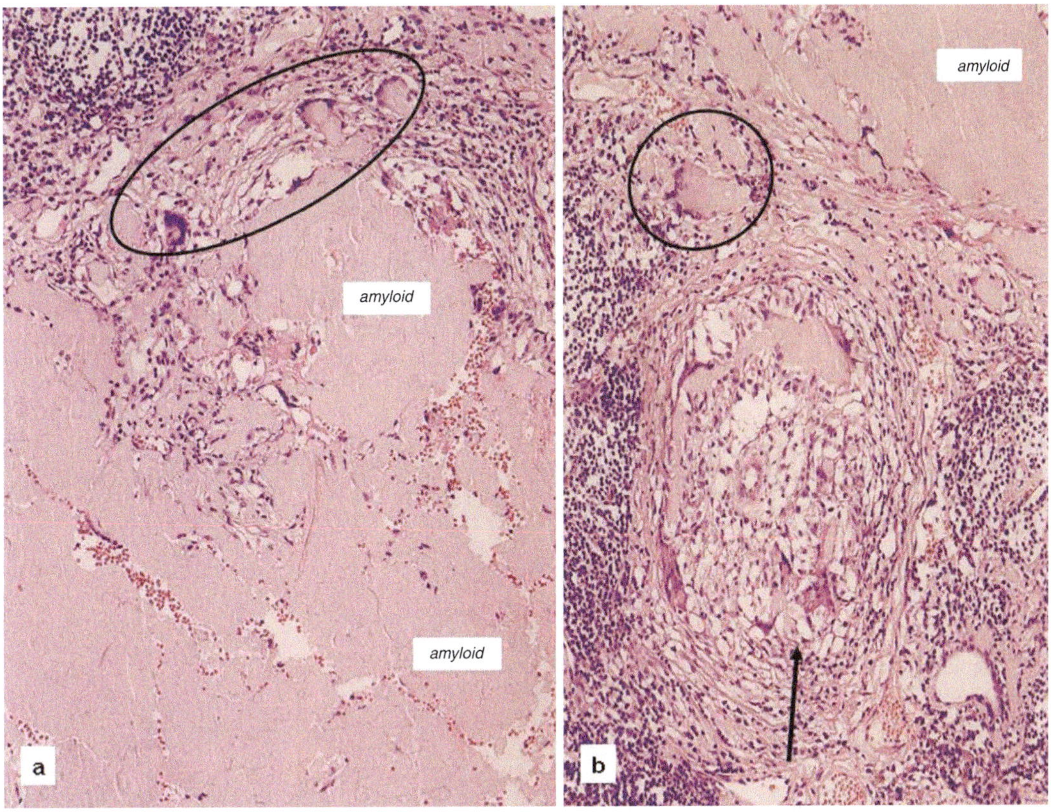

Fig. 18.91 Granulomatous inflammation of foreign bodies. Granulomatous reaction of the type of foreign bodies around amyloid masses. (**a**) Granulomatous reaction around amyloid masses circled by an oval frame; (**b**) granulomatous reaction around amyloid masses (circled by a round frame), subtotally obliterated vessel with signs of granulomatous inflammation near the amyloid site (the vessel is indicated by an arrow). Stained with hematoxylin and eosin. ×400

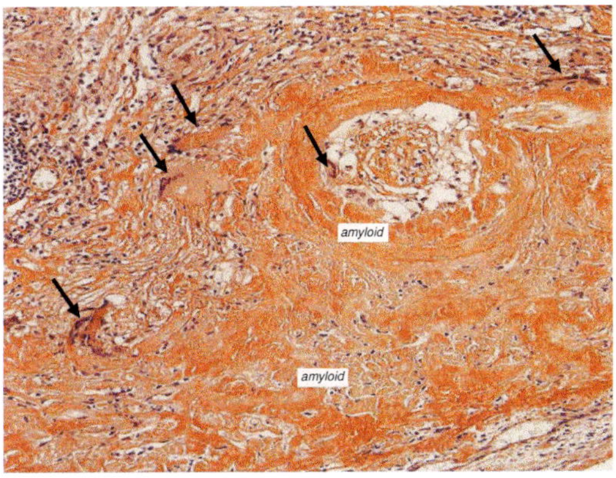

Fig. 18.92 Granulomatous inflammation of foreign bodies. Granulomatous reaction of the type of foreign bodies around amyloid masses (fragment shown in Fig. 18.91b). Giant multinuclear cells around amyloid masses and in the vessel wall with amyloid deposits are indicated by arrows. Stained by Congo red. ×400

References

1. Kradin RL, editor. Diagnostic pathology of infectious diseases. Elsevier; 2018. 698 p.
2. Procop GW, Pritt BS, editors. Pathology of infectious diseases. Elsevier; 2015. 706 p.
3. Leslie KO, Wick MR, editors. Practical pulmonary pathology. A diagnostic approach. 2nd ed. 2011. 828 p.
4. Zinserling VA, Starshinova AA, Karev VE, et al. Granulomatous inflammation of mycoplasma and chlamydia etiology. J Infektologii. 2015;7(4):5–9. (In Russian).

19 Conclusion. Questions Stay To Be Investigated

In spite the long-term history of study of respiratory infections and certain achievements, we see there are a lot of theoretical and pure practical questions which have to be solved.

One of the most intriguing questions in the modern medicine is the problem of new infections, which are regularly described, partly becoming very important as medical and social problems, such as HIV, Zika, SARS, MERS, and recently SARS-CoVi2. Not discussing items related to the appearance of the pathogens and their propagation, one has to consider that in many newly detected infections, the morphological picture has not been described. It is evident that these data are important not only for understanding of the pathogen but also for elaborating of treatment strategy.

Not satisfactory results of treatment and prevention of many respiratory diseases (coronavirus, tuberculosis, influenza) partly can be explained by the leak of knowledge of their pathogenesis based upon corresponding studies, including pathologic.

Recently appeared numerous researches where intimate interactions between different pathogens and the host have been studied predominately on cell cultures, rarer on animal models. Among the most popular research topics are the cell death mechanisms [1]. Very valuable is the conclusion that different pathogens have their own strategies in interaction with the host's cells and it apparently leads to different tissue inflammatory reactions, helping us in routine histopathological diagnostics. Due to objective circumstances, there are practically no studies provided on human tissues in course of severe death-threatening disease, thus real histopathological pictures do not always totally correspond to the pathogenesis assumed in in vitro studies. One has also to consider that in clinical practice we meet pathogens belonging to the same species, but with different expression of pathogeny factors. In order to meliorate the strategy of pathogenic treatment basing upon regulations of cellular defense and alterative mechanisms, comparative studies on tissue level are necessary.

There are certain unclarified discrepancies between results obtained by different methods. Thus, there are numerous data that Klebsiella, basing upon cell studies, is considered as obligate intracellulary pathogen [2], but in the meantime we see it in tissue sections, at least occasionally, lying free.

In clinical pathology in certain percentage, it is extremely difficult to determine exactly etiology of granulomatous and diffuse interstitial lesions. Modern molecular biological technologies not always are helpful. One may suppose that in pathogenesis of many acute and especially chronic pulmonary diseases, pathogens have to play a certain role. If the mechanisms of acute infections are more or less known (but still with a lot of unresolved questions), most of the issues related to chronic ones are practically in the

V. Zinserling, *Infectious Pathology of the Respiratory Tract*,
https://doi.org/10.1007/978-3-030-66325-4_19

darkness. One of the most remarkable examples is tuberculosis. During the whole history of mankind being its important enemy, tuberculosis became a hero of millions of contributions. We can be satisfied that the progress in many fundamental and clinical sciences in collaboration with healthcare institutions allowed to achieve outstanding results in prevention and treatment of this disease. But we have to assume that we are extremely far from complete victory. It depends also from our unsatisfactory knowledge of its pathogenesis. The fundamental studies in this field were provided only in the mid of XX century and cannot be fully accepted nowadays. In recent decades, a series of researches has been provided under the title "study of pathogenesis," but in reality were devoted only to particular issues, such as in vitro relation between mycobacteria and isolated cells. Many important issues have not been discussed for more than 50 years. As the result, we do not possess adequate pathogenetic classification and in majority of world manuals in phthisiatry, the chapter "pathogenesis" doesn't exist and many peculiarities of clinical course are not explained. We sure that complex modern studies of tuberculosis are necessary and have to include obligatory pathological studies of clinical and autopsy specimens.

The existence of numerous infections caused by different Mycoplasma and Chlamydia species is known for about half of century, but many issues still stay unclear, among them the fact that morphological appearance of the lesions caused by them is "terra incognita" for human pathologists, contrary to veterinary ones. We have to consider that nearby entities more or less detail described clinically and relative seldom being life-threatening, a wide spectrum of noninfectious complications exist.

It is hardly believable for people standing far from pulmonology that we have no exact determination of the term "pneumonia" and it frequently leads to misunderstandings. We do not have exact statistics of pneumonia etiology on clinical and autopsy materials. There is no need to explain the importance of such data and nowadays nobody can be satisfied with mortality from different pneumonias, including SARS-CoV-2. We are absolutely sure that better results can be achieved only when getting more detailed information about etiology and pathogenesis in lethal cases, which presently we consider as insufficient.

There is only fragmentary information about the influence of individual properties of the pathogen's strain (viruses, bacteria, fungi, mycoplasma) upon the clinical course and morphological appearance of the disease. Importance of this issue seems to be evident and has to be introduced in clinical and laboratory practice.

There is practically no information about interference between different pathogens in respiratory tract and lungs, in spite of usual appearance of multiple species at the same time, especially in patients with immunodeficiency of different origin. By the way, we can assume that majority of healthy people with normal resistance are the carriers of different pathogens. In such cases host-pathogen relations are practically unknown till due the action of unfavorable factors occurs the activation of infection.

Assuming that the properties of the host do play an important role in the development and course of the disease, we know not much about genetical predisposition, local immunity, and probable autoimmune mechanisms, which differ in various age, although interesting reviews appeared recently [2].

There is leak of information related to the persistence of biological pathogens and its role in the development of chronic lesions, partly which are considered as chronic infections, partly as "inflammatory disease of unclear origin," partly as noninfectious illnesses and syndromes. In spite of numerous literature, devoted to many problems, their structural background stays unclear, especially seldom the investigators are interested in revealing pathogen (or its components) and appropriate tissue and cell reactions.

Perinatal infections in many cases are due to transplacental challenge of the pathogen. The involvement of the lungs is practically obligatory in course of generalized intrauterine infections, which in many cases appear to be of not big danger. Outcomes of perinatal infections are hardly known and probably can lead not only to chronic infectious lesions but also to secondary immunopathological complications. Pathology of perinatal infection is described in the world literature only to a very small extent.

In many respiratory infections of different etiology (such as due to influenza and coronaviruses, pneumococcus, etc.) extrapulmonary manifestations exist, their nature in majority of cases needs to be clarified and studied by methods of pathology.

There is no concordance between specialists of different profiles and scientific schools in the terminology and principles of formulation of clinical and postmortem diagnoses. Not only in textbooks and manuals all over the world but also in mind of clinicians of different profiles and pathologist's certain archaic and never proved views are still alive.

If we consider respiratory infections with special attention, we cannot find among them "common" (banal) not demanding further complex study. Certain aspects of pathogenesis of many respiratory infections still need experimental studies, better in form of animal nosological models. We presented some of our data, we have got in different years, still being actual till nowadays.

Only few researches try to combine traditional routine screening methods with detailed clinicopathological analysis using the most modern and perfect morphological and molecular–biological methods.

Our task in preparing this manual was to share the results of long-term practical and research work of our scientific schools, many aspects of which remained not widely known till yet, but also to evaluate the main direction for the further complex study. We found unnecessary trying to perform complete review of the literature; unfortunately, the majority of modern contributions do not discuss life-time and postmortem morphological diagnostics of infectious lung lesions—main aim we put before us while preparing the manual. Existing manuals include practically complete list of the modern literature on the related topics [2–5]. It appeared also necessary to cite Russian publications of the former century, especially when they present reliable results, the topic remains actual and there are no modern contributions at all.

References

1. FitzGerald ES, Luz NF, Jamieson AM. Competitive cell death interactions in pulmonary infection: host modulation versus pathogen manipulation. Front Immunol. 2020;11:814. https://doi.org/10.3389/fimmu.20.00814.
2. Quinton LJ, Walkey AJ, Mizgerd JP. Integrative physiology of pneumonia. Physiol Rev. 2018;98(3):1417–64. https://doi.org/10.1152/physrev.00032.2017.
3. Kradin RL, editor. Diagnostic pathology of infectious diseases. Elsevier; 2018. 698 p.
4. Procop GW, Pritt BS, editors. Pathology of infectious diseases. Elsevier; 2015. 706 p.
5. Leslie KO, Wick MR, editors. Practical pulmonary pathology. A diagnostic approach. 2nd ed. 2011. 828 p.